MAINSTREAM M

Cardiology

Titles in the series:
Cardiology
Communicable and Tropical Diseases
Endocrinology
Gastroenterology
Haematology
The Liver and Biliary System
Nephrology
Neurology
Respiratory Medicine

Series Editors:
P. W. Brunt
Consultant Physician, Woodend Hospital, Aberdeen
M. S. Losowsky
Professor of Medicine, University of Leeds
A. E. Read
Professor of Medicine, University of Bristol

MAINSTREAM MEDICINE

Cardiology

RICHARD G. CHARLES, BSc, FRCP, FACC
Consultant Cardiologist, Regional Adult Cardiothoracic Unit, Broadgreen Hospital, Liverpool
Clinical Lecturer in Medicine, University of Liverpool

ANDREW J. MARSHALL, MD, FRCP
Consultant Physician and Cardiologist, Plymouth Health District
Honorary Consultant Cardiologist, Royal Naval Hospital, Plymouth

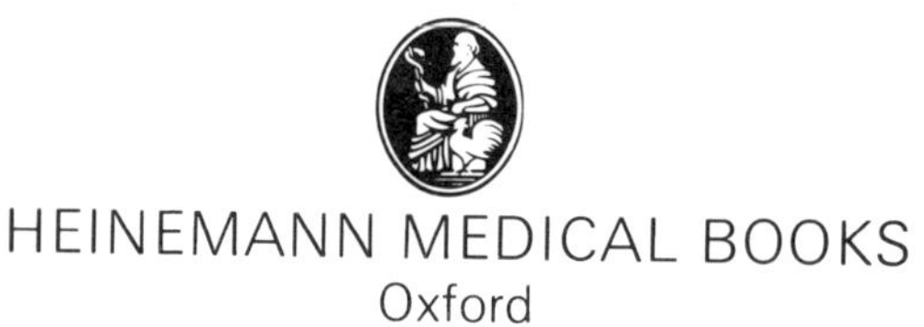

HEINEMANN MEDICAL BOOKS
Oxford

Heinemann Medical Books
An imprint of Heinemann Professional Publishing Ltd
Halley Court, Jordan Hill, Oxford OX2 8EJ

OXFORD LONDON SINGAPORE NAIROBI
IBADAN KINGSTON

First published 1989

British Library Cataloguing in Publication Data

Charles, Richard G.
Cardiology.
1. Man. Heart. Diseases
I. Title II. Marshall, Andrew J.
III. Series
616.1′2

ISBN 0-433-05483-2

Typeset by Latimer Trend & Co. Ltd, Plymouth,
and printed in Great Britain by Biddles Ltd, Guildford

Contents

Series Preface

This is one of a series of small books with two objectives. The main aim is to help postgraduates both from the UK and overseas who are preparing for higher medical examinations; the MRCP (UK) is the primary target but we believe that trainee surgeons will also find it useful. The second is to provide assistance in the clinical situation by summarising relevant information at rather more length than is possible in a general textbook of medicine.

The books are short, with only the essential diagrams and references, and the series seeks to cover comprehensively the field of internal medicine. The authors and editors are all experienced teachers. The approach is similar in each book, and the series will provide a valuable basis of factual knowledge for higher medical examinations. It is assumed that the examination candidate is already an experienced and conscientious physician—these books cannot, of course, compensate for clinical deficiencies.

Each book provides a factual and up-to-date review of clinical information and underlying concepts, avoiding complex discussion of matters where there is uncertainty or difference of opinion. Some material is tabulated for ease of scanning and learning. References are to review articles rather than to original data.

We have no qualms about producing a series of books with examination candidates in mind. The postgraduate has the greatest difficulty in keeping up with advances in the many specialties that make up internal medicine, and examinations may require knowledge of areas where postgraduate experience has been minimal. Our sympathy is with the candidates.

P. W. Brunt
M. S. Losowsky
A. E. Read

Preface

Cardiovascular disease continues to cause premature death and disability at unprecedented levels in the industrialized world. This concentrated review of modern clinical cardiology is offered to meet the needs of postgraduate examination candidates, particularly for the MRCP(UK), and other serious students of the subject. Some basic knowledge is assumed but a revision of essential background is provided in all major sections. Despite enormous technological advances during the past few years much of the fun and fascination of cardiology is still derived from a sound detailed grasp of bedside clinical diagnosis. The candidate will quickly discover that this fact has not eluded his examiners. Accordingly, this volume strives to provide a balanced summary, clinical and technological, of cardiology today.

Acknowledgements

The authors wish to express their profound gratitude to Mrs Mary J. Palmer and Mrs Carol Postle-Hacon for typing the manuscript.

RGC wishes to acknowledge the unique skills of Dr Derek Rowlands in teaching electrocardiography, exemplified in his volumes *Understanding the Electrocardiogram*. While extensive reference has been made to these volumes, with the author's permission, Derek Rowlands bears no responsibility whatsoever for the accuracy or presentation of material in the present chapters on electrocardiography or arrhythmias.

Dr Norman Coulshed generously supplied ECG tracings from his collection.

Chapter One

Arrhythmias

Definition

Arrhythmia is a cardiac rhythm other than normal sinus rhythm.

Background

Arrhythmias are conventionally divided into disorders of impulse formation and disorders of impulse conduction. Since most of the events underlying these disorders are not depicted on the surface electrocardiogram their presence must be deduced from analysis of the morphology and timing of the atrial and ventricular myocardial depolarisation waves—the P waves and QRS complexes. Invasive electrophysiological studies have explained the mechanism of many abnormal cardiac rhythms but clinical electrocardiography remains an essentially empirical discipline from which much information can be derived by adherence to basic principles.

A systematic approach to the analysis of abnormal cardiac rhythms will assist in their identification (Table 1.1). This chapter summarises the recognition and management of the common arrhythmias.

SINUS RHYTHMS

Sinus Rhythm

Definition

This is the normal rhythm of the heart which has a regular rate of 60–100 beats per minute.

Table 1.1

A SIMPLE SYSTEMATIC APPROACH TO RHYTHM ANALYSIS

The P wave
- are P waves present?
- what is the P wave rate?
- are they normal sinus P waves?
- if atrial activity is present but abnormal
  - are there ectopic P waves?
  - is depolarisation retrograde in the atria (negative P waves in leads II, III, aVF)?
  - is there atrial flutter or fibrillation?

The QRS complex
- is the QRS rhythm regular?
- what is the QRS rate?
- is the QRS complex narrow (< 120 ms) or wide (> 120 ms)? A narrow QRS virtually guarantees a supraventricular origin

What is the relationship between P and QRS?
- is the P wave related to the QRS?
- is each P wave followed by a QRS?
- is the P–R interval normal and constant?

Intervals
- measure P–P, R–R, P–R, Q–T intervals carefully

The term 'normal' sinus rhythm implies a normal site impulse formation in the sinus node, a normal P-wave axis ar normal atrioventricular conduction. In some abnormal rhythr the cardiac impulse may be formed in the sinus node but oth criteria for normal sinus rhythm are not fulfilled, for exampl complete atrioventricular block, or atrioventricular dissociatio This is commonly termed 'sinus rhythm in the atria'.

Sinus Bradycardia

Definition

This is sinus rhythm at a P-wave rate below 60 beats per minut

Sinus Tachycardia

Definition

This is sinus rhythm at a P-wave rate above 100 beats per minute.

The causes of both sinus bradycardia and sinus tachycardia are shown in Table 1.2.

Table 1.2

CAUSES OF SINUS BRADYCARDIA AND SINUS TACHYCARDIA

Sinus bradycardia (rate ⩽60 beats/min)	*Sinus tachycardia (rate ⩾100 beats/min)*
Sleep	Exercise
Athletes	Mental stress
Myocardial infarction	Hypovolaemia
Sick sinus syndrome	Cardiac failure
Beta-adrenergic blockers	Idiopathic
Hypothyroidism	
Jaundice	
Raised intracranial pressure	

Sinus Arrhythmia

Definition

This is sinus rhythm displaying an alternating increase and decrease in rate. The most common form is respiratory sinus arrhythmia due to cyclical variation in vagal tone. The rate increases with inspiration. It is a common normal finding in children, young adults and athletes, and may be accentuated by digoxin.

Sinus Arrest

Sinus arrest (Fig. 1.1) is a transient cessation of impulse formation within the sinus node resulting in an absence of P-waves. The duration of sinus arrest is unpredictable and is not a multiple of

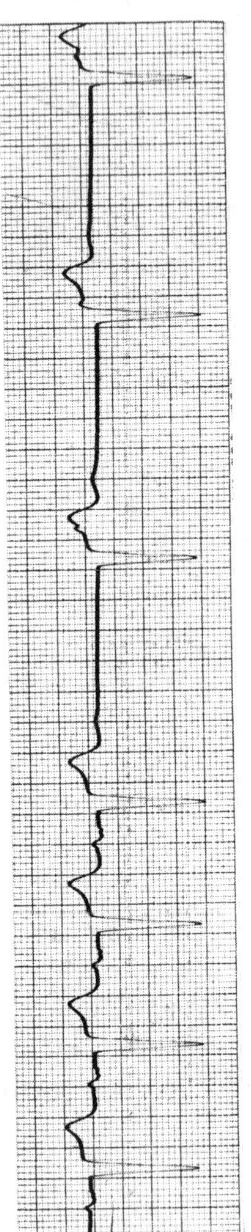

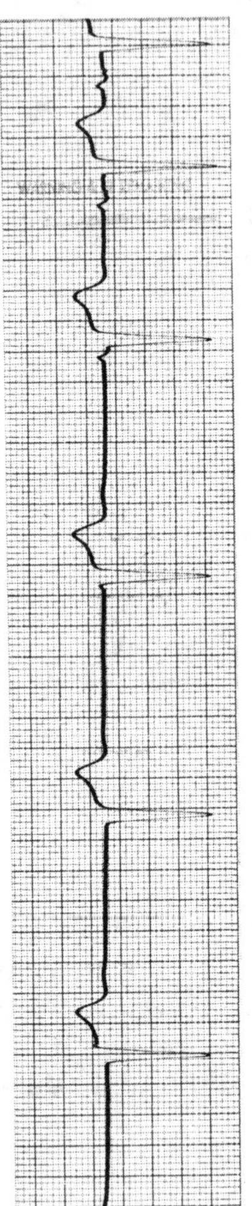

Fig. 1.1. Sinus arrest. The first four beats show sinus rhythm 74 beats/min with first degree atrioventricular block, P–R interval 240 ms. Sinus arrest is terminated after 1.6 s by a junctional escape rhythm, 38 beats/min.

the preceding sinus cycle length. Often it lasts less than 1 s but if prolonged an escape rhythm usually emerges. In sick sinus syndrome (page 36) subsidiary pacemakers may also be depressed resulting in prolonged asystole.

Sinoatrial Block

Impulse formation in the sinus node is normal but there is a failure of impulse conduction to the adjacent atrial myocardium (Fig. 1.2). In this case the P–P intervals are a multiple of the preceding sinus cycle length.

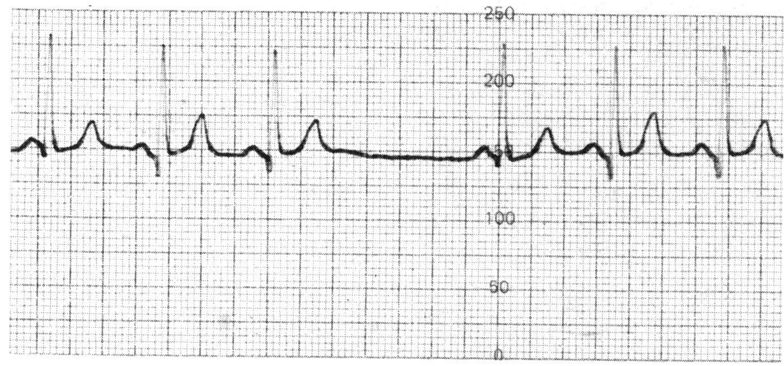

Fig. 1.2. Second degree sinoatrial block. The duration of the pause is equal to twice the sinus node cycle length.

Electrophysiologically sinoatrial block can be classified as first, second or third degree. Only second degree sinoatrial block can be recognised electrocardiographically since sinus node activity is not recorded on the electrocardiogram (ECG).

ECTOPIC BEATS

Definition

An impulse arising outside the sinus node (in the atria, atrioventricular junction, or ventricles) which is premature in the cardiac cycle.

Terminology

The terms ectopic beat, extrasystole and premature contraction are synonymous for practical purposes.

Coupling interval

The interval between the ectopic beat and the preceding beat. An ectopic beat is premature by definition so the coupling interval is shorter than the R–R interval (cycle length) of the basic rhythm. Ectopic beats arising from the same site (unifocal) have a constant coupling interval.

Compensatory pause

This is the duration of the pause after an extrasystole:

(i) A *complete compensatory pause* is present when the sum of the coupling interval and the compensatory pause is equal to twice the sinus cycle length; it is characteristic of a ventricular ectopic beat which fails to conduct retrogradely to the atria, thus leaving the sinus node undisturbed.
(ii) An *incomplete compensatory pause* arises if the sinus node is discharged early by an atrial ectopic beat or by a retrogradely conducted ventricular ectopic beat.

Atrial Ectopic Beat

This is shown in Fig. 1.3 and criteria are shown in Table 1.3.

Most atrial ectopic beats pass normally through the atrioventricular node and distal conducting system. Atrial ectopics arising early in the cardiac cycle may find part of the conducting system still completely or partially refractory:

(i) *Blocked atrial ectopic*: the atrioventricular node is completely refractory so the ectopic P-wave is not followed by a QRS complex. This is the commonest cause of a pause interrupting regular sinus rhythm.
(ii) *Prolonged P–R interval*: the atrioventricular node is partially refractory.

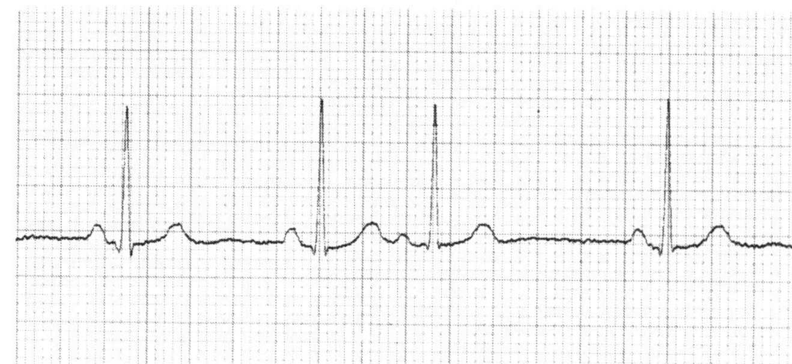

Fig. 1.3. The third P wave is an atrial ectopic beat conducted normally to the ventricles.

Table 1.3

Criteria	*Comment*
Premature P wave	By definition
Abnormal shaped P wave	Abnormal direction of atrial activation
Incomplete compensatory pause	Invasion of sinus node by ectopic impulse disturbs the dominant sinus rhythm
Normal QRS complex	Impulse passes normally through atrioventricular (AV) node and conducting system. If aberrant conduction occurs the ectopic beat usually shows right bundle branch block (RBBB) morphology

(iii) *Phasic aberrant ventricular conduction*: a bundle branch, usually the right, is refractory. The QRS complex following the ectopic P-wave shows a wide, bundle branch block (BBB) morphology, simulating a ventricular ectopic beat. A similar phenomenon may occur in atrial fibrillation. The duration of the refractory period of the bundle branches is proportional to the length of the preceding R–R interval. Aberrantly conducted beats may occur when a short R–R interval follows a long R–R interval. This is termed the Ashman phenomenon (see Fig. 1.8). The aberrantly conducted beat may be misdiagnosed as a ventricular ectopic beat.

Atrioventricular Junctional Ectopic Beat

The criteria are shown in Table 1.4.

Table 1.4

Criteria	*Comment*
Premature QRS; morphology as in sinus rhythm	Ectopic arises in atrioventricular junctional area or bundle of His
P wave precedes, follows or coincides with QRS complex	Depending on relative speed of conduction to atria and ventricles
Incomplete compensatory pause	Sinus node reset by ectopic depolarisation

Ventricular Ectopic Beat

This is shown in Fig. 1.4 and the criteria in Table 1.5.

Sometimes retrograde conduction of a ventricular ectopic to the atria occurs. In this case an abnormal, inverted P-wave follows the ectopic QRS complex. The sinus node is invaded and the compensatory pause is incomplete.

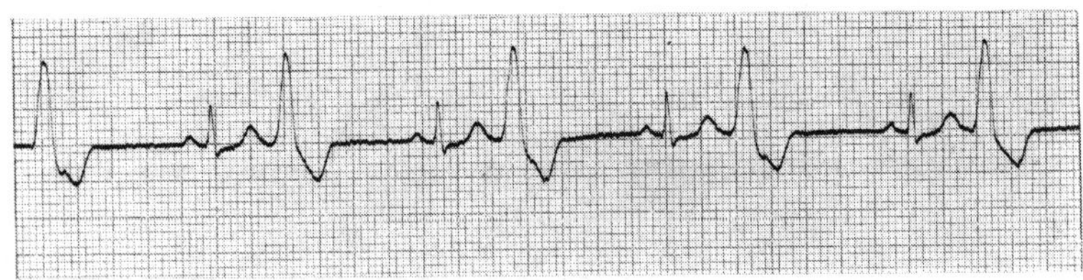

Fig. 1.4. Coupled unifocal ventricular ectopic beats.

Table 1.5

Criteria	*Comment*
Premature, abnormally wide QRS (> 120 ms)	Ectopic arises in Purkinje cell of left or right ventricle. An ectopic arising in the right ventricle will have left bundle branch block configuration and vice versa
ST segment and T wave abnormal (usually opposite in polarity to QRS)	Abnormal pattern of depolarisation results in abnormal pattern of repolarisation
Complete compensatory pause	Usually the ectopic does not conduct back into the atria, so sinus rhythm is not disturbed
P wave of next sinus beat is normal in timing and morphology; usually seen distorting the ST segment or T wave of the ventricular ectopic beat	Sinus rhythm is undisturbed but the P wave finds the ventricle still refractory from the ectopic QRS and is not conducted

Significance of Ectopic Beats

Atrial or ventricular ectopic beats may occur in the normal heart. Their frequency may be increased by nicotine, alcohol, smoking, caffeine, excessive fatigue or anxiety. If organic heart disease is excluded, suppression by drugs is indicated only for unacceptable symptoms.

Atrial and ventricular ectopic beats occur frequently in ischaemic, valvular, hypertensive, inflammatory and heart muscle diseases. Atrial ectopic beats may herald supraventricular arrhythmias including atrial fibrillation. Ventricular ectopic beats, especially if they are frequent, multifocal or consecutive may predict an increased risk of sudden death. However, it is uncertain whether they are an independent risk factor or related mainly to the severity of left ventricular damage. In acute myocardial infarction the concept of 'warning arrhythmias' preceding ventricular tachycardia or fibrillation is now relatively discredited and the drug suppression of ventricular ectopic beats in this context is of uncertain value.

ESCAPE BEATS

When the dominant rhythm fails, for example sinus node arrest, a subsidiary pacemaker site takes over. Escape beats terminate a transient pause in the dominant rhythm and arise in that part of the specialised conducting tissue which has the next highest rate of spontaneous depolarisation, usually the atrioventricular junctional area (see Fig. 1.1). Ventricular escape beats are less common. The site of origin of escape beats, as with ectopic beats, is recognised by their morphology. Management involves correction of the underlying bradycardia.

TACHYCARDIA OF SUPRAVENTRICULAR ORIGIN

Definition

A tachycardia which arises above the bifurcation of the bundle of His (Table 1.6). The term may strictly speaking be used generically for any of the tachycardias listed in Table 1.6. Its common usage is generally restricted to tachycardias of atrial or junctional origin that are difficult to distinguish electrocardiographically.

Table 1.6

TACHYCARDIAS OF SUPRAVENTRICULAR ORIGIN

Site of origin	*Electrocardiographic term*
Sinus node	Sinus tachycardia Sinoatrial re-entry tachycardia
Atrium	Atrial tachycardia Atrial flutter Atrial fibrillation
Atrioventricular junction	Junctional tachycardia

Mechanism of Tachycardias

At each site of origin a tachycardia may be initiated and sustained by one of two mechanisms

(i) A local re-entry circuit.
(ii) Enhanced automaticity of the site of origin.

An exception is atrial fibrillation in which disorderly depolarisation at multiple sites occurs throughout the atrial myocardium. Whatever the site of origin or the mechanism of the tachycardia the electrocardiographic diagnosis may be further complicated by coincidental ventricular pre-excitation due to the presence of an anomalous atrioventricular bypass tract. Clues to the mechanism of a tachycardia of supraventricular origin may sometimes be obtained from the ECG (Table 1.7).

Table 1.7

ECG CLUES TO THE MECHANISM OF A TACHYCARDIA OF SUPRAVENTRICULAR ORIGIN

Mechanism	*ECG clue*
Local re-entry	Common Paroxysmal Initiated by an ectopic beat Sudden onset Sudden cessation* Relatively higher atrial rate
Enhanced automaticity	Less common 'Non-paroxysmal' or sustained Warm-up phenomenon (gradual increase to maximum rate) Relatively lower atrial rate

*This may not be noticed by the patient since paroxysmal tachycardia is commonly followed by a period of sinus tachycardia.

Re-entry mechanism

The anatomical substrate of re-entrant or 'circus movement' depolarisation is the presence of a *re-entrant loop*. The loop comprises two limbs of excitable tissue in electrical continuity, and from this loop depolarisation spreads to adjacent excitable myocardium. It is required that each limb has different electrophysiological properties (longitudinal dissociation).

(i) One limb has a *slow conduction velocity* and a *short refractory period.*

(ii) The other limb has a *fast conduction velocity* and a *long refractory period.*

A readily familiar example is the tachycardia which may occur in patients with Wolff–Parkinson–White syndrome. In this case, one limb of the loop comprises the atrioventricular node (slow conduction velocity, short refractory period) and bundle of His, while the other limb is an anomalous pathway of myocardial tissue (fast conduction velocity, long refractory period) connecting the ventricular myocardium to the atrial myocardium. Let us assume that the depolarisation wave of an atrial ectopic beat arrives simultaneously at the atrioventricular node and at the atrial end of the anomalous pathway. Because of its long refractory period the anomalous pathway has not recovered after the preceding beat and cannot conduct the ectopic depolarisation. The atrioventricular node, however, has recovered and conducts the ectopic depolarisation to the ventricular myocardium. By this time the anomalous pathway has recovered excitability and now conducts the depolarisation wave back up to the atria. Atrial myocardium is depolarised and the wavefront is again presented to the atrioventricular node, completing the re-entry loop. A re-entry or 'circus movement' tachycardia is thus initiated. In this example the limbs of the loop involve large anatomical structures (macro re-entry). In many cases re-entry loops occur in small

Table 1.8

ANATOMICAL RE-ENTRANT LOOPS IN SUPRAVENTRICULAR TACHYCARDIAS

Site	*Components of loop*
Sinus node	Sinoatrial node and adjacent atrial myocardium
Atrium	Atrial myocardium
Atrioventricular node (AVN)	Limbs wholly within AVN but functionally different electrophysiological properties
AVN plus atrioventricular bypass tract	Conduction antegrade through AVN and bundle of His, retrograde through bypass tract

localised areas (micro re-entry) and are the underlying mechanism for most supraventricular and ventricular tachyarrhythmias. The anatomical re-entrant loops in supraventricular tachycardias are shown in Table 1.8.

Ventricular response in supraventricular tachycardias

In the presence of atrial tachycardia the ventricular rate depends principally on

(i) The atrial cycle length (atrial rate).
(ii) The atrioventricular nodal refractory period.

The P wave rate and ventricular response are expressed as a conduction ratio (1:1, 2:1, 3:1, etc.) (Fig. 1.5). An increase in atrioventricular nodal refractory period will decrease the ventricular response. The refractory period is increased by many antiarrhythmic drugs (digoxin, verapamil, beta-adrenergic blocking agents etc.), many disease processes involving the atrioventricular node, and by increased vagal tone (carotid sinus massage, Valsalva manoeuvre, eyeball pressure etc.). If the ventricular rate exceeds 200 beats/minute the presence of an accessory atrioventricular conduction pathway should be suspected.

QRS complex configuration

In supraventricular tachycardias the ectopic atrial depolarisations are conducted to the ventricles in the same manner as sinus depolarisations in that individual, so QRS complexes are normally narrow. Equally, a pre-existing QRS abnormality such as bundle branch block will be present during both sinus rhythm and supraventricular tachycardia.

Functional bundle branch block (aberrant ventricular conduction) may occur during supraventricular tachycardia if a depolarisation arrives in the bundle of His at a time when one bundle branch has recovered but the other has not. Usually the right bundle branch recovers more slowly than the left, so aberrant ventricular conduction usually displays a right bundle branch block pattern.

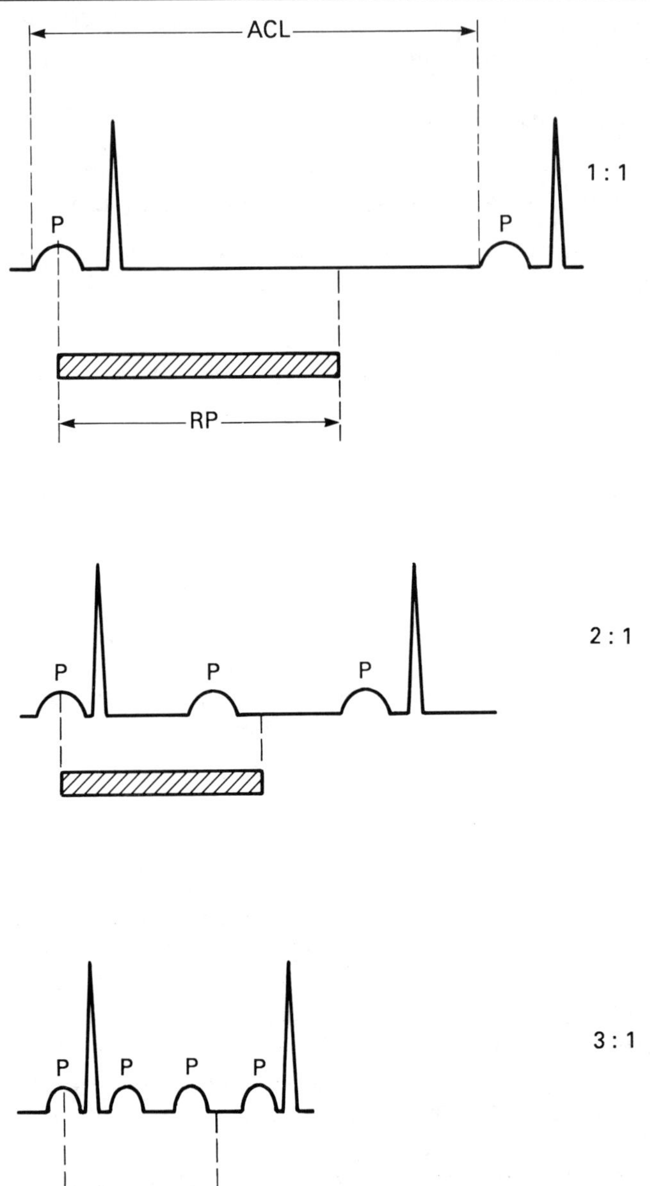

Fig. 1.5. Ventricular response in supraventricular tachycardia. T waves are omitted for clarity. ACL = atrial cycle length, P = P wave, RP = atrioventricular nodal refractory period.

ECG diagnosis of tachycardias of supraventricular origin

Criteria for the diagnosis of sinoatrial nodal re-entrant tachycardia, atrial tachycardia, atrial flutter and atrial fibrillation are given in Table 1.9. Junctional tachycardia is discussed below.

Table 1.9

CRITERIA FOR THE ECG DIAGNOSIS OF TACHYCARDIAS OF ATRIAL ORIGIN

Sinoatrial nodal re-entrant tachycardia	Rare P waves identical to normal sinus rhythm Sudden onset and cessation
Atrial tachycardia	Regular P waves, upright in II, III, aVF Rate 160–250 beats/min Regular QRS complexes with 1:1, 2:1, 3:1 or varying ratio to P waves QRS configuration similar to sinus rhythm except where aberrant ventricular conduction occurs
Atrial flutter	Regular atrial rate, usually 300 beats/min (250–350 beats/min) 'Saw-tooth' configuration of atrial activity Atrioventricular conduction ratio usually 2:1 (may be 3 or 4:1, or variable)
Atrial fibrillation	Chaotic atrial activity No relationship between successive R–R interval durations

Sinoatrial nodal re-entrant tachycardia

This is rarely seen. The re-entrant loop involves the sinoatrial node and its adjacent atrial myocardium. Paroxysmal sinus tachycardia of abrupt onset and termination is seen.

Atrial tachycardia

Atrial tachycardia (Fig. 1.6) originates in atrial myocardium by local re-entry or by enhanced automaticity. The mechanism can be determined only by observing the onset of tachycardia. An abrupt onset, often preceded by an atrial ectopic beat, confirms a re-entrant mechanism.

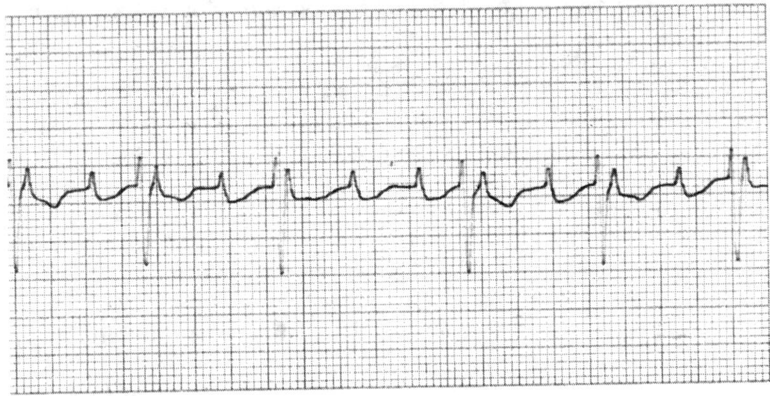

Fig. 1.6. Atrial tachycardia with variable atrioventricular block. The atrial rate is 165 beats/min.

Atrial flutter

Atrial flutter (Fig. 1.7) is a variety of atrial tachycardia. In both rhythms the rate of ventricular response will depend on factors discussed above (page 13).

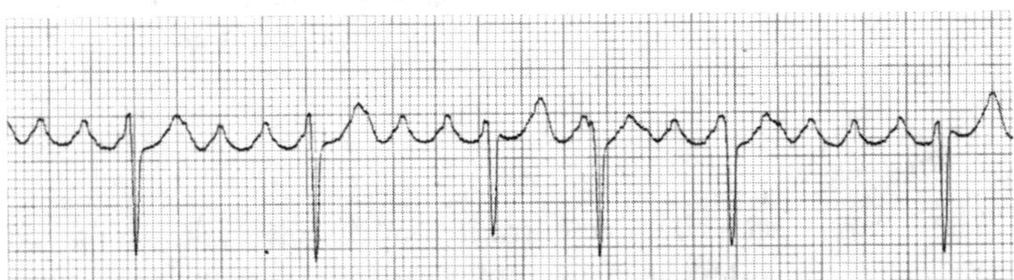

Fig. 1.7. Atrial flutter with variable atrioventricular block. The atrial rate is 300 beats/min.

Atrial fibrillation

This occurs when multiple sites in the atrial myocardium depolarise in an unrelated and chaotic way (Fig. 1.8). An irregular baseline of fibrillation (f) waves is seen. In long-standing atrial fibrillation the amplitude of f waves may be too low for ECG inscription, the baseline then appearing flat. The diagnosis remains apparent from the completely irregular R–R intervals. In atrial fibrillation complete irregularity of the R–R intervals is due to 'decremental conduction' in the atrioventricular node. This relates to the rapid bombardment of the atrioventricular node by fibrillation impulses many of which enter the node but are unable to propagate all the way through. They nevertheless reset the refractory period within the node. The success of an impulse in propagating through the atrioventricular node to reach the ventricular myocardium depends upon its 'strength' and the state of refractoriness in the node at the time of its arrival. R–R intervals are thus subject to large and unpredictable variations.

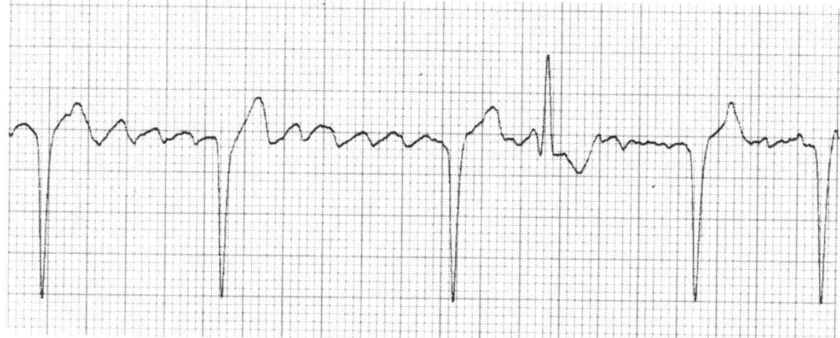

Fig. 1.8. Atrial fibrillation (lead V_1). The fourth beat shows aberrant intraventricular conduction of right bundle branch block (RBBB) configuration; a short R–R interval has followed a long R–R interval (Ashman phenomenon).

Junctional tachycardia

This is a supraventricular tachycardia arising in the atrioventricular junctional region. The characteristics of junctional tachycardias are summarised in Table 1.10. Tachycardias may be paroxysmal or non-paroxysmal according to their mechanism and may arise within or close to the atrioventricular node.

Table 1.10

JUNCTIONAL TACHYCARDIAS: A SUMMARY

Clinical type Mechanism Incidence	Anatomical Site of origin	*ECG Characteristics*		
		During tachycardia		
		Specific features	*Common to all*	*During sinus rhythm*
Non-paroxysmal Enhanced automaticity 10%	Low atrium Atrioventricular node Bundle of His	Gradual onset Rate 60–130 beats/min 1:1 conduction usual but atrioventricular block may occur. Carotid sinus massage increases block but does not terminate	*All junctional tachycardias appear basically similar on ECG* P waves: inverted in II, III, aVf can be before, after or within the QRS complex	*QRS complex normal* (or shows pre-existing abnormalities, for example, left bundle branch block, infarction, hypertrophy)

Paroxysmal Re-entry 90%	Low atrium* Bundle of His* *Atrioventricular node (AVNRT)*: re-entry entirely within the atrioventricular node	Abrupt onset and offset Rate 150–250 beats/min 1:1 conduction; atrioventricular block never occurs	as in sinus rhythm may show aberrant ventricular conduction at higher rates (usually AVRT)	
	Atrioventricular node + anomalous bypass tract (AVRT)	Carotid sinus massage—no change or terminates		
	(i) *Concealed* bypass tract: Conducts retrograde *only* No ventricular pre-excitation			
	(ii) '*Revealed*' bypass tract Antegrade and retrograde conduction possible Ventricular pre-excitation present		In AVRT with 'revealed' bypass tract the QRS complex during tachycardia is almost always normal (see text)	Wolff–Parkinson–White syndrome Lown–Ganong–Levine syndrome

AVNRT = atrioventricular nodal re-entry tachycardia
AVRT = atrioventricular re-entry tachycardia
*occurs rarely

Atrioventricular nodal re-entry tachycardia (AVNRT), which accounts for about three-quarters of all supraventricular tachycardia, and atrioventricular re-entry tachycardia (AVRT) are the commonest.

(i) *Atrioventricular nodal re-entry tachycardia* (Fig. 1.9). The re-entry pathway lies wholly within the atrioventricular node. An episode of tachycardia is initiated by an atrial ectopic beat. If 'longitudinal dissociation' between the limbs of the re-entry pathway is present a tachycardia will ensue. When P waves are seen they are inverted in leads II, III and aVF, and are never subject to atrioventricular block.

(ii) *Atrioventricular re-entry tachycardia*. The re-entry pathway consists of the atrioventricular node and an anomalous extranodal bypass tract, which may be:

(a) *concealed*: it can conduct only in a retrograde direction (ventricle to atrium), so ventricular pre-excitation cannot occur.

(b) *'revealed'*: it is capable of bidirectional conduction. During antegrade conduction an impulse from the atria is conducted rapidly down the bypass tract causing ventricular pre-excitation, and at a

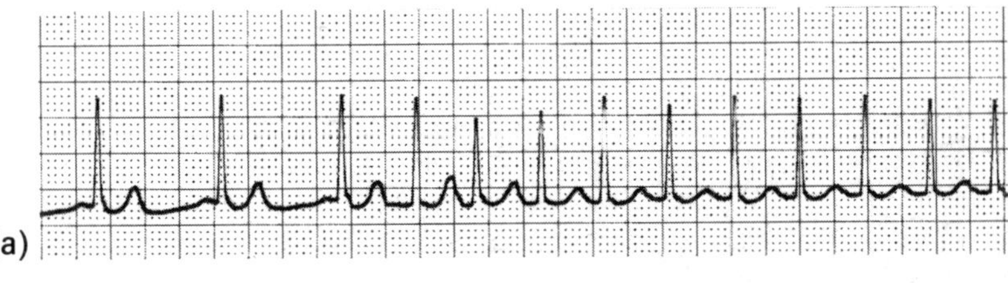

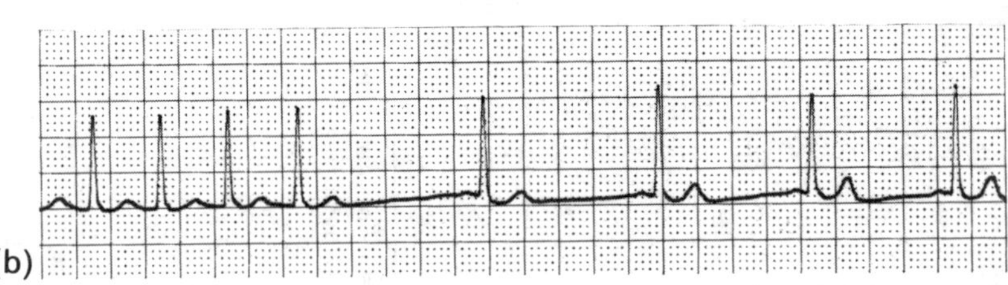

Fig. 1.9. Paroxysmal atrioventricular nodal re-entrant tachycardia. (a) Sudden onset initiated by an extrasystole. (b) Sudden spontaneous termination.

normal velocity through the atrioventricular node. The bypass tract reveals its presence by the inscription of a delta-wave on the upstroke of the QRS complex, following a short P–R interval (Wolff–Parkinson–White syndrome, see below). As in AVNRT an episode of tachycardia is initiated by an atrial ectopic beat and longitudinal dissociation between the limbs of the re-entry pathway sustains a tachycardia. During tachycardia the bypass tract almost always acts as the retrograde limb of the loop, so the QRS complex is normalised. Rarely the bypass tract conducts antegrade during tachycardia and delta waves will be seen. This tachycardia is 'wide-complex' and simulates ventricular tachycardia.

Wolff–Parkinson–White (W–P–W) syndrome

Wolff–Parkinson–White (Fig. 1.10) syndrome is a form of ventricular pre-excitation due to the presence of an anomalous atrioventricular bypass tract (Kent bundle). The ECG features are shown in Table 1.11. Pre-excitation due to anomalous bypass tracts connecting the atrium to the atrioventricular node (James fibres), the bundle of His or the bundle branches produce a short P–R interval and a normal QRS complex (Lown–Ganong–Levine syndrome) (Fig. 1.11).

Up to 80% of patients with W–P–W syndrome are prone to recurrent tachycardia. Also, atrial tachycardia, atrial flutter (Fig. 1.12) or atrial fibrillation may occur in patients who coincidentally have W–P–W syndrome. Antegrade 1:1 conduction through the bypass tract allows very rapid ventricular rates which may exceed 300 beats/minute in atrial fibrillation, with possible induction of ventricular fibrillation.

Management of supraventricular arrhythmias

Treatment modes are summarised in Table 1.12. Many factors must be considered when deciding how or whether to treat. Urgent termination may be indicated for impaired mental, haemodynamic or metabolic status. The possible benefits of prophylactic drug treatment must be weighed against the risks of

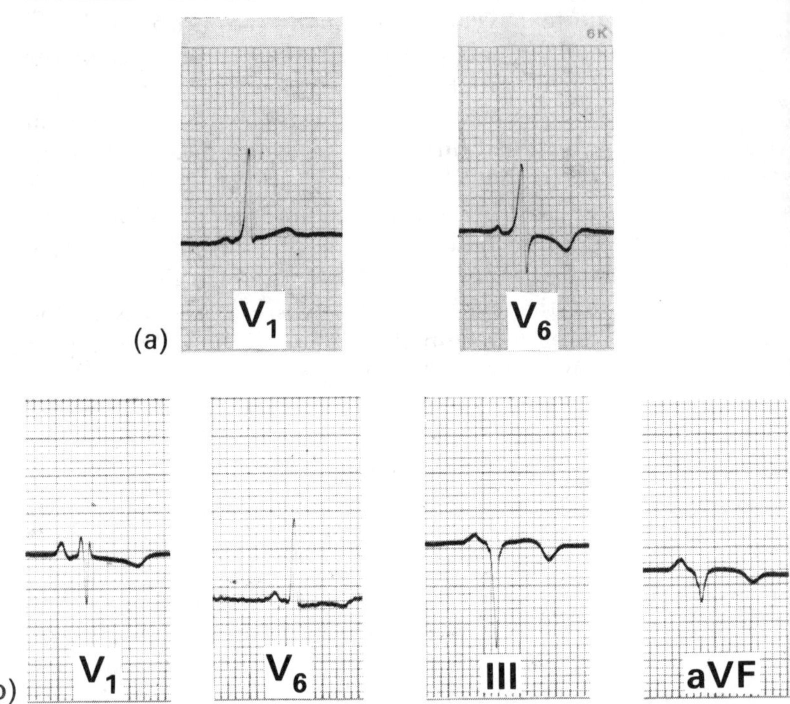

Fig. 1.10. Wolff–Parkinson–White (W–P–W) syndrome. The delta wave causes a short P–R interval and a broad QRS complex. (a) Type A: the dominant R-wave in lead V_1 simulates RVH, RBBB and true posterior myocardial infarction. (b) Type B: the negative delta-wave in leads III and aVf simulate inferior myocardial infarction.

Table 1.11

FEATURES OF WOLFF–PARKINSON–WHITE (W–P–W) SYNDROME

P–R interval	Short, less than 100 ms
Delta wave	Slurred QRS upstroke
QRS complex	Duration greater than 100 ms
type A (left-sided bypass)	QRS complex predominantly positive in right precordial leads; simulates RBBB, RVH or true posterior infarction
type B (right-sided bypass)	QRS often wide and negative in leads II, III, aVF; simulates inferior infarct

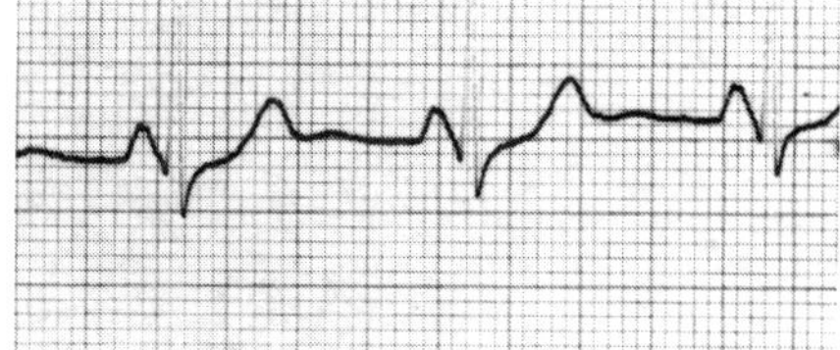

Fig. 1.11. Lown–Ganong–Levine syndrome. Lead V_5. Short P–R interval with a normal QRS complex.

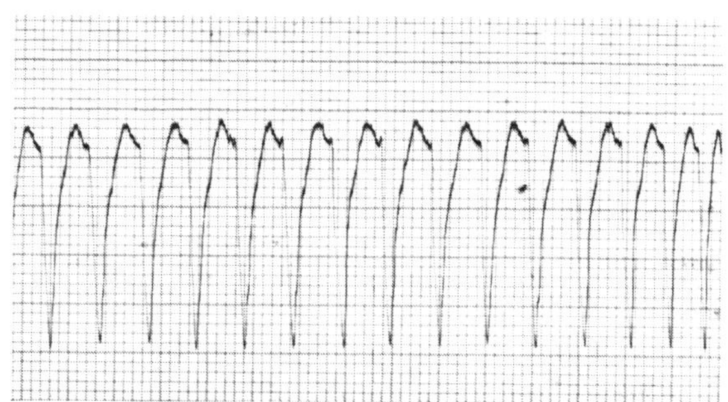

Fig. 1.12. Atrial flutter with 1:1 atrioventricular conduction resulting in a ventricular rate of 300 beats/min (lead I) in W–P–W syndrome (same patient as in Fig. 1.10b). Antegrade conduction through the bypass tract causes a 'wide-complex' simulating ventricular tachycardia.

potentially serious drug side-effects. Reassurance and explanation is an important part of the management of otherwise harmless recurrent supraventricular tachyarrhythmias.

VENTRICULAR ARRHYTHMIAS

Ventricular tachycardia

Definition

Three or more ventricular ectopic beats in regular rapid succession. The rate is usually between 140–250 beats/minute.

Pathogenesis

Ventricular tachycardia (Figs 1.13 and 1.14) is due to a local re-

Table 1.12

MANAGEMENT OF SUPRAVENTRICULAR ARRHYTHMIAS

Re–entrant tachycardias including W-P-W	*Atrial, junctional tachycardia (enhanced automaticity)*	*Atrial flutter*	*Atrial fibrillation*	*Atrial fibrillation in W-P-W syndrome*
Termination Sedation Vagal manoeuvres ● carotid sinus massage ● Valsalva manoeuvre ● 'diving reflex' Verapamil 5–10 mg i.v. over 1 min (propranolol, disopyramide) Underdrive pacing in RV Overdrive pacing in RA D.C. cardioversion	Stop digoxin if toxicity suspected Otherwise, digoxin is useful to increase atrio–ventricular block Disopyramide or flecainide decrease enhanced automaticity (atrial stabilizing agents)	D.C. cardioversion Atrial overdrive pacing ± concurrent i.v. disopyramide	Digoxin Verapamil or propranolol assist rate control D.C. cardioversion after anticoagulation	Avoid digoxin which enhances conduction in bundle of Kent D.C. cardioversion
Prophylaxis Reassurance Drugs (verapamil, quinidine, disopyramide, digoxin, amiodarone Anti-tachycardia pacing Surgical division of by–pass tract	D.C. cardioversion		Quinidine or amiodarone help prevent paroxysmal atrial fibrillation	Amiodarone, disopyramide and quinidine slow conduction in bundle of Kent and prevent atrial fibrillation Surgical division of by–pass tract

RA = right ventricle
RA = right atrium

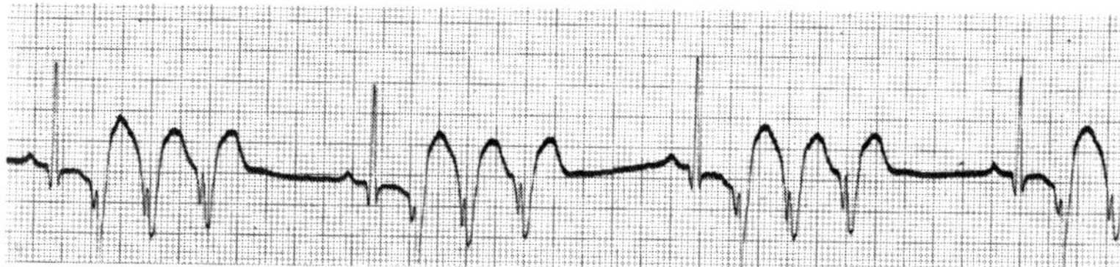

Fig. 1.13. Episodes of self-limiting ventricular tachycardia, rate 170 beats/min, initiated by 'R-on-T' ventricular ectopic beats.

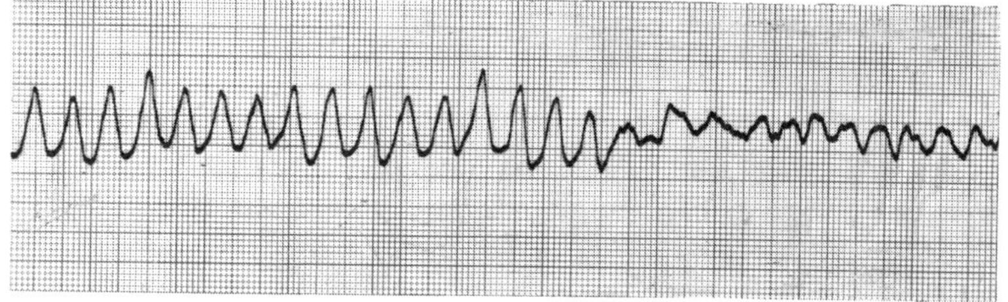

Fig. 1.14. Ventricular tachycardia terminating in ventricular fibrillation.

entry mechanism involving the Purkinje network. As in supraventricular re-entry tachycardias, it is initiated by an appropriately timed ectopic beat (ventricular) and is paroxysmal.

Relationship of P wave and QRS complexes

In at least half of all cases of ventricular tachycardia the abnormal ventricular depolarisation does not pass back through the atrioventricular node to the atria. Sinus rhythm is undisturbed and atrioventricular dissociation is seen, confirming that the wide-complex tachycardia is ventricular in origin and not supraventricular with aberrant conduction. If the abnormal ventricular depolarisation is conducted retrogradely to the atria an inverted P wave is seen following each QRS complex. The distinction between a ventricular or supraventricular origin for the tachycardia is then more difficult.

Capture and fusion beats

If P waves cannot be seen during the tachycardia indirect evidence of independent atrial activity is provided by *capture beats*. Their occurrence during a wide complex tachycardia is diagnostic of a ventricular origin.

A capture beat occurs when an atrial impulse is so timed that it is conducted to the ventricles, arriving before the next expected beat of the ventricular tachycardia. It appears as a normal, narrow QRS complex interrupting the sequence of ventricular tachycardia. If the atrial impulse arrives a little later it may coincide with the next expected beat from the ventricular ectopic focus resulting in a *fusion beat*, intermediate in form between the normal QRS complex and the ventricular ectopic depolarisation.

QRS complex

The QRS complex is always abnormally wide—greater than 120 ms. If the QRS complex is wider than 160 ms ventricular tachycardia is virtually assured. The QRS rate is 140–250 beats/min and the rhythm regular, although minor variations in R–R interval may occur. Since QRS morphology is constant the rhythm is termed *monomorphic* ventricular tachycardia.

Distinction between ventricular tachycardia and supraventricular tachycardia with aberrant conduction

Careful scrutiny of the 12-lead ECG of a wide-complex tachycardia will in most cases allow the distinction to be made. Sometimes it can be necessary to seek independent atrial activity by recording from an electrode placed in the oesophagus or the right

Table 1.13
USE OF THE ECG TO DIFFERENTIATE VENTRICULAR TACHYCARDIA (VT) FROM SUPRAVENTRICULAR TACHYCARDIA WITH ABERRANT VENTRICULAR CONDUCTION (SVT–AVC)

	SVT–AVC	*VT*
QRS duration	< 140 ms	> 140 ms
QRS complex configuration	Right bundle branch block (RBBB)	Left axis deviation in the frontal plane
Atrioventricular dissociation	Very rare	Occurs in 50% of patients
Capture and fusion beats	Never	Diagnostic

atrium. As discussed above, demonstration of independent atrial activity proves a ventricular origin but P wave activity related to each QRS complex is compatible with either ventricular or supraventricular origin. Distinguishing ECG features are shown in Table 1.13.

Clinical significance of ventricular tachycardia

Underlying pathology includes ischaemic heart disease, cardiomyopathies, mitral valve prolapse and digitalis toxicity. Ventricular tachycardia may be relatively or completely asymptomatic but usually presents with haemodynamic collapse, syncope, dizzy spells or cardiac arrest. It may degenerate to ventricular fibrillation.

Management

Cardioversion is required for shock or cardiac arrest. If the patient is stable lignocaine remains the drug of first choice, followed by procainamide, mexiletine or disopyramide. Cardiac pacing, single or dual chamber, can be very effective in preventing recurrent paroxysmal ventricular tachycardia. The simplest method is ventricular overdrive pacing which can also terminate the tachycardia.

If recurrent ventricular tachycardia occurs outside the context of an acute situation, such as in myocardial infarction, and is likely to recur then long-term prophylaxis is required. Several oral agents can be used. Amiodarone is the most effective but has significant long-term unwanted effects. Under certain circumstances an artificial implantable cardioverter-defibrillator (AICD) or surgery to ablate the ectopic focus may be considered.

Torsade de pointes ('twisting of the points')

This is polymorphic ventricular tachycardia in which there is a rhythmic change in cardiac axis so that complexes appear upright for several seconds before twisting around to an inverted appearance in sinusoidal fashion. It is commonly associated with a prolonged Q–T interval, often induced by antiarrhythmic drugs, tricyclic antidepressants, phenothiazines, hypokalaemia, sick sinus syndrome or congenital prolongation of the Q–T interval

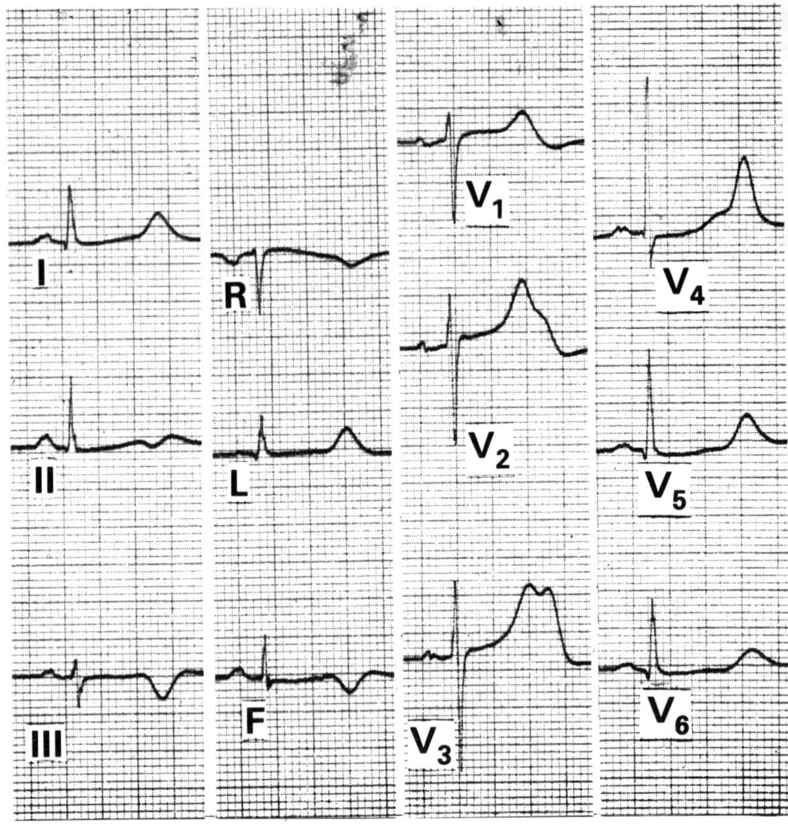

Fig. 1.15. Sinus rhythm. P–R interval 180 ms. Axis + 15°. The Q–T interval is grossly prolonged, for example, approximately 760 ms in V_5. From a 50-year-old patient with hereditary long Q–T syndrome.

(Fig. 1.15) (Romano–Ward and Jervell, Lange–Nielsen syndromes).

Treatment is usually by correction of the precipitating cause.

Accelerated idioventricular rhythm (AIVR)

AIVR (Fig. 1.16) is due to enhanced automaticity of a focus in the Purkinje network. It is non-paroxysmal and commonly emerges as an escape rhythm during underlying sinus bradycardia in the course of acute myocardial infarction. AIVR is a benign rhythm. Treatment consists of correcting the underlying

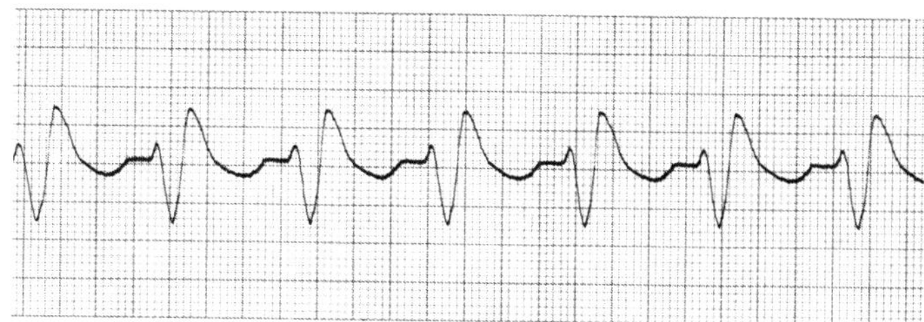

Fig. 1.16. Accelerated idioventricular rhythm, rate 80 beats/min.

bradycardia. The QRS rate is usually between 60 and 130 beats/min but the criteria for its ECG diagnosis are otherwise those of ventricular tachycardia.

Ventricular parasystole

In ventricular parasystole there are two independent foci of impulse formation:

(i) The sinus node (usually).
(ii) A ventricular ectopic focus.

The ventricular parasystolic focus has three properties:

(i) *Entrance block*: it cannot be penetrated electrically and reset by impulses originating from the sinus node. Its inherent rhythm therefore continues undisturbed.
(ii) *Constant rate*: the parasystolic focus has a constant inherent rate although minor variations are seen. The interectopic intervals are thus mathematically related. Some parasystolic discharges are not manifest on the ECG since they occur when the ventricular myocardium is still refractory from the preceding sinus beat. Since the parasystolic focus is autonomous the sinus beats and the ectopic beats bear no relationship to each other and the *coupling intervals vary*.
(iii) *Exit block*: impulse formation in the parasystolic focus is regular but conduction to the adjacent myocardium may intermittently fail.

The combined effects of intermittent exit block and refractoriness of the myocardium may conspire to prevent parasystolic beats appearing in the ECG for prolonged periods. Long ECG strips are often required confidently to analyse parasystolic rhythm since many multiples of the basic parasystolic cycle length may intervene between two beats. The fortuitous coincidence of sinus and parasystolic beats may result in *fusion beats*.

Clinical significance

Ventricular parasystole is uncommon. It occurs in a variety of serious underlying myocardial diseases and in digitalis intoxication. It may precede ventricular tachycardia or fibrillation. The treatment is that of the underlying condition.

Ventricular fibrillation

Ventricular fibrillation (Fig. 1.14) is a rapid, irregular chaotic rhythm seen usually as a terminal event. Since coordinated contraction of the ventricular myocardium is impossible there is circulatory arrest. It is frequently precipitated by a ventricular ectopic beat of very short coupling interval such that the ectopic depolarisation falls in the vulnerable period of the preceding T-wave (R on T ectopic).

Clinical significance

Ventricular fibrillation occurs most commonly in ischaemic heart disease. Cardiac arrest in acute myocardial infarction is due to ventricular fibrillation in 90% of cases. Other causes include chronic ischaemic heart disease, digitalis toxicity, anaesthetic agents, myocardial muscle disease and electrocution. The context in which ventricular fibrillation occurs has prognostic significance. Its occurrence due to electrical instability of the heart early in otherwise uncomplicated myocardial infarction is termed *primary fibrillation.* Defibrillation is usually successful and the prognosis excellent. *Secondary fibrillation* complicating cardiogenic shock, cardiac failure or other serious myocardial disease is less successfully treated and implies a poor subsequent prognosis.

Treatment

Treatment is by immediate defibrillation and cardiopulmonary resuscitation. In recurrent ventricular fibrillation bretylium tosylate may be a valuable adjunct to standard management.

ATRIOVENTRICULAR (AV) BLOCK

Background

In atrioventricular block there is a delay or failure of impulse conduction from the atria to the ventricles. The site of block may be in the atrioventricular node, the bundle of His, simultaneously in both bundle branches or any combination of these sites.

Atrioventricular block is classified as:

(i) *First degree*: there is a delay in conduction but all atrial depolarisations reach the ventricles. Every P-wave is followed by a QRS complex (Fig. 1.17).

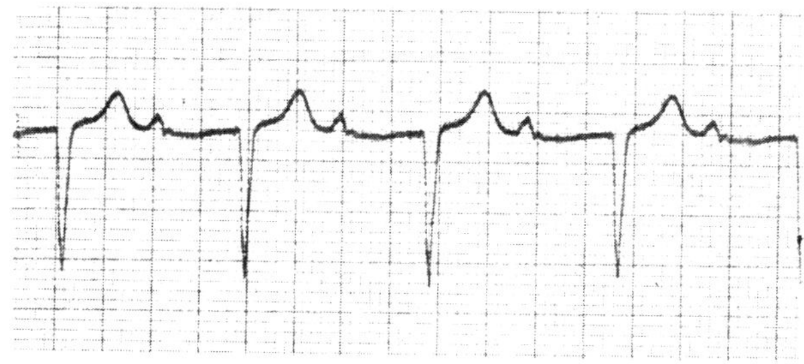

Fig. 1.17. First degree atrioventricular block, P–R interval 400 ms.

(ii) *Second degree*: there is intermittent failure of impulse conduction. Some P waves are followed by a QRS complex and some are not (Figs 1.18, 1.19).

(iii) *Third degree*: there is complete failure of impulse conduction. P waves are completely dissociated from QRS complexes (Fig. 1.20).

Depending on the period of observation an individual subject may display normal sinus rhythm and any or every degree of

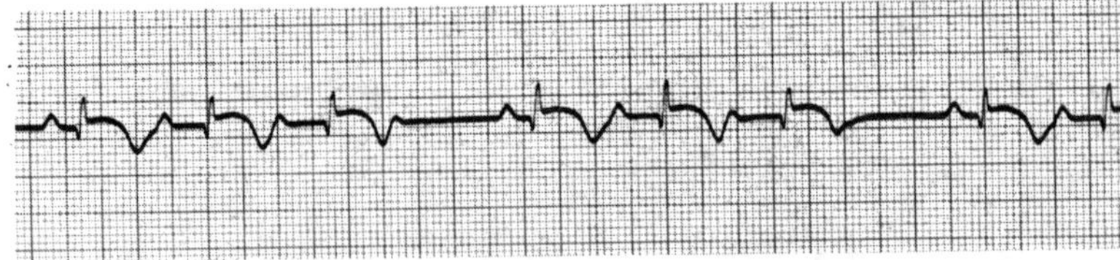

Fig. 1.18. Mobitz type I (Wenckebach) second degree atrioventricular block in a patient with acute inferior myocardial infarction (lead II).

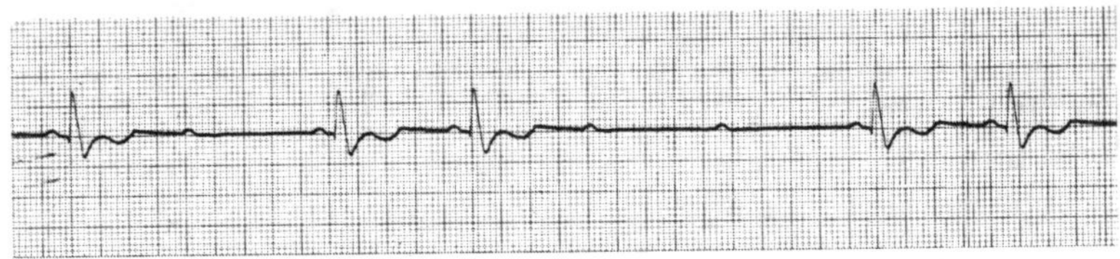

Fig. 1.19. Mobitz type II second degree atrioventricular block. The conduction ratio varies between 2:1 and 3:1.

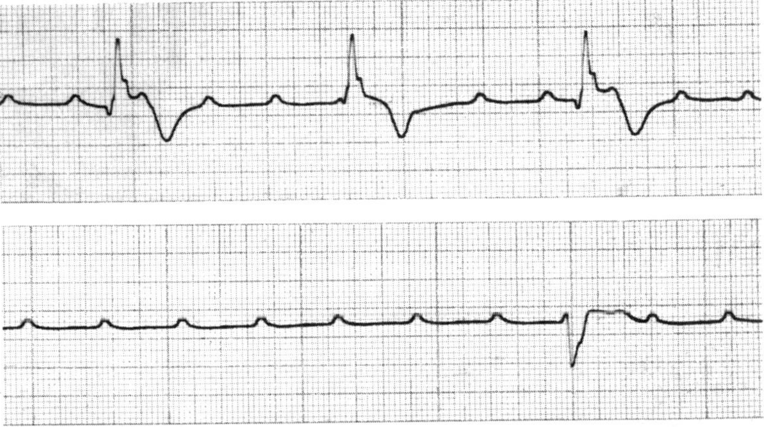

Fig. 1.20. Third degree (complete) atrioventricular block culminating in prolonged ventricular asystole during a Stokes–Adams attack.

atrioventricular block. The causes of atrioventricular block are shown in Table 1.14 and its ECG criteria in Table 1.15.

Clinical features

First degree and Mobitz type I second degree block are asymptomatic. Symptoms arising from the low heart rate in Mobitz type

Table 1.14
CAUSES OF ATRIOVENTRICULAR BLOCK

Congenital
- isolated atrioventricular block
- associated with structural lesions (corrected transposition, endocardial cushion defects)

Acquired
- idiopathic conduction system disease
- acute myocardial infarction
- chronic ischaemic heart disease
- calcific aortic stenosis
- cardiac surgery
- connective tissue disease (polymyositis, rheumatoid arthritis, ankylosing spondylitis, scleroderma)
- infiltrations (tumour, amyloidosis, sarcoidosis)
- myxoedema
- heredofamilial neuromuscular diseases
- Chagas disease
- rheumatic fever
- diphtheria
- transient disturbances (electrolyte intolerance, digitalis toxicity)

II and third degree block include effort intolerance, heart failure, dizzy spells and syncope. Syncopal (Stokes–Adams) attacks are typically sudden in onset and of short duration. More prolonged attacks lead to anoxic muscular twitching and fits, but incontinence is unusual. Spontaneous restoration of rhythm is accompanied by facial flushing and rapid clinical recovery. During an attack there may be profound slowing of the rate, ventricular asystole, ventricular tachycardia or fibrillation. Sudden death is common.

Management

Cardiac pacing is mandatory in symptomatic atrioventricular block. Urgent implantation is required because of the ever-present risk of sudden death. Asymptomatic second degree (Mobitz type II) and third degree block are definite indications for permanent cardiac pacing because the poor prognosis is corrected. The use of long-acting isoprenaline has long been obsolete.

Table 1.15
ATRIOVENTRICULAR BLOCK

Degree	*ECG criteria*	*Site of block*	*Comment*
First	P–R interval constant. Duration > 200 ms	Atrioventricular node	Can be normal in subjects with high vagal tone. Asymptomatic
Second			
Mobitz type I (Wenckebach)	Progressive prolongation of P–R interval until complete block occurs. After a single dropped QRS atrioventricular conduction is restored and the cycle repeated	Atrioventricular node	Occasionally seen in young athletes with high vagal tone. Usually pathological but rarely progresses to high degree block Rarely symptomatic Good prognosis
Mobitz type II	Constant P–R interval (normal or prolonged). Intermittent single beat atrioventricular block.	His bundle, bundle branches	More frequently progresses to third degree block; prognosis poor

	2:1 atrioventricular block (more common)	Atrioventricular node, His bundle, bundle branches	2:1 block may be an extreme form of Wenckebach (Type I) and occur in the atrioventricular node; the prognosis is thus less certain
Third	No relationship between P waves and QRS complexes. QRS complexes may be		Subsidiary pacemaker in His bundle is reliable. Rate 50–60 beats/min.
	(i) narrow	Atrioventricular node	Common in acute inferior infarction. Stokes–Adams attacks/asystole are rare
	(ii) wide	His bundle, bundle branches	Subsidiary pacemaker in Purkinje system is unreliable. Rate 20–35 beats/min. Stokes–Adams attacks/asystole common

Congenital atrioventricular block has a high mortality in the neonatal period but a good prognosis in later childhood and early adult life. An asymptomatic patient with a ventricular rate above 50 beats/min at rest and a further rise on exercise may be observed, but symptoms or a resting rate below 50 beats/min should indicate pacemaker implantation.

The management of atrioventricular block complicating acute myocardial infarction is discussed on p. 27.

SICK SINUS SYNDROME

Background

Sick sinus syndrome (sinoatrial disorder) is a clinical entity based on impaired sinus node impulse formation and conduction. Impaired A–V nodal conduction may also be present.

Electrocardiogram

Rhythm disturbances include:

(i) Persistent inappropriate sinus bradycardia with impaired ability to increase the heart rate on exercise (chronotropic incompetence).
(ii) Sinus arrest and/or sinoatrial block.
(iii) Combined sinoatrial and atrioventricular conduction system abnormalities.
(iv) Alternating bouts of bradyarrhythmia and paroxysmal tachycardias of supraventricular origin (bradycardia–tachycardia syndrome).

Causes

Idiopathic fibrosis of the sinus node and atrial myocardium is the commonest cause. The process may also involve the distal conducting system. As in idiopathic atrioventricular block the incidence rises with age. Sick sinus syndrome may also develop in association with a wide variety of underlying cardiac diseases, after cardiac surgery (especially repair of an atrial septal defect), and with antiarrhythmic drug toxicity.

Clinical features

Palpitations and dizzy spells are common; syncope is less frequent. Systemic embolic occur in up to 15% of patients with bradycardia–tachycardia syndrome.

Treatment

Cardiac pacing is required for symptomatic bradycardia. Failure of the sinus node to recover promptly after a bout of tachycardia may cause symptomatic bradycardia in which case antiarrhythmic drugs may obviate the need for pacing. In practice it is usually necessary to implant a pacemaker if drugs are required because the sinus node may be further depressed.

If there is no evidence of atrioventricular conduction disease it is preferable to use atrial pacing. This preserves atrioventricular synchrony during pacemaker operation, and may help to prevent the emergence of supraventricular arrhythmias. The incidence of embolism may also be reduced. Where paroxysmal atrial tachyarrhythmias persist anticoagulants should be used if not otherwise contraindicated.

Sick sinus syndrome has a good long-term prognosis which is not further improved by pacing or drug therapy. Cardiac pacing is therefore indicated only for symptomatic bradyarrhythmias.

HYPERSENSITIVE CAROTID SINUS SYNDROME

Background

Carotid sinus stimulation normally causes a vagally mediated fall in sinus rate. A hypersensitive response to carotid sinus massage may be of two types:

(i) *Cardioinhibitory*: promotes ventricular asystole exceeding 3 s in duration (Fig. 1.22a). Sinus arrest or sinoatrial block are usual, but additional impairment of atrioventricular conduction is not unusual.

(ii) *Vasodepressor*: a fall of 50 mmHg in systolic blood pressure or a fall of 30 mmHg associated with typical symptoms, without a fall in heart rate. The pure vasodepressor type is rare, but a vasodepressor component

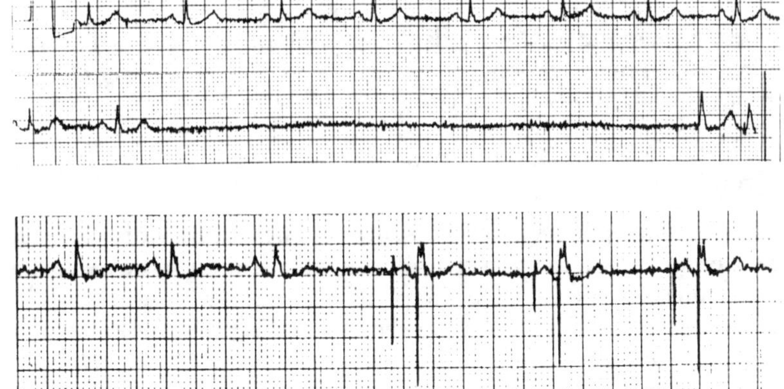

Fig. 1.21. Hypersensitive carotid sinus syndrome. (a) Right carotid sinus massage causes sinus node arrest and ventricular asystole lasting 5.4 s. The presenting symptoms were reproduced. (b) The 4th, 5th and 6th beats show dual chamber (atrioventricular sequential) pacing during carotid sinus massage. The patient's symptoms were abolished.

may commonly be unmasked by cardiac pacing when symptoms persist due to a fall in blood pressure despite maintenance of cardiac rate.

Treatment

Recurrent syncope due to cardioinhibitory hypersensitive carotid sinus syndrome requires cardiac pacing. Dual chamber pacing is probably more effective in preventing persistent symptoms due to hypotension since atrioventricular synchrony is preserved (Fig. 1.21b).

INVESTIGATION OF CARDIAC ARRHYTHMIA

Symptoms

A cardiac arrhythmia is usually suspected because palpitations, dizziness, syncope, chest discomfort or other episodic symptoms are described. Patients can often illustrate the sensation of palpitations by tapping the desk top, providing useful clues to the mode of onset, rate and regularity of the rhythm. Trigger factors such as caffeine, alcohol or drug usage should be considered.

Physical examination

A general and cardiac physical examination provides evidence of underlying disease. If the arrhythmia is present the priority will be to record an electrocardiogram.

The response to *carotid sinus massage* can provide useful information (Table 1.16). The patient is examined supine with the neck extended and rotated away from the side of examination. The carotid pulse is palpated at the angle of the jaw. Light pressure may cause immediate asystole in hypersensitive carotid sinus syndrome. If no change occurs firm rotational massage is continued for 5 s. The procedure is repeated on the opposite side. Carotid sinus massage must always be performed after auscultation to exclude carotid artery stenosis, and under ECG and blood pressure control.

Table 1.16
RESPONSES TO CAROTID SINUS MASSAGE

Cardiac rhythm	*Response*
Normal sinus rhythm	Slows sinus rate Increases atrioventricular nodal conduction time and refractoriness
Sinus tachycardia	Rate slows during massage
Junctional re-entry tachycardias	No change or slight slowing or abrupt termination
Atrial tachycardia	Increases degree of atrioventricular block
Atrial flutter	Does not terminate
Atrial fibrillation	Transient slowing of ventricular rate Does not terminate
Ventricular tachycardia	No effect (very rarely terminates)

Electrocardiography

This is the definitive diagnostic investigation, recording the current rhythm and providing clues, such as ectopic beats or ventricular pre-excitation, to possible abnormal rhythms. Since the 12-lead ECG can provide information for only 1 or 2 min more prolonged monitoring is usually necessary.

Ambulatory electrocardiography (Holter monitoring)

A small ECG amplifier and tape recorder are carried on a waist belt. A continuous multichannel ECG is recorded for up to 24 hours. An event marker is provided for the patient to indicate the occurrence of symptoms. A note of activities and symptoms are recorded in a diary.

Ambulatory electrocardiography can correlate symptoms with rhythm disturbances. Asymptomatic but prognostically important arrhythmias may be recorded in patients at risk, for example, ventricular tachycardia in ischaemic heart disease or cardiomyopathies. No arrhythmia may be recorded during symptoms, a useful 'negative' result.

Patient-activated monitors

If the suspected arrhythmia is associated with symptoms but is very infrequent and unlikely to be recorded during a 24 h monitoring period a patient-activated monitor can be provided, such as the Cardio-Memo. This allows the patient to record a short period (about 40 s) of ECG during the symptoms, which can subsequently be converted to an audio-signal for transmission by telephone to the receiving centre for immediate interpretation or storage.

Exercise stress testing

The physiological demands of exercise and accompanying changes in autonomic tone may usefully induce arrhythmias in a controlled environment. Full cardiopulmonary resuscitation facilities must be available.

Intracardiac electrography

Using standard cardiac catheterisation techniques electrode catheters are introduced via femoral and antecubital veins and positioned to record from the high and low right atrium, the bundle of His (by careful positioning across the tricuspid valve), the right ventricle and the left atrium (by placing an electrode in the coronary sinus). The technique is used

(i) To record the sequence of cardiac activation.
(ii) To introduce accurately timed single or multiple extra-stimuli; these are used:
    (a) to measure conduction times and refractory periods in the specialised conducting system;
    (b) to initiate and terminate supraventricular and ventricular re-entry tachycardias.

Such electrophysiological studies have provided a wealth of information about the mechanisms of cardiac arrhythmias. Their main clinical applications are to assess the patient's suitability for specialised antitachycardia pacemakers or implantable cardio-verter–defibrillators, and to assess the efficacy of antiarrhythmic drug therapy of life-threatening arrhythmias.

CARDIAC PACEMAKERS

Background

The cardiac pacemaker is an electronic device used to stimulate the heart. Symptomatic bradycardia is the principal indication for pacing.

The implantable cardiac pacemaker weighs about 40 g, and consists of

(i) *A power source*: a lithium–iodine battery with a potential lifetime of approximately 10 years.
(ii) *Circuitry*: a 'hybrid' circuit using a silicon chip and some discrete components. Its functions include:
    (a) *Timing*: to deliver stimulation pulses at predetermined intervals.
    (b) *Sensing*: to inhibit the pacemaker output when the native cardiac rate is satisfactory.

    Other functions which may be provided are:

    (c) *Programmability*: the ability to alter pacemaker

rate, output, sensitivity and refractory periods non-invasively using an external electromagnetic programmer.

(d) *Telemetry*: data such as the current pacemaker programme, battery impedance, pacing impedance and intracardiac electrograms can be telemetred from the pacemaker and received externally.

Indications for pacing

The indications for implantation of a permanent pacemaker are shown in Table 1.17. Other indications are more controversial. Prophylactic permanent pacing for newly acquired but persistent conduction defects following acute myocardial infarction are of uncertain benefit.

Table 1.17

DEFINITE INDICATIONS FOR PERMANENT PACEMAKER IMPLANTATION

Symptomatic
- third degree atrioventricular block
- second degree atrioventricular block (type I and type II)
- atrial fibrillation with a slow ventricular response
- sick sinus syndrome
- hypersensitive carotid sinus syndrome

Asymptomatic
- third degree atrioventricular block
- second degree atrioventricular block, type II

Specialised pacemakers may also be used to terminate certain tachyarrhythmias by interference with re-entry pathways if drug therapy has failed.

Pacing Modes

The majority of pacemakers implanted to date have been designed to pace and sense in a single chamber, either the ventricle or the atrium. Of these the vast majority are employed in the ventricle.

Ventricular 'demand' pacing has been outstandingly successful in abolishing Stokes–Adams attacks and prolonging life expectancy in patients with third degree atrioventricular block. However this mode of pacing has two major disadvantages:

(i) Atrioventricular synchrony, with its known haemodynamic benefits, is not restored.

(ii) A rate response to exercise is not possible.

To overcome these disadvantages the 'dual chamber' pacemaker has been developed. This device can sense and pace in both the atrium and the ventricle. The pacemaker senses the P-wave and if there is no native QRS complex sensed within a predetermined atrioventricular interval (analogous to the P–R interval) a ventricular pacing stimulus is triggered (Fig. 1.22(a)). If the sinus rate falls below a predetermined value the atrium can also be paced (see Fig. 1.22b). Atrioventricular synchrony is maintained, and since the ventricular paced rate can follow the P-wave rate within preset safety limits a ventricular rate response to exercise is restored.

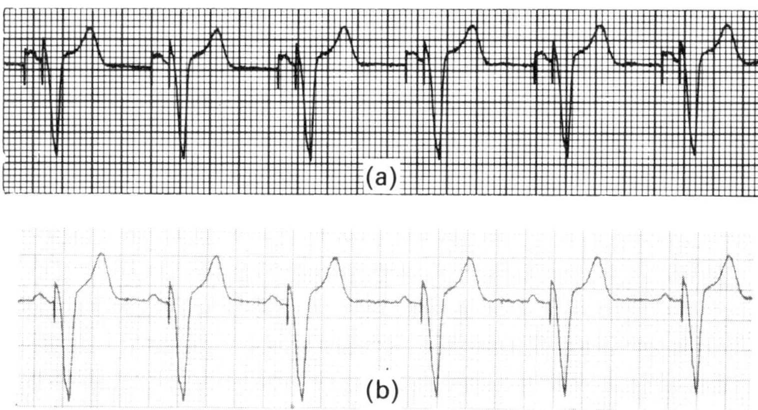

Fig. 1.22(a). Complete heart block treated by dual chamber (DDD) pacing. The sinus node rate is 67 beats/min. A paced ventricular complex follows each intrinsic P wave. (b) Atrio-ventricular sequential (DVI) pacing A paced atrial complex is followed after a preset (A–V) interval by a paced ventricular complex.

The complexity of such pacing modes has necessitated the development of a descriptive code. In its simplest form the code consists of three letters (Table 1.18). The first and second letters refer to the chamber paced and sensed respectively. The third letter refers to the response of the pacemaker to a sensed event. It can be seen that the ventricular demand pacemaker would be

Table 1.18
THE THREE-LETTER PACEMAKER CODE

First letter *Chamber paced*	*Second letter* *Chamber sensed*	*Third letter* *Mode of response*
	O = no sensing	O = no response
V = ventricle	V = ventricle	I = inhibited
A = atrium	A = atrium	T = triggered
D = double (atrium and ventricle)	D = double (atrium and ventricle)	D = atrial triggered and ventricular inhibited

designated 'VVI' while the dual chamber pacemaker described above would be designated 'DDD'. This code is now in universal common usage.

Many other pacemaker operational modes are available. Their description is beyond the scope of this text.

Rate-responsive Pacing

The use of dual chamber pacemakers to restore an exercise rate response entirely depends on the presence of normal and stable sinus rhythm in the atria. When this does not obtain it has proved possible to use other biological parameters as an index of metabolic need. These include the sensing of blood temperature, respiratory rate, the vibrations of body activity and the catecholamine-induced shortening of the Q–T interval, all of which have been used to drive ventricular paced rate on exercise. New biosensors and their incorporation into dual chamber pacemaker systems are currently under development.

FURTHER READING

Bennett D.H. (1981). *Cardiac Arrhythmias. Practical Notes on Interpretation and Treatment.* Bristol: John Wright.

Rowlands D.J. (1987). *Understanding the Electrocardiogram. Section 3: Rhythm Abnormalities.* London, Gower Medical Press.

Schamroth L. (1971). *The Disorders of Cardiac Rhythm.* Oxford: Blackwell Scientific Publications.

Chapter Two

The Electrocardiogram

The aim of this chapter is to summarise the criteria by which the normal and abnormal electrocardiogram (ECG) can be recognised. It cannot provide a comprehensive account of electrocardiography and a basic familiarity with the subject is assumed.

ELECTROPHYSIOLOGICAL BASIS OF THE ECG

Voltage differences between activated and resting tissue are generated by ion fluxes across the cell membrane. Figure 2.1 shows the action potential from a single myocardial cell.

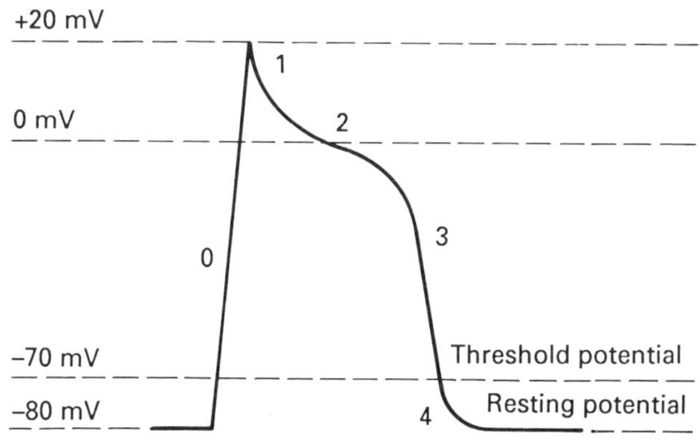

Fig. 2.1. Phases of the action potential.

Phases

Phase 0: rapid depolarisation

This is sudden increased permeability to Na^+ through 'fast' channels (-80 mV to -40 mV) and Ca^{2+} through 'slow' channels (-40 mV to $+20$ mV).

Phase 1: early rapid repolarisation

This is inactivation of the rapid Na^+ influx, and possible intracellular influx of Cl^-.

Phase 2: plateau phase

This has low membrane conductance to all ions, but slow inward K^+ current occurs.

Phase 3: final rapid repolarisation

This has outward K^+ current and inactivation of inward currents.

Phase 4: resting membrane potential

The behaviour here depends on the cell type.

(i) Myocardial cell: the potential remains steady throughout diastole.
(ii) Specialised conduction or 'pacemaker' cell: This displays *phase 4 diastolic depolarisation.* If the threshold potential is reached spontaneous depolarisation occurs initiating an action potential. The diastolic depolarisation rate is normally fastest in sinoatrial nodal cells which therefore dominate the cardiac rhythm.

The ECG is the surface manifestation of the combined action potentials generated in the atrial and ventricular myocardium. The QRS complex, ST segment and T waves are the surface ECG manifestations of action potential phases 0, 1, 2 and 3 respectively. Phase 4 corresponds to the isoelectric baseline. Electrical activity from the sinoatrial node and specialised conducting tissue is not recorded on the conventional ECG.

Spread of Cardiac Activation

The sequence of activation depends upon its site of initiation, the

Table 2.1

ANATOMICAL FEATURES OF THE SPECIALISED CONDUCTING SYSTEM
(DIMENSIONS ARE APPROXIMATE AVERAGE VALUES)

Structure	*Anatomical features*
Sinoatrial node	Site: right atrium, mouth of superior vena cava Size: 15 × 6 × 2 mm
Atrioventricular node	Site: right side of lower interatrial septum Size: 5 × 2 × 1 mm
Bundle of His	Site: traverses the central fibrous body to reach the upper interventricular septum Size: 15 mm long, 2 mm diameter
Right bundle branch	A direct continuation of the bundle of His to the endocardial surface of the right ventricle; upper part does not give rise to Purkinje fibres
Left bundle branch	Left side of upper interventricular septum, to which it supplies Purkinje fibres; bifurcates almost immediately
Left anterosuperior division (fascicle) Left posteroinferior division (fascicle)	Supplies anterosuperior left ventricle Supplies posteroinferior left ventricle
Purkinje network	Arises from main left bundle, the lower right bundle and both left divisions to supply the endocardial surfaces of the ventricles

distribution of excitable myocardium and the normal function of the specialised conduction system. The anatomy of the specialised conducting system is summarised in Table 2.1.

The normal cardiac impulse is formed in the sinoatrial node and spreads throughout the atrial myocardium at a velocity of 1000 mm/s. Since the sinoatrial node lies in the upper right atrium the predominant direction of spread is downwards and leftwards. The only electrical connection between atria and ventricles is the atrioventricular node and bundle of His. The atrial myocardium and ventricular myocardium are separated electrically by the non-conducting fibrous atrioventricular ring. The impulse is delayed by the atrioventricular node which conducts at a velocity of 200 mm/s. Activation of the ventricular myocardium starts on the upper left side of the interventricular septum, spreading through it from left to right. The right ventricular free wall is then activated fractionally earlier than the left ventricular free wall. Conduction through specialised tissue distal to the atrioventricular node occurs at 4000 mm/s. Since the left ventricle contains the greatest myocardial mass the predominant direction of activation in the ventricles is downwards and to the left.

In the intact heart depolarisation proceeds from endocardium to epicardium, but repolarisation occurs in the opposite direction. The reason for this is uncertain. It means, however, that an electrode sensing from the epicardial surface of the heart will record a depolarisation waveform and a repolarisation waveform of the same polarity, that is, when the QRS complex is positive the T wave will also be positive.

Theoretical Aspects of the ECG Leads

A basic understanding of the ECG leads requires appreciation of the following points:

(i) *Depolarisation is a vector quantity*: the activation wave has magnitude and direction, and is therefore a vector quantity. Its magnitude depends on the mass of myocardium depolarised. Its direction depends on its site of initiation and subsequent spread. A lead records maximum voltage when its direction of sensing is parallel to the direction of activation at any moment during the cardiac cycle.

(ii) *Linear and volume conductors*: the limbs are *linear* conductors and there is no significant voltage drop along their length. Wherever the electrode is placed on the limb the waveform recorded is the same as that recorded at the point where the limb joins the trunk. The trunk is a *volume* conductor. Voltages vary considerably with the recording position on a volume conductor, so the positioning of chest leads materially affects the waveform obtained.

(iii) *The Einthoven triangle hypothesis* presents four assumptions which provide a basis for understanding the limb leads and the cardiac axis. The assumptions, all approximations, are

(1) The trunk is a homogeneous volume conductor.
(2) The electrical forces generated by the heart are regarded as originating from a point source at the centre of the heart.
(3) The effective sensing positions of the right arm, left arm and left foot leads (R, L and F) form an equilateral triangle with the heart (assumed to be a point source generator) at its centre.
(4) The limb leads record in the frontal plane only.

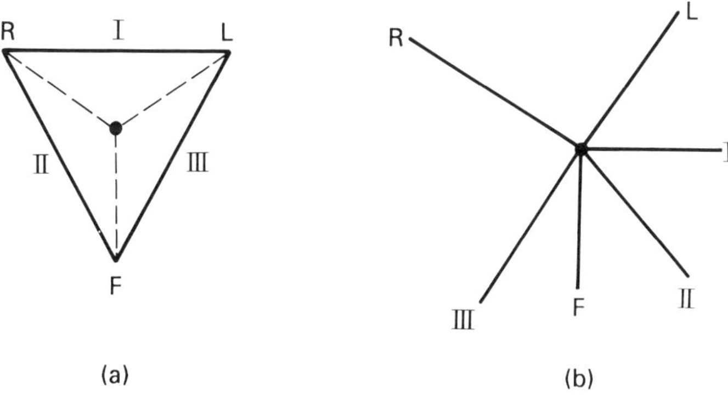

Fig. 2.2(a). The heart is represented as a point at the centre of an equilateral triangle. The sensing direction of the bipolar leads I, II, III and the unipolar leads (dotted) R, L, F are indicated. (b) The sensing direction is more easily appreciated if the figure is rearranged. Leads I and L sense the anterolateral aspect of the heart, leads II, III and F the inferior aspect. Lead R looks into the cavity of the ventricles.

Figure 2.2a shows the heart as a 'point source' within an equilateral triangle representing the torso, with the left arm, right arm and left foot connections indicated. The direction in which each lead senses cardiac activity is more easily appreciated if the diagram is rearranged as in Figure 2.2b.

ECG Lead Connections

ECG leads are either bipolar or unipolar (Table 2.2). The *bipolar limb leads* record the potential difference between two limbs, one connected to the positive terminal and the other to the negative terminal of the recording galvanometer. The right leg connection is an earth lead to minimise electrical interference in the recording.

The *unipolar limb leads* are constructed by joining R, L and F together and connecting them to the negative terminal of the galvanometer to form an 'indifferent electrode' which is considered to have zero potential. The positive 'exploring electrode' is placed on the right arm, left arm or left foot and records the potential from the respective limb. The letter V signifies a unipolar lead. A rather low amplitude waveform is recorded

Table 2.2

ECG LEAD CONNECTIONS

Lead	*Connection*
I	LA^+, RA^-
II	LL^+, RA^-
III	LL^+, LA^-
V1	4th interspace, right of sternum
V2	4th interspace, left of sternum
V3	Midway between V_2 and V_4
V4	5th interspace, midclavicular line
V5	Anterior axillary line, level of V_4
V6	Midaxillary line, level of V_4

L(R)A = left (right) arm
LL = left leg
+ (−) = lead connected to positive (negative) terminal of the galvanometer

which can be 'augmented' by disconnecting from the central terminal the extremity from which the recording is being made. These leads are thus named aVR, aVL and aVF. The exploring lead location for the precordial leads is shown in Table 2.2.

QRS Axis

Since depolarisation is a vector quantity the series of instantaneous vectors which constitute total cardiac activation may be expressed as a *mean QRS vector*. If this vector is then related to the triangle formed, according to Einthoven's hypothesis, by the frontal plane leads and the voltage in each of the leads is known, the *mean frontal plane QRS axis* is obtained. The mean frontal plane QRS axis is of crucial importance in deciding whether the ECG is normal or abnormal.

Determination of the Mean Frontal Plane QRS Axis

The mean frontal plane QRS axis (the axis) is easily obtained by inspection of the six frontal plane ECG leads and use of the hexaxial reference system (Fig. 2.3). This system is derived simply from the disposition of the leads as shown in Fig. 2.2b and divides the circle into angles of 30°. Each line is marked in degrees, positive or negative, with lead I chosen arbitrarily as zero degrees. The following steps give the axis in degrees:

(1) Find the frontal plane lead in which the QRS complex is most nearly equiphasic (that is, the algebraic sum of the positive and negative QRS components is most nearly zero). This is not necessarily the smallest QRS complex. The axis is approximately at right angles to this lead.

(2) If the lead at right angles to the most nearly equiphasic lead is predominantly positive the axis must point in the same direction as this lead. If it is predominantly negative the axis must point in the opposite direction to this lead.

Steps 1 and 2 give the axis to the nearest 30°.

(3) The axis is obtained to within 15° (the most accurate possible according to the Einthoven hypothesis) as follows. Inspect again the most nearly equiphasic lead and

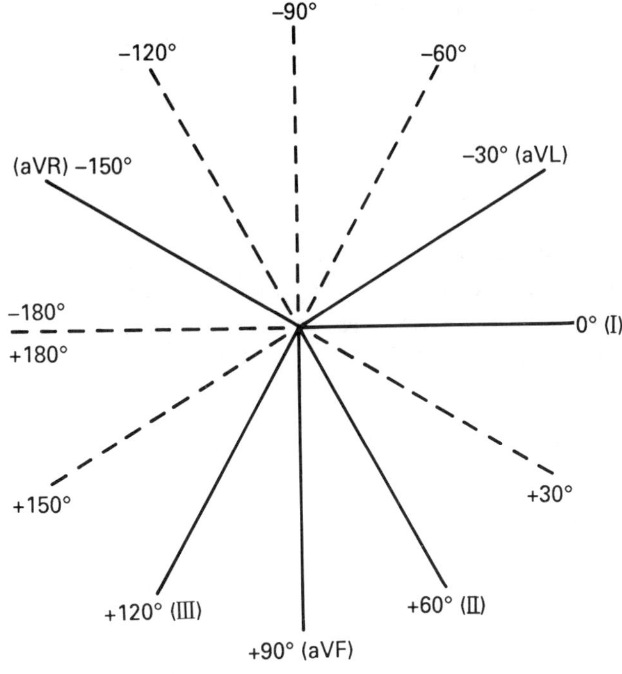

Fig. 2.3. Hexaxial reference system.

decide whether the QRS complex is (a) exactly equiphasic, (b) slightly more positive than negative, (c) slightly more negative than positive:

(a) if the QRS is exactly equiphasic the axis already obtained need not be altered;

(b) if the QRS is more positive than negative the axis must point a little more towards the first lead. Alter the axis obtained in step 2 by 15° around the hexaxial reference system *towards* the first lead;

(c) if the QRS axis is more negative than positive the axis must point a little more away from the first lead. Alter the axis obtained in step 2 by 15° *away from* the first lead.

An exactly similar procedure may be used to determine the mean frontal plane T wave axis. The difference between the QRS axis and T wave axis is called the *ventricular gradient*. It does not normally exceed 60°. The estimation of ventricular gradient is useful in deciding whether the T waves in the frontal plane leads are normal or abnormal.

Nomenclature of the QRS Complex

The 'QRS complex' is a generic term denoting the surface electrocardiographic manifestation of ventricular myocardial depolarisation. By convention different QRS waveforms are labelled as shown in Fig. 2.4.

THE NORMAL ELECTROCARDIOGRAM

Criteria by which the normal ECG complex is recognised are summarised in Tables 2.3 and 2.4. Normal sinus rhythm, standard calibration (1 mV = 10 mm) and normal paper recording speed (25 mm/s) are assumed. Certain identification of the normal ECG is the most difficult skill in basic ECG interpretation.

Reporting the 12-Lead ECG

It is the authors' experience that the presence of a glaring ECG abnormality will deflect the student's attention from equally important but less obvious abnormalities in the record. This is avoided by adhering to a system for reporting any 12-lead ECG. The identity of the patient, the date of the recording and its calibration are first established. The following questions must then be answered:

(i) What is the cardiac rhythm?
(ii) What is the cardiac rate?
(iii) What is the mean frontal plane QRS axis?
(iv) Is the P wave, the QRS complex and the T wave normal for the lead under consideration?
(v) Is the P–R interval, the S–T segment and the Q–T interval normal or abnormal?

Table 2.3

CRITERIA FOR NORMAL P, QRS AND T WAVES

	Any lead	*Limb leads*	*Precordial leads*
P wave Atrial myocardial depolarisation	Height and duration ≯ $2\frac{1}{2}$ mm	Best lead II Axis + 15° to + 75°	Best lead V_1 Upright in V_1 to V_6; may be biphasic in V_1 and V_2 but negative component must be smaller than positive
QRS complex Ventricular myocardial depolarisation	Size: q ≯ 25% of R wave Duration: q ≯ 40 ms QRS ≯ 100 ms	(i) Axis − 30° to + 90° (ii) R aVl ≯ 13 mm R aVf ≯ 20 mm	(i) rS in V_1 progresses to qR in V_6 (ii) Transitional zone (R = S) Usual: V_4 Clockwise rotation: V_5 to V_6 Anticlockwise rotation: V_1 to V_3 (iii) Size: (a) at least one R > 8 m (b) tallest R > 27 mm (c) deepest S ≯ 30 mm
T wave Ventricular myocardial repolarisation		Direction usually concordant with QRS Ventricular gradient ≯ 60°	V_1 upright in 80% V_2 upright in 95% V_3 to V_6 upright Height: 42/3 R, ≮ 1/8 R in any one lead
U wave Origin uncertain	Direction concordant with T wave Size (~ 10% of T wave) Varies with T wave size		

Abbreviations: ≯ not greater than; ≮ not less than

Table 2.4

CRITERIA FOR NORMAL ECG INTERVALS

Interval	*Duration*	*Comment*
P–R interval or	120–200 ms	Shortens with increasing heart rate
S–T segment	Not important	Deviation of ± 1 mm from isoelectric (T–P) line is pathological
Q–T interval R-R Q-T	Corrected Q–T interval (Q–Tc) $= \frac{\text{measured Q–T (s)}}{\sqrt{\text{R–R interval (s)}}}$ Normal < 0.47 s	Represents duration of depolarisation and repolarisation (electrical systole) Shortens with increasing heart rate

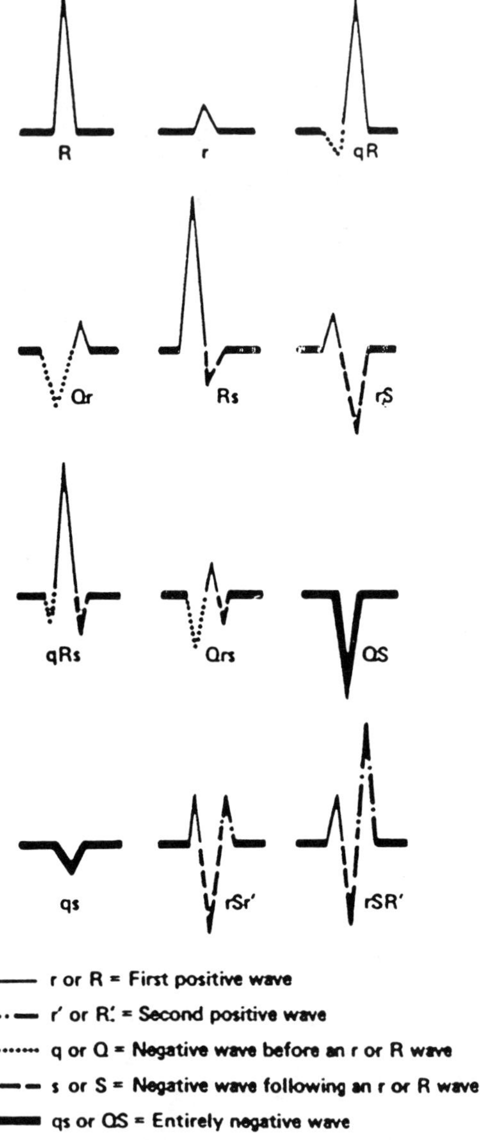

Fig. 2.4. Nomenclature of the QRS complex. From Rowlands (1983), reproduced with permission of Oxford University Press.

THE ABNORMAL ELECTROCARDIOGRAM

Left Ventricular Hypertrophy (LVH)

This is shown in Fig. 2.5 and criteria are shown in Table 2.5.

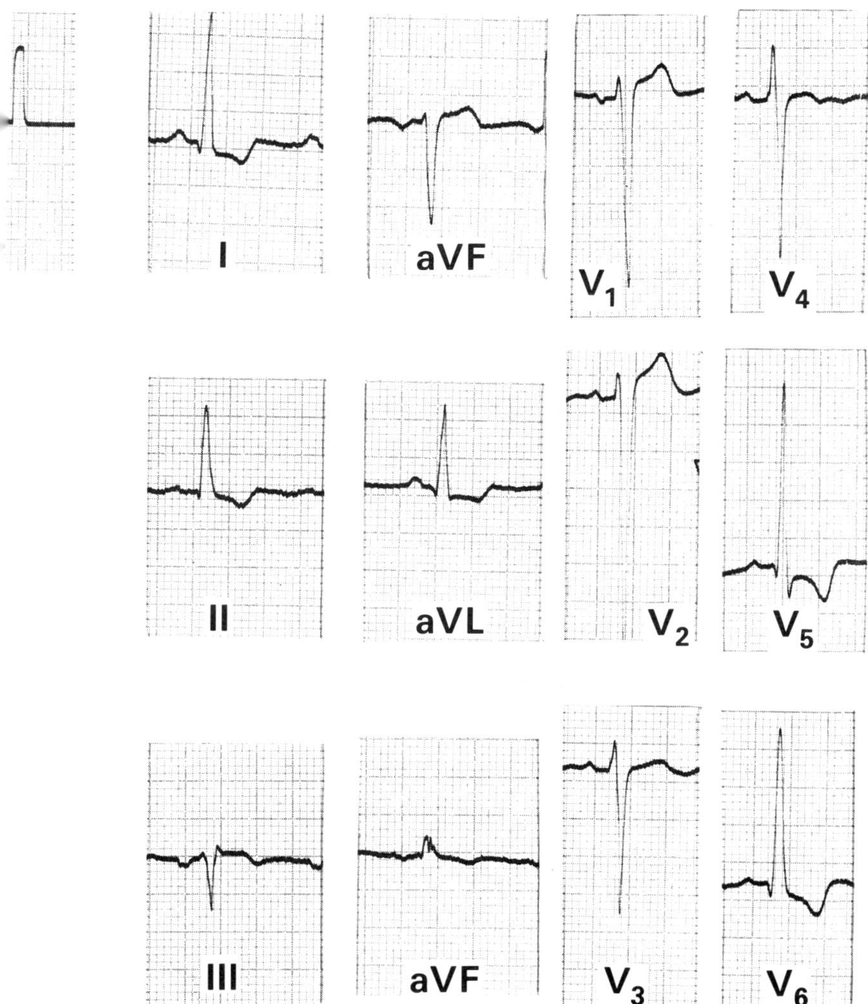

Fig. 2.5. Sinus rhythm. Axis + 15°. Severe left ventricular hypertrophy. The recording is from a patient with severe calcific aortic stenosis.

Table 2.5

Criteria	*Comment*
(1) $SV_1 + RV_5$ or $V_6 > 35$ mm (2) R in V_4, V_5 or $V_6 > 27$ mm (3) S in V_1, V_2 or $V_3 > 30$ mm (4) R in $aV_1 > 13$ mm (5) QRS width > 40 ms S–T depression, T wave flattening or inversion in leads V_4, V_5, V_6, I, aVL	Criterion (1) is the single most useful. The more criteria fulfilled the more likely is LVH to be present. In young/thin chest wall patients SV1 + RV5 or V6 must exceed 40 mm. Repolarisation changes alone are not sufficient to diagnose LVH; when accompanying the voltage criteria for LVH they are called the 'strain pattern' indicating severe LVH. Left axis deviation is not a necessary finding

Table 2.6

Criteria	*Comment*
(1) R > S in V_1 (2) Axis more positive than + 90° (3) ST depression/T wave inversion in V_1, V_2, V_3	Right bundle branch block (RBBB) must be excluded. Other causes for a dominant R wave in V_1 are (i) Type A Wolff–Parkinson–White syndrome, (ii) true posterior myocardial infarction, (iii) Duchenne muscular dystrophy

Fig. 2.6. Sinus rhythm. P–R interval 240 ms (first degree atrioventricular block). Right axis deviation +105°. Severe right ventricular hypertrophy. The recording is from a young woman with primary pulmonary hypertension.

Right Ventricular Hypertrophy (RVH)

This is shown in Fig. 2.6 and criteria are shown in Table 2.6.

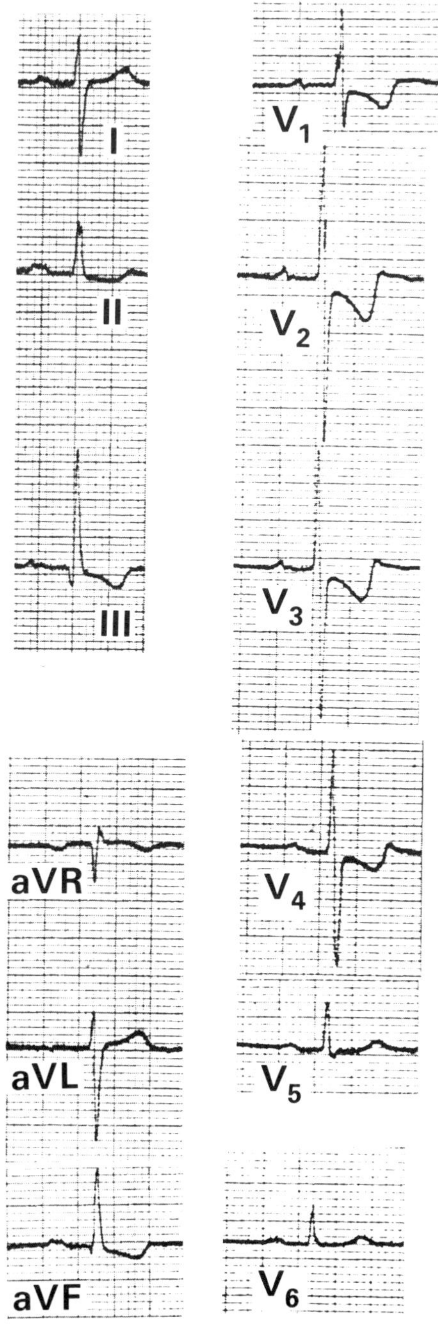

Left Atrial Abnormality

This is shown in Fig. 2.7 and the criteria in Table 2.7.

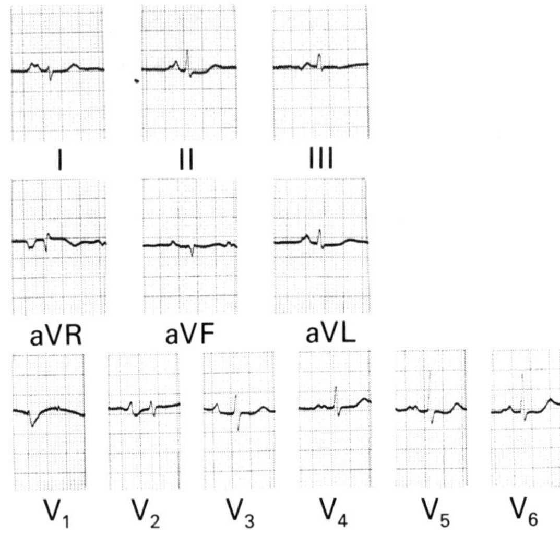

Fig. 2.7. Sinus rhythm. P–R interval 200 ms. Right axis deviation +105°. Left atrial abnormality. The recording is from a woman with severe mitral stenosis.

Table 2.7

Criteria	*Comment*
(1) P wave bifid in limb leads and duration > 120 ms (2) P wave biphasic in V_1, the terminal negative component larger than the initial positive component	The term left atrial 'abnormality' is preferred to hypertrophy. The criteria are present in atrial dilatation, ischaemia, infarction, intra-atrial conduction defect or inflammation. The presence of LVH makes true left atrial hypertrophy more likely

Right Atrial Abnormality

This is shown in Fig. 2.8 and the criteria in Table 2.8.

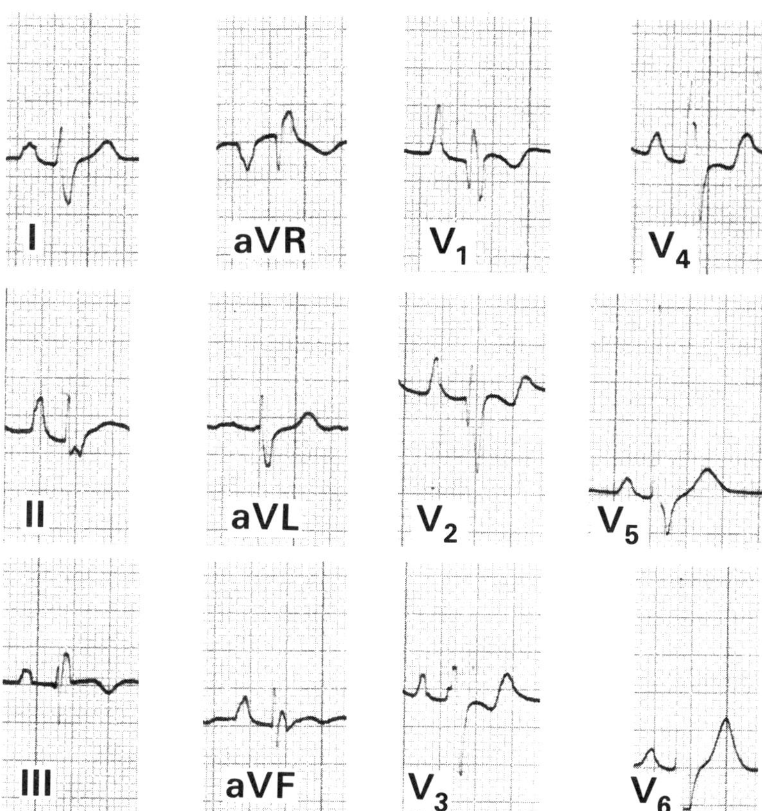

Fig. 2.8. Sinus rhythm. P–R interval 210 ms (first degree atrioventricular block). Axis indeterminate. Marked right atrial abnormality. The total QRS duration is prolonged at 120 ms. There is a broad, slurred S wave in V6 suggestive of right bundle branch block, but the QRS complex in V_1 is not typical. The recording is from a 15-year-old girl with Ebstein's anomaly.

Table 2.8

Criteria	*Comment*
P wave height greater than 3 mm in II, III, or aVF	The term 'abnormality' is preferable to hypertrophy (see left atrial abnormality)

Bundle Branch Block

The term bundle branch block implies 'complete' bundle branch block which is present when the total QRS duration exceeds 120 ms. It is then usually sufficient to inspect leads V1 and V6 to determine which bundle is blocked. 'Incomplete' bundle branch block is present when the total QRS duration is less than 120 ms but the other criteria for bundle branch block are present. An abnormal frontal plane QRS axis is not an expected feature of bundle branch block but may be present as an additional abnormality.

The clinical significance of bundle branch block is summarised in Table 2.9.

Table 2.9
CLINICAL SIGNIFICANCE OF BUNDLE BRANCH BLOCKS

Right bundle branch block	*Left bundle branch block*
Can occur in otherwise normal hearts	Always pathological
Ischaemic heart disease	Ischaemic heart disease
Rheumatic heart disease	Aortic stenosis
Hypertensive heart disease	Hypertensive heart disease
Cardiomyopathies	Cardiomyopathies
Pericarditis	Infiltrative myocardial disease
Myocarditis	Idiopathic conduction system disease
Idiopathic conduction system disease	Cardiac tumours
Atrial septal defect	Syphilis
Tetralogy of Fallot	Surgical trauma
Chagas' disease	Congenital heart disease

Left bundle branch block

This may be due to a lesion affecting the main left bundle or to lesions affecting both the left anterior–superior and the left posterior–inferior fascicles.

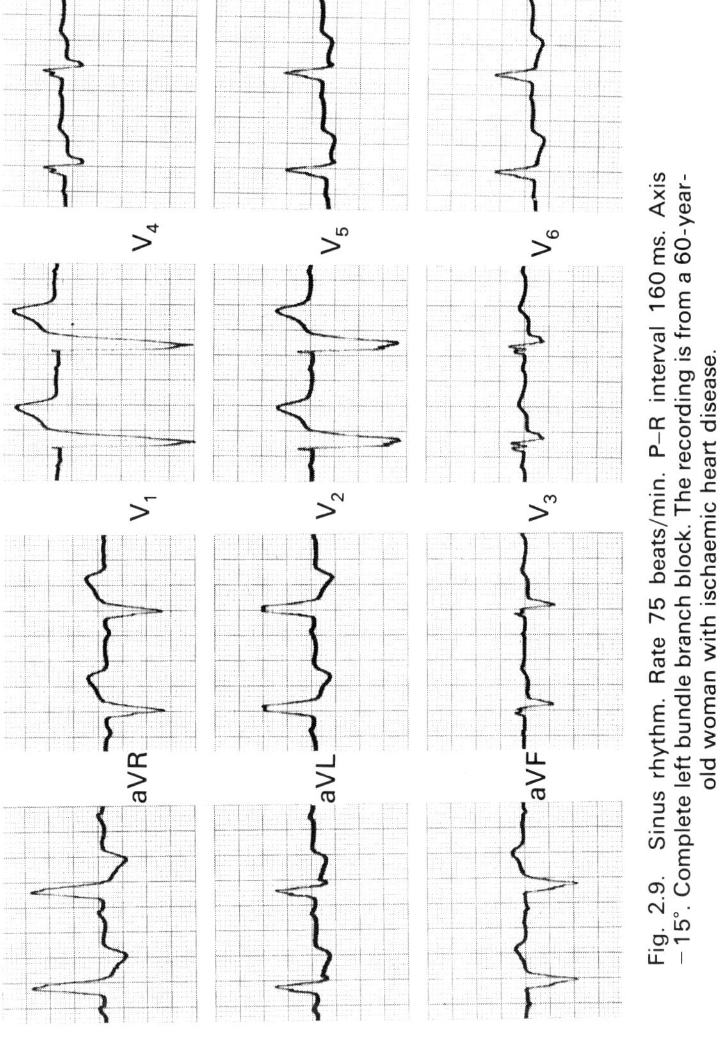

Fig. 2.9. Sinus rhythm. Rate 75 beats/min. P–R interval 160 ms. Axis −15°. Complete left bundle branch block. The recording is from a 60-year-old woman with ischaemic heart disease.

It is a safe rule of practice to assume that once the heart rate, rhythm, and cardiac axis have been established the identification of complete left bundle branch block precludes any further analysis of the ECG.

Complete left bundle branch block (LBBB)

This is shown in Fig. 2.9 and criteria in Table 2.10.

Table 2.10

Criteria	*Comment*
(1) QRS duration > 120 ms (2) V_1 is typically QS and V_6 is monophasic R (3) Absence of initial (septal) q wave in V_5, V_6, I and aVL (4) No secondary R wave in V_1 to indicate RBBB	LBBB is always pathological. Left ventricular hypertrophy and myocardial infarction cannot be diagnosed when LBBB is present. 'Notching' of the QRS complex may or may not be present. Precordial T-wave direction is usually opposite to dominant QRS direction

Complete right bundle branch block (RBBB)

This is shown in Fig. 2.10 and criteria in Table 2.11.

Table 2.11

Criteria	*Comment*
(1) QRS duration > 120 ms (2) Secondary R wave in V_1 ('M' shape), and slurred S wave in V_6	Only the last part of the QRS complex is abnormal. Therefore, unlike in LBBB, it is still possible to diagnose left ventricular hypertrophy, myocardial infarction, etc.

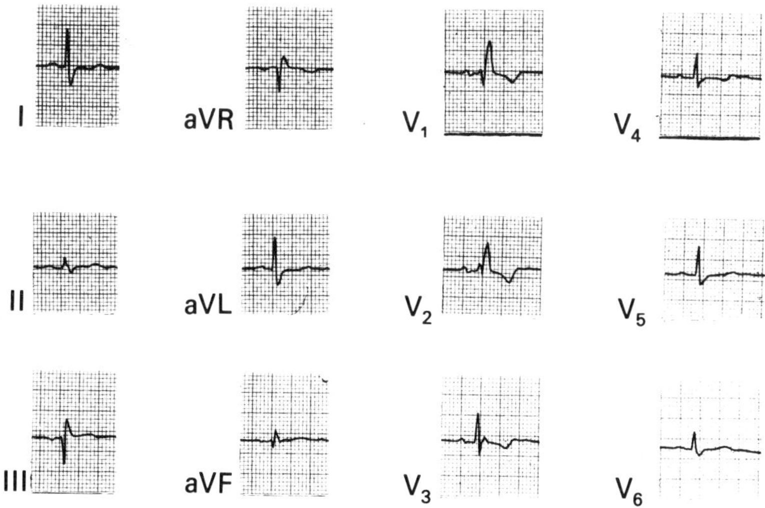

Fig. 2.10. Sinus rhythm. P–R interval 170 ms. Axis −15°. Complete right bundle branch block.

Fascicular Blocks

Division of the bundle of His into three fascicles is an extremely useful concept in clinical electrocardiography but may be an anatomical oversimplification. The three fascicles are:

(i) Right bundle branch: a direct continuation of the bundle of His.

(ii) Left bundle branch which divides almost immediately into:

  (a) anterior–superior fascicle, in which conduction is mainly downwards and to the right;

  (b) posterior–inferior fascicle in which conduction is mainly upwards and to the left.

In left anterior fascicular block (LAFB) excitation of the left ventricle is effected by the left posterior fascicle in an upward and leftward direction. In left posterior fascicular block (LPFB) activation is effected by the left anterior fascicle in a downward and rightward direction. The ECG manifestation is thus a shift in mean frontal plane QRS axis. LAFB and LPFB may be caused by any process in the left ventricular myocardium involving their fibres, for example, fibrosis, ischaemia, carditis. The posterior fascicle is a broader, more robust structure which is less frequently damaged.

Left anterior fascicular block

This is shown in Fig. 2.11 and the criteria in Table 2.12.

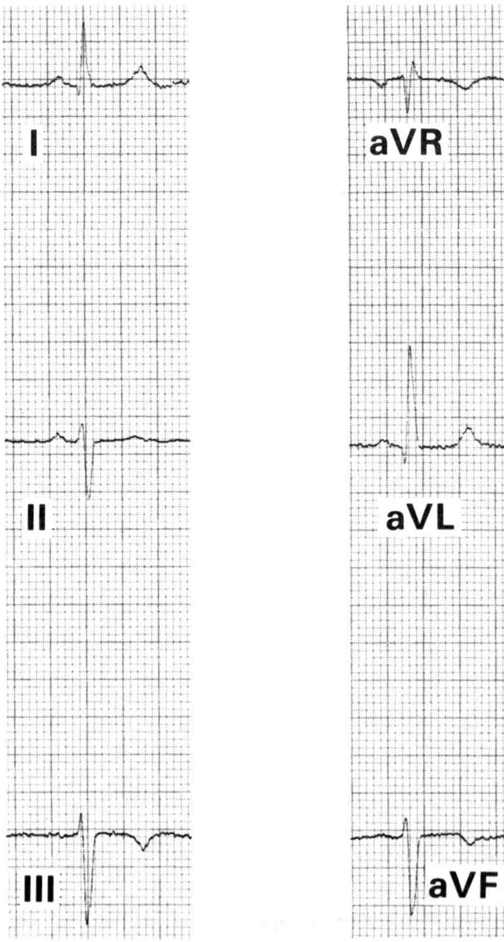

Fig. 2.11. Left anterior fascicular block. Sinus rhythm, P–R interval 140 ms. Axis −45°.

Table 2.12

Criteria	*Comment*
(1) Mean frontal plane QRS axis more negative than − 30° (2) Initial r waves present in inferior leads	Other causes of left axis deviation (Table 2.13) must be excluded. Inferior infarction is excluded by small r waves in leads II, III and aVF

Table 2.13
CAUSES OF LEFT AXIS DEVIATION

Left anterior fascicular block
Inferior myocardial infarction
Ostium primum atrial septal defect
Wolff–Parkinson–White (W–P–W) syndrome
Hyperkalaemia
Tricuspid atresia

Left posterior fascicular block

Criteria are shown in Table 2.14.

Table 2.14

Criteria	*Comment*
Mean frontal plane QRS axis between + 90° and + 120°	LPFB is a diagnosis made on the exclusion of other causes of right axis deviation (Table 2.15)

Table 2.15
CAUSES OF RIGHT AXIS DEVIATION

Tall, thin subject
Right ventricular hypertrophy
Emphysema
Ostium secundum atrial septal defect
Extensive anterolateral myocardial infarct

Bifascicular block and trifascicular block

The following combinations are termed 'bifascicular block'

LAFB + RBBB
LPFB + RBBB
Complete LBBB, if LAFB or LPFB were known to predate complete LBBB

Trifascicular block is strictly equivalent to complete heart block, especially if fascicular blocks were known to predate the complete block. The term is also used where bifascicular block coexists with a P–R interval exceeding 200 ms (first degree atrioventricular block), implying that conduction is delayed in the remaining fascicle.

The causes of fascicular blocks are listed in Table 2.16.

Table 2.16
CAUSES OF FASCICULAR BLOCKS

Idiopathic conduction system disease
Ischaemic heart disease
Cardiomyopathies and specific heart muscle diseases
Calcific aortic stenosis
Endocardial cushion defects

Myocardial Infarction

The electrocardiography of myocardial infarction is discussed in detail on p. 0. The general criteria for myocardial infarction are shown in Table 2.17.

Poor R wave progression or QS complexes may be found in a

Table 2.17

Criteria	*Comment*
(1) Pathological Q waves greater than 40 ms duration greater than 25% of the succeeding R wave	QS complexes are normal in lead aVR, and can be normal in leads III and aV_1 depending on axis. QS complexes in lead III alone are often erroneously interpreted as suggesting inferior infarction
(2) Loss of R wave voltage in the infarct region	R wave reduction must involve two or more leads

Table 2.18
CONDITIONS WHICH MAY CAUSE A PSEUDOINFARCTION PATTERN ON THE ECG

Hypertrophic cardiomyopathy
Wolff–Parkinson–White (W–P–W) syndrome
Chronic airways disease
Pulmonary embolism
Mitral valve prolapse
Severe hyperkalaemia
Severe left ventricular hypertrophy
Subarachnoid haemorrhage

variety of other conditions leading to an erroneous diagnosis of myocardial infarction. Conditions giving rise to 'pseudoinfarction' patterns are shown in Table 2.18.

MISCELLANEOUS CONDITIONS

Pericarditis

Transient S–T segment elevation is the commonest finding. The S–T segment change is generalised in pericarditis whereas in myocardial ischaemia the S–T segment change is localised, reflecting the distribution of the pathological processes. Upward concavity of the S–T segment is a common but less reliable distinguishing feature of pericarditis.

Hypothermia

Progressive hypothermia is associated with the following ECG changes:

(i) Muscle tremor artefact due to shivering.
(ii) Sinus bradycardia.
(iii) Prolonged P–R and Q–T intervals.
(iv) J wave—a broad secondary hump commencing on the downslope of the QRS deflection and encroaching into the S–T segment; it is seen only in severely reduced body temperature.

Hypothyroidism

Chronic severe hypothyroidism (Fig. 2.12) may result in:

(i) Sinus bradycardia.
(ii) Low voltage P–QRS–T complexes.
(iii) Prolonged P–R and Q–T intervals.
(iv) Rarely second or third degree atrioventricular block.

Other causes of generalised low voltage are shown in Table 2.19.

Table 2.19
CAUSES OF GENERALISED LOW ECG VOLTAGE

Obesity
Emphysema
Pericardial effusion
Constrictive pericarditis
Hypothyroidism
Incorrect calibration

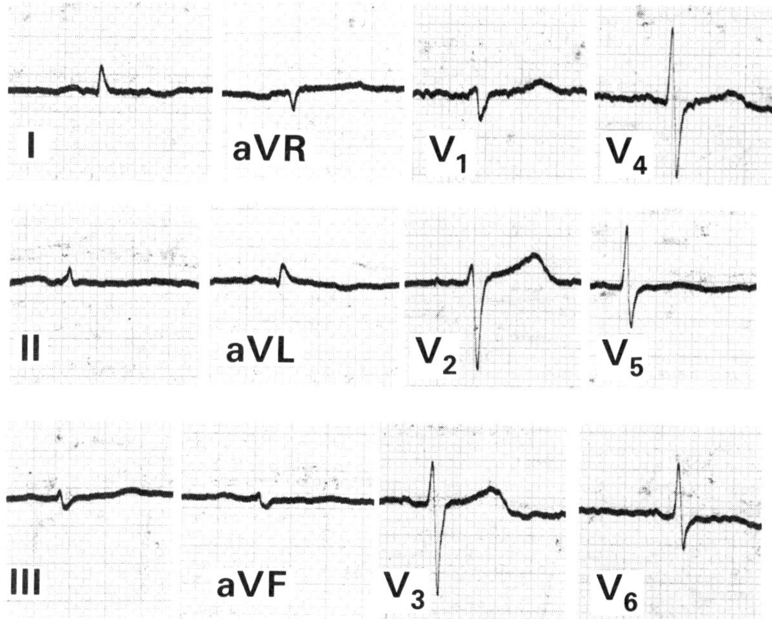

Fig. 2.12. Sinus bradycardia (the heart rate was 50 beats/min). P–R interval 180 ms. Axis 0°. Low voltage tracing with muscle tremor artefact. The recording is from a 72-year-old man with untreated myxoedema.

Table 2.20

ECG CHANGES DUE TO ABNORMAL SERUM POTASSIUM

Hyperkalaemia	*Hypokalaemia*
Tall, narrow ('tented') T waves	Decreased T wave amplitude, increased V wave S–T segment depression
Decreased R wave voltage. Widening of QRS complex	Wide QRS complex
Fascicular and bundle branch blocks	Atrial and ventricular arrhythmias
Wider QRS of bizarre morphology	Atrioventricular
Long Q–T interval Marked S–T depression	Ventricular fibrillation
Ventricular arrhythmias, ventricular fibrillation (usually when $K^+ > 7.5$ mmol/l)	

Hyperkalaemia and Hypokalaemia

Gross changes in serum potassium are associated with increasingly marked ECG changes. The ECG should never be used to monitor serum potassium. Serum potassium must always be checked in any patient with unexplained cardiac arrhythmia. Typical changes are shown in Table 2.20.

Digitalis

Effects are shown in Fig. 2.13.

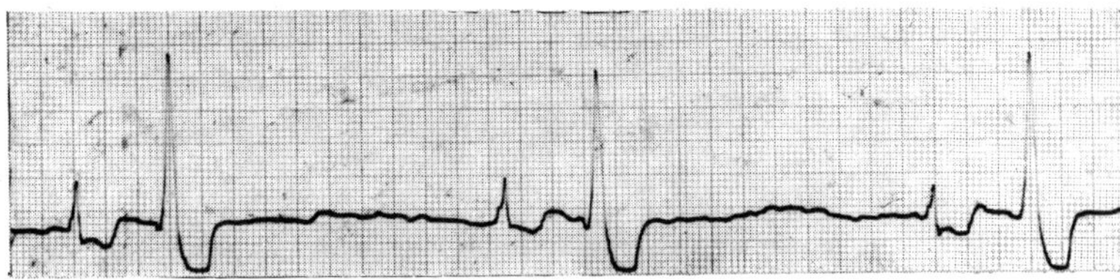

Fig. 2.13. Digoxin toxicity. There is atrial fibrillation. The QRS complexes are regular due to junctional bradycardia. There are coupled ventricular ectopic beats. The patient had taken an intentional overdose of 17.5 mg digoxin. The serum digoxin was 8.0 ng/ml.

Table 2.21

ECG CHANGES INDUCED BY THERAPEUTIC LEVELS AND BY TOXIC LEVELS OF DIGITALIS

Digitalis effect	*Digitalis toxicity*
Decreased T-wave voltage	Ventricular ectopic beats, especially coupled beats
Downsloping S–T segment depression ('left-handed tick')	Junctional rhythm or junctional tachycardia
Increased U-wave voltage	Paroxysmal atrial tachycardia with atrioventricular block
Short Q–T interval	Sinus bradycardia, sinoatrial block, sinus arrest
	First, second or third degree atrioventricular block
	Ventricular tachycardia, ventricular fibrillation

(i) *Digitalis effect*: a patient receiving digitalis may or may not show characteristic ECG changes. These mean only that digitalis is being taken by the patient, not that toxicity is present.

(ii) *Digitalis toxicity*: cardiac arrhythmias due to digitalis always indicate toxicity. Digitalis toxicity presents clinically with anorexia, nausea, vomiting and visual disturbances sometimes affecting colour vision. The ECG may show almost any atrial or ventricular arrhythmia and any degree of atrioventricular block.

ECG changes induced by digitalis are shown in Table 2.21.

FURTHER READING

Rowlands D.J. (1980). *Understanding the Electrocardiogram: Section 1: The Normal ECG*. London, Gower Medical Press.

Rowlands D.J. (1982). *Understanding the Electrocardiogram: Section 2: Morphological Abnormalities*. London, Gower Medical Press.

Rowlands D.J. (1983). In *Oxford Textbook of Medicine*, eds D.J. Weatherall, J.G.G. Ledingham and D.A. Warrell, pp. 13–49. Oxford: Oxford University Press.

Schamroth L. (1976). *An Introduction to Electrocardiography*. Oxford: Blackwell Scientific Publications.

Chapter Three

Special Investigations in Cardiology

EXERCISE STRESS TESTING

Background

Exercise stress testing is a widely used, safe and relatively sensitive investigation used principally in the diagnosis and evaluation of ischaemic heart disease. Its role in the screening of asymptomatic members of the general population is more controversial because of the higher incidence of false positive tests in asymptomatic individuals. The indications for exercise stress testing are shown in Table 3.1.

Table 3.1
INDICATIONS FOR EXERCISE STRESS TESTING

Diagnosis of chest pain (suspected IHD)
Assessment of severity of IHD
Evaluate the benefit of therapy (medical, CABG, PTCA)
Evaluation of postmyocardial infarction patients
Evaluate functional disability in valvular heart disease
Evaluate individuals with multiple IHD risk factors
Screen high risk professionals (such as airline pilots)
Asymptomatic population screening (insurance medicals, routine health screening)

IHD = ischaemic heart disease
CABG = coronary artery bypass grafting
PTCA = percutaneous transluminal coronary angioplasty

Exercise physiology

Physical exercise rapidly increases metabolic demand and oxygen consumption. A closely coordinated physiological response is required to increase oxygen uptake and to deliver more oxygen and metabolic substrates to the exercising muscle.

Increased oxygen uptake

Oxygen consumption ($\dot{V}o_2$) is increased in direct proportion to the muscular work done up to maximal work capacity ($\dot{V}o_{2max}$), the point at which no further increase in oxygen uptake is possible. Oxygen uptake depends on age, fitness, body weight and muscle mass. Resting oxygen consumption, defined as 1 metabolic equivalent (MET) is 3.5 ml O_2/kg bodyweight/min and can be increased on exercise up to 15-fold in a normal healthy individual. $\dot{V}o_{2max}$ is achieved by increases in respiratory rate, tidal volume and alveolar oxygen diffusion.

Increased oxygen delivery

The increased oxygen uptake during exercise is delivered to the exercising muscle mass by increasing the cardiac output. Cardiac output is determined by the relationship

$$\text{Cardiac output (ml/min)} = \text{heart rate (beats/min)} \times \text{stroke volume (ml/beat)}$$

Heart rate is increased by diminished vagal tone and increased sympathetic stimulation. Stroke volume is increased by enhanced diastolic filling of the ventricles (Frank–Starling mechanism) and by increased ventricular myocardial contractility. Heart rate is the major contributor to increased cardiac output, the ability to increase stroke volume being relatively limited. The maximal heart rate at $\dot{V}o_{2max}$ is an important determinant of effort tolerance and decreases with age. The predicted maximal heart rate of an individual can be estimated by the formula

$$\text{Maximum heart rate} = 220 - \text{age in years}$$

The rate of fall in heart rate after exercise is an index of cardiorespiratory fitness which reflects repayment of the oxygen debt accumulated during exercise.

The release of oxygen to the tissues is facilitated by an increase in oxygen extraction from oxyhaemoglobin, increasing the arteriovenous oxygen difference. At high levels of exercise the increased H^+ ion concentration, $P\text{CO}_2$ and temperature in active muscle shift the oxyhaemoglobin dissociation curve to the left. This mechanism of increasing oxygen delivery to the tissues is particularly important in patients with a reduced ability to increase cardiac output.

The cardiorespiratory responses to exercise are summarised in Table 3.2. They are assisted by the peripheral circulatory responses of vasodilatation, decreased peripheral vascular resistance and a shift of blood volume away from less vital vascular beds, for example, the splanchnic circulation.

Table 3.2

CARDIORESPIRATORY RESPONSES TO EXERCISE

Increased oxygen uptake
↑ respiratory rate
↑ tidal volume
↑ number of alveoli ventilated
Increased oxygen delivery
↑ heart rate
↑ stroke volume
↑ oxygen extraction

Myocardial oxygen consumption

Unlike skeletal muscle myocardial muscle metabolism is almost exclusively aerobic. The heart extracts 70% of the oxygen transported by the blood. The increased oxygen demand during exercise must be met wholly by an increased oxygen supply provided by increased coronary arterial blood flow, achieved by coronary vasodilatation. If coronary blood flow is restricted by the presence of obstructive atheromatous coronary stenoses oxygen supply will be inadequate to meet the demand and myocardial ischaemia will ensue.

The main factors increasing myocardial oxygen demand are

(i) Heart rate.
(ii) Myocardial contractility.
(iii) Ventricular wall tension.

Thus myocardial oxygen consumption is proportional to heart rate × systolic blood pressure—the 'peak double product'. A patient with coronary artery disease develops angina pectoris at a relatively constant double product whatever the type or duration of exercise.

The effects of myocardial ischaemia

(i) *Chest pain*: angina pectoris is a relatively insensitive indicator of myocardial ischaemia. Many patients with coronary artery disease develop ischaemic ECG changes on exercise in the absence of chest pain (silent myocardial ischaemia).
(ii) *ECG S–T segment changes*: a positive test is defined by a horizontal or downsloping S–T segment which is depressed by at least 1 mm below the isoelectric line at the 'J' point (the junction of the QRS complex and S–T segment) and persists for 80 ms.
(iii) *Left ventricular dysfunction* is indicated by a poor overall exercise duration, failure of blood pressure to rise, or a drop in systolic blood pressure of 15–20 mmHg during exercise. The latter excludes the small drop in systolic blood pressure seen at maximal exercise due to general vasodilatation.
(iv) *Ventricular arrhythmias* accompanying S–T segment depression in patients with ischaemic heart disease indicate a worse prognosis than repolarisation changes alone. A

Table 3.3
FEATURES OF A 'STRONGLY POSITIVE' EXERCISE STRESS TEST

Greater than 3 mm S–T segment depression
Early onset (within 3 min) of S–T segment depression
Persistence (more than 8 min) of S–T segment depression during the recovery phase
Systolic blood pressure fails to rise or falls
Poor overall exercise duration

'strongly positive' exercise test predicts a high probability of serious coronary artery disease, for example, left main stem stenosis, three-vessel coronary disease (Table 3.3).

Test protocols

Numerous dynamic (isotonic) exercise protocols using the treadmill or bicycle ergometer have been proposed. Most involve multistage increments of exercise workload. Perhaps the most widely used in the evaluation of ischaemic heart disease is the Bruce treadmill protocol (Table 3.4).

Table 3.4

BRUCE TREADMILL PROTOCOL

Stage	*Duration (min)*	*Speed (mph)*	*Gradient (%)*
I	3	1·75	10
II	3	2·5	12
III	3	3·4	14
IV	3	4·2	16
V	3	5·0	18

Table 3.5

SENSITIVITY, SPECIFICITY AND PREDICTIVE VALUE: DEFINITION AND APPLICATION TO EXERCISE STRESS TESTING (EST)

Term	*Definition*	*Level in EST*
Sensitivity	$\frac{\text{Number of true positive tests}}{\text{Total number of positives in group}}$	65%
Specificity	$\frac{\text{Number of true normal tests}}{\text{Total number of normals in group}}$	85%
Predictive value	$\frac{\text{True positive tests}}{\text{True positive tests + false positive tests}}$	80%

Predictive value of exercise stress testing

No diagnostic test is 100% sensitive (that is, positive in every patient known to be abnormal) or 100% specific (that is, always negative in every patient known to be normal). The predictive value (the likelihood that an abnormality is present if the test is positive) of a test varies with the prevalence of the disease in the population being tested. These terms are defined in Table 3.5. Using coronary angiography as the 'gold standard' for the presence or absence of coronary artery disease the sensitivity, specificity and predictive value of exercise stress testing can be determined. Approximate values are shown in Table 3.5.

Safety of exercise stress testing

Exercise stress testing must be supervised by a physician trained and fully equipped for cardiopulmonary resuscitation. If the contraindications to testing (Table 3.6) are observed the mortality rate of stress testing is less than 0.01% and the morbidity rate (non-fatal complications) is 0.025%.

Table 3.6
CONTRAINDICATIONS TO EXERCISE STRESS TESTING

Acute myocardial infarction
Unstable angina pectoris
Severe aortic stenosis
Uncontrolled arrhythmias
Second or third degree atrioventricular block
Severe hypertension
Known left main coronary stenosis
Congestive cardiac failure
Active systemic illness
Lack of informed consent

ECHOCARDIOGRAPHY

Background

Echocardiography utilises ultrasound to examine the motion and position of cardiac structures. The velocity and direction of blood flow in the heart and great vessels can be examined using Doppler methods.

Ultrasound frequencies used in adults are 2–3.5 MHz (mega-Hertz = million cycles/s). Higher frequencies of 3.5–7.0 MHz are used in children. Lower frequencies are used in adults to penetrate the thicker chest wall but only at the expense of resolution (the ability to separate objects close together) which varies directly with frequency.

Ultrasound is produced by the application of an electrical pulse to a piezoelectric transducer. The transducer is placed on the chest wall where it transmits a 1 μs burst of ultrasound then for 999 μs acts as a receiver for echoes reflected back from the underlying boundaries between materials of different acoustic impedance, such as blood in the cardiac chambers and solid intracardiac structures. The echoes received by the transducer are converted to electrical signals and displayed on an oscilloscope. Since the velocity of sound in tissue and the time taken for the ultrasound to leave and return to the transducer are known the distance between the transducer and the reflecting structure can be determined. In this way a map is constructed of the relative position of cardiac structures and the change in their position with time throughout the cardiac cycle. The information is differently displayed according to the technique employed.

M-mode Echocardiography

In M-mode echocardiography the received echoes are displayed on the oscilloscope as dots of varying brightness according to their amplitude (loudness) which are swept along a time-base. The M-mode (motion-mode) presentation is a one-dimensional recording of the dimensions and motion of structures along the axis of the narrow ultrasound beam employed.

Technique

The transducer is placed on the chest wall at the left sternal edge in the 4th or 5th intercostal spaces. The mitral valve is first identified from its characteristic M-shape and strong, bright echoes. Inferior and lateral angulation of the transducer displays the cavity and walls of the left ventricle while superior and medial angulation displays the aortic root, aortic valve and left

Table 3.7

APPLICATIONS OF M-MODE ECHOCARDIOGRAPHY

Application	*Limitation*
Cardiac chamber dimensions; interventricular septal and left ventricular posterior wall thickness	Narrow beam may miss regional abnormality, for example, left ventricular aneurysm Endocardial echoes on each side of chamber may be difficult to image simultaneously
Left ventricular function: stroke volume, ejection fraction	Calculations inaccurate in IHD—narrow beam misses regional wall motion variations
Cardiac valves: cusp thickness, mobility, calcification; diagnostic morphology in certain disorders	Severity of stenosis cannot be quantified Normal valve echo can coexist with severe regurgitation Pulmonary and tricuspid valves can be difficult to image
Pericardial effusion	Loculated effusions missed Confusion with pleural effusion
Myxomas, vegetations	Size and motion pattern not assessed
Septal defects	Suspected only on secondary haemodynamic (ASD) or left (VSD) ventricular volume overload Direct visualisation very unreliable

IHD = ischaemic heart disease
ASD = atrial septal defect
VSD = ventricular septal defect

atrium. Many structures can be recognised by their anatomical relationships.

Since the sampling rate is 1000 pulses/s the technique permits an extremely accurate recording of the amplitude and rate of motion of structures. Table 3.7 shows categories of information which can reliably be obtained from M-mode echocardiography. It must be emphasised that measurements and calculations must be made only from optimal quality recordings in which the relevant structures are correctly identified by the observer.

Two-dimensional Echocardiography

The limitations of M-mode echocardiography stem mainly from its inability to depict cardiac shape and motion lateral to the single beam. In two-dimensional echocardiography the single beam is moved rapidly through a sector of up to 90° constructing a real time, cross-sectional image of a 'slice' of the heart. From the one-dimensional 'map', unrecognisable as a heart, produced by M-mode recordings comes a two-dimensional image which is immediately recognisable.

Rapid movement of the beam is achieved by one of two transducer systems:

(i) Mechanical: a series of transducers is rotated.
(ii) Phased array: the beam is electronically steered by a computer-controlled firing sequence of multiple ultrasonic elements.

Technique

Two-dimensional echocardiography depicts 'slices' of the heart. In practice three standard orthogonal imaging planes are recognised:

(i) Long axis plane: parallel to the long axis of the heart and perpendicular to the body surface.
(ii) Short axis plane: perpendicular to the long axis plane and to the body surface.
(iii) Four-chamber view: transects the heart approximately parallel to the body surface.

Recordings are most frequently made from the parasternal and apical approaches using a selection of imaging planes. Subcostal and suprasternal views may also be useful.

Advantages of two-dimensional echocardiography

M-mode and two-dimensional echocardiography are complementary. M-mode is certainly superior for quantitative measurements. The advantages of the two-dimensional technique are mostly predictable from the limitations listed in Table 3.1, but are summarised in Table 3.8.

Table 3.8
ADVANTAGES OF TWO-DIMENSIONAL ECHOCARDIOGRAPHY

- Direct visualisation of
  - cardiac chamber shape
  - ventricular regional wall motion abnormalities
  - valve orifice size
  - loculated pericardial effusions
  - size and motion pattern of intracardiac masses
  - atrial and ventricular septal defects
- Anatomical analysis of congenital heart defects
- More sensitive diagnosis of
  - mitral valve prolapse
  - bicuspid aortic valve
- Improved visualisation of
  - pulmonary and tricuspid valve
  - right atrium

Doppler Echocardiography

The Doppler principle states that when a sound wave is reflected from a moving object its frequency is altered, the frequency being increased if the object is approaching the sound source and decreased if it is moving away. The change in frequency is the Doppler shift.

Ultrasound back-scattered from moving red blood cells undergoes a Doppler shift which can be used to determine the direction and velocity of blood flow. Three techniques are in current clinical use:

(i) *Continuous wave (CW) Doppler*: the ultrasound beam is transmitted as a continuous wave. Mean instantaneous blood flow velocity and direction of flow are determined. The method allows measurement of high flow velocities, for example, through stenotic valves, but the site at which the velocity change occurs cannot be localised.

(ii) *Pulsed Doppler*: since the time taken for the pulse to return to the transducer is known the depth from which the velocity has been measured can be determined. This position is termed the 'sample volume'. Using pulsed Doppler in conjunction with a two-dimensional echocardiographic image the sample volume can be located with accuracy at a site of interest, such as a stenotic valve. The limitation of pulsed Doppler is in the maximum velocity that can be recorded. If the frequency of the backscattered sound wave exceeds the pulse repetition rate of the pulsed Doppler it will not be possible to measure the frequency of the reflected wave—a phenomenon termed 'aliasing'.

(iii) *Doppler colour flow mapping*: Doppler velocity information is obtained simultaneously from multiple sites. The different velocities are colour-encoded to give a two-dimensional representation of intracardiac blood flow velocity, direction and turbulence. In combination with a two-dimensional image an anatomical-physiological picture superficially resembling a contrast angiogram is obtained. Stenotic and regurgitant jets through valves, flows through septal defects and normal intracardiac flow distribution have been studied. The technique, introduced commercially early in the 1980s, remains under intensive evaluation.

Clinical application of Doppler echocardiography

Current clinical applications are summarised in Table 3.9.

Table 3.9
CLINICAL APPLICATION OF DOPPLER ECHOCARDIOGRAPHY

Clinical requirement	*Application*
(1) Assessment of valve disease	
valve stenosis	Valve gradient can be calculated from modified Bernoulli equation gradient = $4V^2$ where V = velocity CW Doppler is essential
valve regurgitation	Retrograde flow detection is sensitive by pulsed and colour flow Doppler Quantitation relatively inaccurate
(2) Intracardiac shunt assessment	Abnormal flow and turbulence due to VSD and ASD localised by pulsed and colour flow Doppler
(3) Cardiac output and/or pulmonary flow measurement	Velocity patterns in aorta and pulmonary artery reflect cardiac output; may be useful in serial monitoring of intensive care patients
(4) Non-invasive haemodynamics	Methods for intracardiac pressure, exercise flow velocity and left ventricular function measurements, and haemodynamic analysis of complex congenital heart lesions are all under current assessment

CW = continuous wave
ASD = atrial septal defect
VSD = ventricular septal defect

NUCLEAR CARDIOLOGY

Background

Nuclear cardiology is the study of the heart and great vessels using radioactive tracers (radionuclides). A radionuclide is an atom with an unstable nucleus which will decay spontaneously to a more stable form, emitting radiation as it decays. Radionuclide techniques are safe, relatively non-invasive and quantitative. Their main applications are summarised in Table 3.10.

Table 3.10

COMMON APPLICATIONS OF RADIONUCLIDE TECHNIQUES

Detection of acute myocardial infarction
Detection and localisation of reversible myocardial ischaemia
Detection and quantitation of viable myocardium
Quantitation of overall and regional left ventricular function
Detection of intracardiac shunts

Principle of instrumentation

The gamma radiation emitted from the intravenously administered radionuclide is received and amplified by a radiation detector (such as a gamma camera) and analysed by computer techniques. The radiation detector consists of three basic components:

(i) *Scintillation crystals*: sodium iodide crystals containing thallium impurity respond to gamma radiation by emitting light.

(ii) *Photomultiplier tube*: light energy from the scintillation crystal is detected and converted into an amplified electrical signal output.

(iii) *Collimator*: the lens of the system which ensures that only gamma rays emitted from the subject in a direction perpendicular to the crystal will enter the radiation detector. Collimators may be general purpose, high resolution or high sensitivity according to the radionuclide administered and the type of investigation performed.

The data acquired may be presented as either

(i) *A scintigram*: an image of the distribution of radioactivity.

(ii) *A time-activity curve*: a graph of the change in disintegration count rate with time.

Radionuclide Techniques

A summary of the most commonly used techniques and their indications is given in Table 3.11.

Myocardial infarct imaging

Two techniques are used for the detection of myocardial infarction or ischaemia.

(i) *'Hot-spot' imaging*: also called infarct-avid imaging or positive imaging. The radionuclide concentrates selectively in acutely necrosed or irreversibly ischaemic myocardial cells. Technetium-99m (^{99m}Tc: that is, the element technetium, atomic mass 99, in its metastable state) is most extensively used.

(ii) *'Cold-spot' imaging*: also called ionic-tracer scanning or negative imaging. The radionuclide behaves like the potassium ion. It is taken up and concentrated by normal myocardial cells in proportion to blood flow and metabolic activity. Thallium-201 (^{201}Tl) is usually used. In addition to myocardial infarct imaging an extension of 'cold-spot' imaging, the thallium exercise stress test, is increasingly used in the evaluation of reversible myocardial ischaemia.

The relative advantages and disadvantages of these techniques in myocardial infarct imaging are shown in Table 3.12.

Assessment of left ventricular function

Two main radionuclide techniques are available for the study of overall left ventricular function (ejection fraction) and regional left ventricular wall motion (see Table 3.11). The same information is obtained invasively by X-ray contrast left ventricular angiography. Radionuclide angiography is non-invasive and allows repeated study with zero morbidity or mortality. Both

Table 3.11

SUMMARY OF COMMON RADIONUCLIDE TECHNIQUES

Clinical requirement	*Technique (radionuclide)*	*Principle*	*Method*	*Indication*
Myocardial infarct imaging	'Hot spot' imaging $99^{m}Tc$—stannous pyrophosphate (Tc-Pyp)	Tc–Pyp complexes with Ca^{2+} in acutely necrotic myocardium Infarct mass must be > 3 g	Image acquired > 2 h after i.v. Tc–Pyp Optimum study 24–96 h postinfarct	(1) Suspected AMI with equivocal ECG, for example, LBBB, old infarction after cardiac surgery (2) Localisation of AMI (3) Prognosis: poor with persistently positive 'hot spot' scan at 10 days post-AMI
	'Cold spot' imaging ^{201}Tl	^{201}Tl taken up by *normal* myocardial cells Infarct mass must be > 7 g	Image acquired 5–10 min after i.v. ^{201}Tl	

Radionuclide stress testing (EST)	'Cold spot' imaging	As above	^{201}Tl given i.v. during maximal exercise Defect present at 10 min but absent at 4 h after exercise shows reversible ischaemia	(1) Increased sensitivity over standard EST (2) Silent myocardial ischaemia* (3) Assess CABG patency (4) Assess functional significance of equivocal lesion at coronary angiography
Assess left ventricular (LV) function	Radionuclide angiography 99^{m}Tc—tagged albumin or own red blood cells (i) 'first pass' study (ii) equilibrium technique (MUGA scan)	(i) Sequential data acquired during 'first pass' of tracer through central circulation (ii) Multiple data acquisitions after complete mixing of tracer in circulating volume; ECG gated	Ejection fraction and wall motion assessment obtained from time-activity curves and from 'cine-cycle' images	Serial non-invasive assessment of left ventricular function in ischaemic, valvular and myocardial disease, at rest and/or on exercise

MUGA = multigated acquisition. Ca^{2+} = calcium ions. AMI = acute myocardial infarction
LBBB = complete left bundle branch block

*In an asymptomatic patient with a positive exercise stress test a positive thallium exercise stress test increases the likelihood that ischaemic heart disease is present, and that the result is not a 'false-positive' exercise test.

Table 3.12

RADIONUCLIDE MYOCARDIAL INFARCT IMAGING: RELATIVE MERITS OF 'HOT' AND 'COLD' SPOT SCANS

	'Hot spot' imaging technetium-99^m	*'Cold spot' imaging thallium-201*
Advantages	Higher sensitivity and specificity Old infarcts not imaged Detects both left and right ventricular infarcts Daily scans possible	Up to 100% sensitivity within 6 h of acute infarct
Disadvantages	Delay of up to 48 h before diagnostic uptake pattern False positive tests in unstable angina ventricular aneurysm cardioversion calcific valve disease myocardial tumour	Expensive Daily scans impossible (long half-life of ^{201}Tl) Does not differentiate old versus new infarction ischaemia versus infarction False positive tests in cardiomyopathy left bundle branch block myocardial tumour

Table 3.13

RADIONUCLIDE ANGIOGRAPHY: RELATIVE MERITS OF 'FIRST PASS' AND EQUILIBRIUM TECHNIQUES

Clinical study	*First pass*	*Equilibrium*
Left ventricular ejection fraction	Accurate	Accurate
Regional left ventricular wall motion	Good	Excellent
Intracardiac shunt detection	Possible	Impossible
Sequential studies/patient monitoring	Inferior	Superior
Interventions causing rapid heart rate changes	Superior	Inferior

techniques employ ^{99m}Tc bound to human albumin or to the patient's own red blood cells to ensure that the tracer remains within the intravascular compartment. The relative merits of the two radionuclide techniques are summarised in Table 3.13. Both first-pass and subsequent equilibrium studies may be performed following a single injection of non-diffusable tracer.

CARDIAC CATHETERISATION

Background

Human cardiac catheterisation was first shown to be feasible by Werner Forssman in Germany. In 1929 at the age of 25 he exposed a vein in his own left arm, inserted a catheter, advanced it for 65 cm then walked to the X-ray department and with the help of a nurse confirmed its position in the right atrium. He predicted that the technique would become clinically important, but it was not until the 1940s that McMichael in England and Cournand in America began formally to establish its decisive role in the modern diagnosis and treatment of heart disease. Precise haemodynamic and cineangiographic data have enabled the development of cardiac surgery. Such data have also provided the 'gold-standard' for the validation of non-invasive methods such as echocardiography and nuclear cardiology. As a result much cardiac disease can be diagnosed and treated without cardiac catheterisation but it still remains the case that most patients considered for cardiac surgery will undergo invasive investigation. Ischaemic heart disease accounts for the great majority, followed by valvular and congenital heart disease. Specific indications are discussed in the appropriate chapters of this text.

Cardiac Catheters

Cardiac catheters are long, flexible tubes with high torque control manufactured to different specifications for special purposes. Commonly used catheters are:

(i) *Single end-hole* (for example, Cournand): for right heart and pulmonary wedge pressure measurement.
(ii) *Balloon-tipped* (flow directed or Swan–Ganz): for bedside right heart and pulmonary wedge catheterisation.

(iii) *Angiographic* (for example, pigtail, N.I.H.): multiple side holes for even delivery of X-ray contrast medium.
(iv) *Coronary arteriographic* (for example, Judkins, Sones, Amplatz): designed and/or preshaped for entry to the coronary artery orifices.
(v) *Electrode tipped*: for stimulating or recording intracardiac electrical activity.
(vi) *Transseptal*: a long needle, curved at its tip, is advanced from the femoral vein to the right atrium. The inter-atrial septum is punctured and a precurved catheter passed over the needle to the left atrium and left ventricle.
(vii) *Therapeutic*: for example, balloon catheters for percutaneous transluminal angioplasty, valvuloplasty and atrial septostomy.

Access to the Circulation

There are two usual routes:

(i) *Femoral vein and artery*: these are approached percutaneously using a hollow (Seldinger) needle. A guide wire and introducer are inserted and the catheter advanced through the introducer.
(ii) *Brachial vein and artery*: the vessels are exposed by direct 'cutdown' in the antecubital fossa.

Right Heart Catheterisation

Under X-ray control the catheter is passed from the peripheral vein via the inferior or superior vena cava to the right atrium, right ventricle, main pulmonary artery and branches to the pulmonary 'wedge' position in a peripheral pulmonary artery branch. If a patent foramen ovale or an atrial septal defect is present the catheter can be passed to the left atrium and left ventricle. A patent ductus arteriosus will allow passage of the right heart catheter from the pulmonary artery to the aorta.

Left Heart Catheterisation

The catheter is passed from the peripheral artery to the aorta and retrograde across the aortic valve to the left ventricle. The left atrium and ventricle may be entered also by the transseptal method.

Table 3.14
INFORMATION DERIVED FROM CARDIAC CATHETERISATION

Technique	*Example of information derived*
Pressure measurement	
Pressure waveform	Cardiac chamber identification Large 'v' wave of atrioventricular valve regurgitation 'Dip-and-plateau' of ventricular diastolic waveform in pericardial constriction
Elevated pressure	High RA and RV pressures in pulmonary arterial hypertension High end-diastolic pressure in RV and LV dysfunction
Pressure gradient	High LV and low aortic pressure in aortic stenosis
Oxygen saturation measurement	Cardiac output (direct Fick principle) Resistance across vascular beds Quantitation of intracardiac shunts
Contrast angiography	
Anatomical	Structural abnormalities of the heart and great vessels in congenital or acquired disease Coronary arteriographic anatomy
Functional	Regional and global ventricular function Quantitation of valvular function

RA = right atrium; RV = right ventricle; LV = left ventricle.

Information Acquired

Three classes of diagnostic information are acquired:

(i) *Pressure measurement*: pressure at various sites is transmitted through the fluid-filled catheter to an external strain-gauge transducer. High fidelity recordings (usually for research purposes) are obtained using catheter tip manometers.
(ii) *Oxygen saturation*: samples obtained through the catheter are measured colorimetrically by oximetry. Cardiac output calculations (Fick principle) and shunt detection are the usual indications.
(iii) *Selective contrast angiocardiography*: radio-opaque contrast media are injected into various sites; structural and functional information is recorded using single or multiple plane cineangiography.

Examples of the specific information derived are summarised in Table 3.14. Normal values are summarised in Table 3.15 and

Table 3.15
NORMAL UPPER LIMIT OF PRESSURES

Site	*Pressure (mmHg)*	
Right atrium	'a'	8
	'v'	5
	mean	6
Right ventricle (systolic/end diastolic)	30/8	
Pulmonary artery	30/12	
	mean	18
Left atrium (or pulmonary wedge)	a	12
	v	14
	mean	12
Left ventricle (systolic/end diastolic)	140/12	
Aorta	140/90	
	mean	105

Table 3.16

CARDIAC CATHETERISATION: COMMONLY USED CALCULATIONS

	Calculation	*Comment*
Cardiac output (ml/min) (direct Fick method)	$\frac{\text{Oxygen uptake/min}}{\text{Arterial } o_2 \text{ content } minus \text{ Venous } o_2 \text{ content}}$ (ml o_2/100 ml blood)	Cardiac output varies with body surface area; normal cardiac index (litres/min/M^2) = 2.6 – 4.2
Pulmonary vascular resistance	$\frac{PAp - LAp}{\text{pulmonary flow}}$ (pulmonary flow = cardiac output if no shunt present)	Equation gives resistance in arbitrary units of mmHg/(L/min) These are usually converted to metric resistance units by a conversion factor of × 80 Normal = 20–130 dynes-s-cm^{-5}
Shunt determination Pulmonary: systemic flow	$\frac{A_0\ o_2 - SVC\ o_2}{A_0\ o_2 - PAo_2}$	In the presence of a left to right shunt the ratio is > 1 (more blood flows through the pulmonary than the systemic circulation). A ratio of 2:1 or greater is haemodynamically significant

PAp = pulmonary artery mean pressure; LA*p* = left atrial (or pulmonary wedge) mean pressure
A_0o_2 = aortic oxygen saturation; $SVCo_2$ = superior vena caval oxygen saturation;
PAo_2 = pulmonary arterial oxygen saturation

calculations in Table 3.16. The derivation of the formulae given is beyond the scope of this text (see Further reading section).

Complications of cardiac catheterisation

The mortality of cardiac catheterisation is 0.1% with higher rates in patients under 1 year of age and over 60. Non-fatal complications include myocardial infarction, cerebrovascular accidents, distal embolism and perforation of the heart or great vessels. Local vascular complications are more common, and there is probably no significant difference between the brachial and femoral approaches. The overall incidence of complications is low especially when the procedure is performed by a fully trained and experienced operator.

FURTHER READING

Bodenheimer M.M., Banks V.S., Helfant R.H. (1980). Nuclear cardiology. *American Journal of Cardiology*, **45,** 661.

Bruce R.A., Hornsten T.R. (1969). Exercise stress testing in evaluation of patients with ischaemic heart disease. *Progress in Cardiovascular Disease*, **11,** 371.

Feigenbaum H. (1984). Echocardiography. In *Heart Disease—A Textbook of Cardiovascular Medicine*, ed. Braunwald E., pp. 88–145. Philadelphia, London: W.B. Saunders (543 references).

Goldschlager N., Selzer A., Cohn K. (1976). Treadmill stress tests as indicators of presence and severity of coronary artery disease. *Annals of Internal Medicine*, **85,** 277.

Grossman W. (1980). *Cardiac Catheterisation and Angiography* (2nd ed.) Philadelphia: Lea and Febiger.

Roelandt J. (1986). Colour-coded Doppler flow imaging: What are the prospects? *European Heart Journal*, **7,** 184.

Sahn D.J., Valdes-Cruz M. (1986). New advances in two-dimensional Doppler echocardiography. *Progress in Cardiovascular Disease*, **28,** 367.

Sami M., Kraemer H., De Busk R.F. (1979). The prognostic significance of serial exercise testing after myocardial infarction. *Circulation*, **60,** 1238.

Smith J.J., Kampine J.P. (1984). *Circulatory Physiology—The Essentials*. Baltimore, London: Williams and Wilkins.

Willerson J.T., Parkey R.W., Buja L.M., Bonte F.J. (1979). In *Nuclear Cardiology (Cardiovascular Clinics)*, ed. J.T. Willerson. Philadelphia: F.A. Davis.

Chapter Four

Cardiomyopathy and Specific Heart Muscle Disorders

Definition

Cardiomyopathy is heart muscle disease of unknown cause. In *specific heart muscle disease* the cause is known or the myocardium is involved in a systemic disorder, such as drug toxicity or collagen disease. A specific cause will be found in fewer than 10% of patients investigated for heart muscle disease. Heart muscle disease caused by ischaemic, hypertensive, valvular, pulmonary, pericardial or congenital heart disease is excluded.

THE CARDIOMYOPATHIES

Background

There are three separate types of cardiomyopathy each with a clearly distinct haemodynamic fault:

(i) Dilated (formerly congestive).
(ii) Hypertrophic.
(iii) Restrictive.

Each has its own clinical presentation and management. In general, the diagnosis of cardiomyopathy should be suspected when the clinical presentation does not obviously fit the commoner types of heart disease. Heart failure or dilatation of obscure cause suggests dilated cardiomyopathy and extensive ECG changes of ventricular hypertrophy suggest hypertrophic cardiomyopathy. Restrictive cardiomyopathy is very rare in temperate climates. The haemodynamic classification of the cardiomyopathies is provided by cardiac catheterisation, but echocardiography is the single most crucial clinical investigation (see Chapter 3).

Dilated Cardiomyopathy

Definition

A chronic, occasionally reversible disorder of the myocardium in which impaired systolic contraction is associated with dilatation of the left or right ventricles or both.

Background

Dilated cardiomyopathy occurs throughout the world and in all age groups but is seen most commonly in middle-aged men. The condition may be the end stage of damage to a predisposed myocardium exposed to a variety of environmental factors including alcohol and infectious agents; 'alcoholic cardiomyopathy' is not a separate entity and heart muscle disease rarely coexists with liver cirrhosis. Familial occurrence is rare. Low output congestive cardiac failure is frequent but not invariable, and arrhythmias are common.

Pathology

All four cardiac chambers are dilated, the ventricles more than the atria. Ventricular hypertrophy is variable and survival is

Table 4.1

CONDITIONS DETECTED BY ENDOMYOCARDIAL BIOPSY

Cardiac transplant rejection
Adriamycin (daunorubicin) toxicity
Myocarditis
Amyloidosis
Sarcoidosis
Haemochromatosis
Endocardial fibroelastosis
Endomyocardial fibrosis
Carcinoid
Glycogen storage disease
Cardiac tumour
Fabry's disease

longer in patients with a greater degree of left ventricular hypertrophy. Thrombi are often found in the ventricles overlying thickened endocardium. The cardiac valves and coronary arteries are normal. Ventricular endomyocardial biopsy shows non-specific interstitial fibrosis and myocardial fibre degeneration. No specific markers establish the diagnosis of dilated cardiomyopathy although endomyocardial biopsy, performed at cardiac catheterisation, is useful to exclude specific heart muscle diseases (Table 4.1).

Symptoms and signs

Asymptomatic cardiomegaly may be a chance discovery. Presentation is usually with:

(i) *Heart failure*: early symptoms may be wrongly ascribed to a 'virus' or respiratory infection.
(ii) *Arrhythmias*: ventricular arrhythmias are common; atrial fibrillation may precipitate heart failure.
(iii) *Embolism*: systemic emboli arise from the dilated left atrium or ventricle; pulmonary embolism is common in established heart failure.

If the condition is mild there may be no abnormal signs. Most patients have signs of:

(i) *Cardiac dilatation*: displaced and diffuse apex beat, palpable third or fourth heart sounds, pansystolic murmurs of mitral and tricuspid regurgitation.
(ii) *Low stroke volume*: low volume and amplitude pulse, normal or low blood pressure with narrow pulse pressure, soft first heart sound.
(iii) *Cardiac failure*.

Differential diagnosis

Dilated cardiomyopathy is a diagnosis of exclusion and must be differentiated from structural heart disease or specific heart muscle disease (Table 4.2).

Table 4.2

DIFFERENTIAL DIAGNOSIS OF DILATED CARDIOMYOPATHY

From structural heart disease	
Ischaemic heart disease	Angina pectoris ECG Coronary angiography
Valvular heart disease	Valve calcification (X-ray) Echocardiography Cardiac catheter
Pericardial effusion	Echocardiography
From specific heart muscle disease	
Myocarditis	Serology Myocardial biopsy
Hypertensive heart failure	Known hypertension (blood pressure may be normal during hypertensive failure)
Sarcoidosis	Ventricular arrhythmias common at presentation Myocardial biopsy
Amyloid	Echocardiography (two-dimensional) Myocardial biopsy
Endocrine disease	Biochemical investigation for thyroid disease, phaeochromocytoma, acromegaly
Haemochromatosis	Systemic physical signs Iron studies Myocardial biopsy
Collagen disease (especially scleroderma)	ESR, rheumatoid factor Immunoglobulins
Neuromuscular disorders	

Investigations

The ECG and chest X-ray show non-specific abnormalities (Table 4.3). The most useful investigations are (see also Chapter 3):

(i) *M-mode echocardiography*: excludes pericardial effusion as a cause of a large, globular heart on chest X-ray. The typical findings are:
  (a) increased left ventricular cavity size;

(b) reduced contraction of the septum and posterior wall;

(c) intrinsically normal cardiac valves with decreased excursion due to low cardiac output.

(ii) *Two-dimensional echocardiography*: images the whole myocardium and usually confirms global dilatation and reduced contractility, although discrete regional wall motion abnormalities may occur as in ischaemic heart disease. Right ventricular function is better preserved in ischaemic and valvular heart disease than in dilated cardiomyopathy. Intracardiac thrombus is accurately detected by two-dimensional echocardiography.

(iii) *Cardiac catheterisation*: left ventricular end-diastolic, left atrial and pulmonary wedge pressures are elevated. Moderate elevation of pulmonary artery and right ventricular end-diastolic pressure is common. Cardiac output is low.

Coronary angiography is typically normal. It excludes left ventricular dysfunction due to atheromatous coronary artery disease, and anomalous origin of the left coronary artery from the pulmonary artery in young patients. Endomyocardial biopsy excludes some forms of specific heart muscle disease (see Table 4.1).

Treatment

There is no specific treatment. The principles of management are:

(i) Modification of contributory factors:

(a) prohibit alcohol;

(b) limit exercise;

(c) control blood pressure;

(d) reduce weight.

(ii) Supportive therapy:

(a) long-term anticoagulants effectively prevent systemic and venous thromboembolism;

(b) diuretics reduce elevated pulmonary venous pressure and help shrink the left ventricle. The value of digitalis in myocardial failure with sinus rhythm is doubtful; the new inotropic agents amrinone and milrinone may prove valuable;

(c) vasodilators, e.g. angiotensin converting enzyme

Table 4.3

INVESTIGATIONS DIFFERENTIATING THE CARDIOMYOPATHIES

	Dilated	*Hypertrophic*	*Restrictive*
ECG	Sinus tachycardia Atrial fibrillation Ventricular arrhythmias ST/T wave changes Left bundle branch block 'Pseudoinfarction' pattern	Left ventricular hypertrophy Left or biatrial P waves Abnormal Q waves ST/T wave changes Ventricular and atrial arrhythmias	ST/T wave changes Conduction defects, especially right bundle branch block Low voltage tracing
Chest X-ray	Cardiomegaly (simulates pericardial effusion) Pulmonary venous congestion Pulmonary oedema	Variable, often normal Mild/moderate left ventricular ± left atrial enlargement	Normal, or mild cardiac enlargement Pulmonary venous congestion

Echocardiogram	Left ventricular dilatation Septal and posterior wall hypokinesia Low amplitude valve excursion due to low stroke volume	Asymmetrical septal hypertrophy (ASH) Systolic anterior motion (SAM) of the mitral valve Midsystolic aortic valve closure Small left ventricle	Normal size left ventricle Normal systolic function Dense endocardial echoes (two-dimensional)
Cardiac catheter	Low cardiac output Raised left and often right ventricular diastolic pressures	Raised left ventricular diastolic pressure Dynamic left ventricular outflow gradient	Diastolic plateau ('square root sign') in ventricular pressure trace Left ventricular diastolic pressure raised more than right
Angiocardiography	Dilated, hypokinetic left ventricle Mitral regurgitation	Hyperdynamic left ventricular contraction Misshapen ventricle Mitral regurgitation	Squared-off left ventricle Normal contractility Atrioventricular valve regurgitation

(ACE) inhibitors, nitrates, prazosin reduce the inappropriately elevated preload and afterload and should be used early in treatment; clinical benefit is confirmed and recent evidence shows that prognosis may be improved.

(d) beta-adrenergic blockers in low doses (metoprolol 12.5–50 mg orally twice daily) may paradoxically benefit some patients. Close observation is mandatory as severe left ventricular failure may occur. The mechanism of benefit is unknown;

(e) antiarrhythmics: 90% of patients have complex ventricular arrhythmias. Ventricular tachycardia is a strong predictor of sudden death especially when episodes are frequent. Amiodarone is the most effective drug.

(iii) Cardiac transplantation (see Chapter 10).

Prognosis

Two-thirds of patients die within 2 years of diagnosis although up to 25% may recover. Four factors predict a poor prognosis:

(i) Age greater than 55 years.
(ii) Cardiothoracic ratio greater than 55%.
(iii) Cardiac index less than 3·0 l/min/m^2.
(iv) Left ventricular end diastolic pressure greater than 20 mmHg.

Unusual forms of dilated cardiomyopathy

Three conditions are difficult to classify but can be regarded as forms of dilated cardiomyopathy.

(i) *Peripartum heart failure*: gradual or sudden heart failure of unknown cause during late pregnancy may result in death, chronic disease or complete recovery. There is a tendency to relapse in subsequent pregnancies.

(ii) *Endocardial fibroelastosis*: diffuse endocardial thickening with dilatation and failure of the left ventricle occurs in early infancy and can complicate other congenital disorders, especially coarctation of the aorta.

(iii) *Right ventricular cardiomyopathy*: dilated cardiomyopathy affecting predominantly or exclusively the right ventricle. Right heart failure and recurrent ventricular tachycardia are typical.

Hypertrophic Cardiomyopathy

Definition

This is unexplained hypertrophy particularly involving the interventricular septum of a non-dilated left ventricle, resulting in abnormal diastolic function due to myocardial stiffness.

Background

Early descriptions emphasised the finding of variable systolic pressure gradients dividing the left ventricle into a high pressure

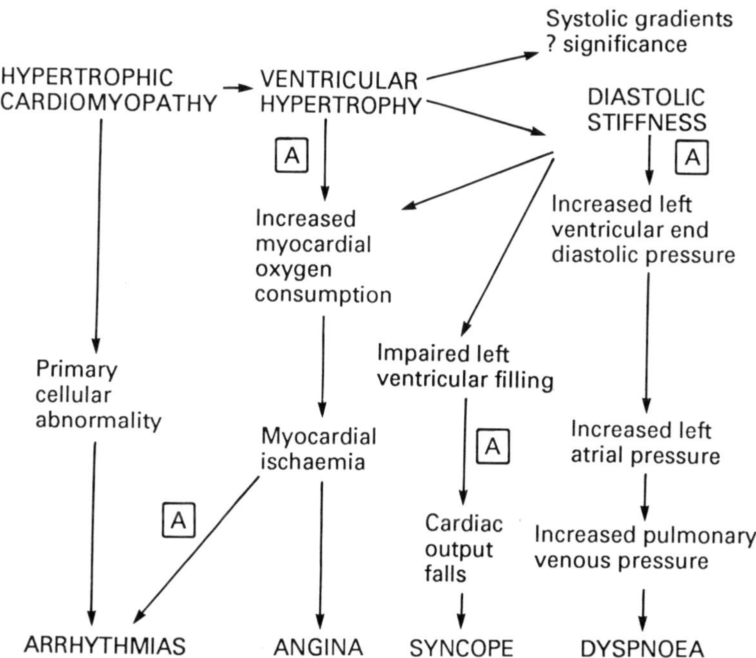

Fig. 4.1. Mechanism of symptoms in hypertrophic cardiomyopathy. Autonomic influences (A), especially tachycardia, may exacerbate the symptoms.

apical region and a low pressure subaortic region. A decrease in left ventricular volume or afterload would increase the gradient, whereas an increase in left ventricular volume would reduce or abolish the gradient. The gradient can reach 150 mg, and it was initially believed that the resulting obstruction to flow was the major cause of symptoms. In fact, most patients do not display intraventricular pressure gradients and their significance is now disputed, so the term 'obstructive' has been dropped.

Abnormal diastolic relaxation rather than systolic obstruction is the important pathophysiological abnormality. Impaired diastolic filling and increased end diastolic pressure in combination with left ventricular hypertrophy result in the typical symptoms of dyspnoea, angina, arrhythmias and syncope (Fig. 4.1).

Hypertrophic cardiomyopathy is inherited by an autosomal dominant gene with variable penetration, sometimes linked to the HLA system, but sporadic cases often occur. First degree relatives often display milder disease and are detected only in family surveys. All ages are affected although symptomatic hypertrophic cardiomyopathy is associated with a variety of conditions including Noonan's syndrome, lentiginosis and acromegaly; it is the commonest cause of death in Friedreich's ataxia.

Pathology

The salient features are both macroscopic and microscopic.

Macroscopic

- (i) Increased ventricular myocardial mass.
- (ii) Asymmetric septal hypertrophy (ASH): may affect the whole septum or just the upper or apical part. ASH is not pathognomonic; concentric hypertrophy of the septum and free wall may occur.
- (iii) Small ventricular cavities.
- (iv) Dilated atria due to:
  - (a) increased resistance to ventricular filling;
  - (b) valvular regurgitation.
- (v) 'Contact lesion': a fibrous plaque where the anterior mitral leaflet or subvalvular apparatus impact upon the interventricular septum. Infective endocarditis may develop on the contact lesion and on the mitral or aortic valves.

Microscopic

(i) whorls of cells: marked myocardial fibre disarray is not diagnostic and may occur in hypertrophy secondary to recognised causes.

Symptoms

Hypertrophic cardiomyopathy may present in three ways:

(i) Most patients are asymptomatic and are detected during incidental medical examination. The systolic murmur is frequently mistaken for either aortic stenosis or mitral regurgitation.
(ii) Sudden death, often in active young people.
(iii) Dyspnoea, angina pectoris and syncope are the classic presenting symptoms (see Fig. 4.1).

Signs

Careful physical examination is very useful in the diagnosis of hypertrophic cardiomyopathy and its differentiation from aortic stenosis or mitral regurgitation:

(i) *Carotid pulse*: normal or high volume, jerky character. This is the most useful sign differentiating fixed aortic valvular stenosis in which the pulse is of small volume and slow rising (anacrotic or 'plateau' pulse).
(ii) *Venous pulse*: small dominant 'a' wave, especially if the right ventricle is involved.
(iii) *Apex beat*: a double impulse is caused by a prominent atrial beat preceding the left ventricular impulse. A triple impulse is virtually diagnostic; the atrial beat is followed by two impulses representing early and late systole, before and after the peak of the left ventricular outflow gradient.
(iv) *Auscultation*: a midsystolic ejection murmur maximal between the apex and the left sternal edge; 50% of patients have an additional pansystolic murmur of mitral regurgitation. The systolic ejection murmur, corresponding to the left ventricular outflow gradient, may be varied in loudness by simple manoeuvres which may

differentiate it from the murmurs of aortic stenosis and mitral regurgitation (Table 4.4).

(v) *Signs of complications*:
   (a) atrial fibrillation;
   (b) congestive cardiac failure;
   (c) thromboembolism (especially in (a) or (b));
   (d) infective endocarditis.

Table 4.4

VARIATION IN THE LOUDNESS OF SYSTOLIC MURMURS BY MANOEUVRES WHICH ALTER LEFT VENTRICULAR (LV) SIZE AND OUTPUT

	Hypertrophic cardiomyopathy	*Aortic stenosis*	*Mitral regurgitation*
Squat from standing position (↑ afterload) (↑ venous return)	↓	↓ or =	↑
Standing	↑	↑ or =	↓
Valsalva strain phase (↓ LV volume)	↑	↓	↓
Amyl nitrite inhalation (↓ afterload)	↑	↑	↓
Postectopic beat (↑ preload) (↑ contractility)	↑*	↑	
Isometric handgrip (↑ afterload)	↓	↓ or =	↑

*pulse volume decreases
= unchanged

Investigations

The most useful are:

(i) *Echocardiography*: the classic findings on M-mode and two-dimensional echocardiography are shown in Table 4.3. No single feature is pathognomonic but a combination of well-marked features is diagnostic.

(ii) *Ambulatory electrocardiography*: this may reveal ventricular arrhythmias which are predictive of sudden death, and should be performed routinely in all patients with hypertrophic cardiomyopathy.

(iii) *Angiography*: a misshapen, typically 'bent banana'-shaped cavity is seen on left ventriculography which may also show mitral regurgitation. Systolic contraction is hyperdynamic. Angina may be due to coexistent atheromatous coronary artery disease demonstrated by selective coronary angiography.

Management

Preventive

(i) Arrhythmias: sudden death is common and predicted by ventricular arrhythmias or ambulatory ECG monitoring. Amiodarone 400–600 mg daily after loading with 1200 mg/day for 1 week is the most effective drug. Atrial fibrillation in hypertrophic cardiomyopathy is also best treated with amiodarone in hypertrophic cardiomyopathy.

(ii) Avoid competitive athletic activity.

(iii) Anticoagulants reduce the incidence of thromboembolism due to atrial fibrillation and heart failure.

(iv) Screen first degree relatives.

Symptomatic

(i) Beta-adrenergic blockers: the main benefit is the suppression of tachycardia (see Fig. 4.1).

(ii) Verapamil has been used to improve ventricular filling and reduce outflow gradients; benefit is inconsistent.

(iii) Surgery to remove hypertrophied septal muscle (myotomyectomy) achieves unpredictable benefit at high operative mortality (5–10%). Mitral valve replacement is sometimes indicated.

Restrictive Cardiomyopathy

Definition

This is fibrosis of the endocardium and inner myocardium, often affecting the atrioventricular valves, causing restriction of diastolic ventricular filling but normal systolic function.

Background

Although a 'restrictive' functional abnormality is found in some specific heart muscle diseases the WHO Classification limits the term restrictive cardiomyopathy to endomyocardial fibrosis (EMF) and eosinophilic endomyocardial disease (Loeffler's endocarditis). Restrictive cardiomyopathy is rare worldwide but is commonest in tropical latitudes, 10° north and south of the equator.

Pathology

Endomyocardial fibrosis is the structural abnormality and there appears to be no pathological difference between the 'tropical' and 'non-tropical' forms. Strong evidence exists that EMF is the end result of cardiac involvement in any disease process which includes abundant and prolonged eosinophilia (Table 4.5) defined as > 1500 eosinophils/mm^2 for at least 6 months or until death confirms the diagnosis.

Table 4.5

CAUSES OF HYPEREOSINOPHILIA

Hypereosinophilic syndrome
Neoplasm
Leukaemia
Filarial infection
Hodgkin's disease
Asthma
Drug hypersensitivity

Clinical features

Hypereosinophilia is most commonly of unknown cause—the hypereosinophilic syndrome. Malaise, fever, weight loss, skin rash, heart failure, embolism and mitral regurgitation are seen leading acutely to death or chronically to restrictive cardiomyopathy. Diagnostic findings are summarised in Table 4.3. Constrictive pericarditis may closely simulate restrictive cardiomy-

Table 4.6
SPECIFIC HEART MUSCLE DISEASE: CLASSIFICATION

Classification	*Clinical forms*
Infective	
Virus	Numerous agents
Bacteria	Diphtheria, meningococcus
Spirochaetes	Leptospirosis
Protozoa	Chagas' disease
Rickettsial	Psittacosis, Q fever, scrub typhus
Fungi	Aspergillosis, candidiasis
Metabolic	
Endocrine	Diabetes
	Hyperthyroidism and hypothyroidism
	Acromegaly
	Phaeochromocytoma
	Addison's disease
Inherited storage disease	Glycogen storage diseases
	Mucopolysaccharidoses
	Fabry's disease
	Refsum's disease
Deficiency states	Kwashiorkor
	Thiamine deficiency
General system disease	
Collagen vascular	Rheumatoid disease
	Systemic lupus erythematosus
	Scleroderma
	Polyarteritis nodosa
Infiltrations and granulomas	Amyloidosis
	Sarcoidosis
	Leukaemias
	Haemochromatosis
Heredofamilial neuromyopathic diseases	
	Progressive muscular dystrophies
	Dystrophia myotonica
	Friedreich's ataxia
Hypersensitivity and toxic reactions	
Drugs	Adriamycin/daunorubicin
	Busulphan
	Vincristine
	Methysergide
Industrial chemicals	Hydrocarbons
	Mercury, phosphorus, cobalt

Table 4.6

SPECIFIC HEART MUSCLE DISEASE: CLASSIFICATION

Classification	*Clinical forms*
Toxins	Snake bite Wasp and spider stings
Physical agents	Radiation Heat stroke Hypothermia

opathy. Left and right ventricular diastolic pressures are usually equal in constrictive pericarditis and unequal in restrictive cardiomyopathy. Endomyocardial biopsy may help differentiate the conditions but sometimes exploratory thoracotomy is the final arbiter.

Management

Steroids or cytotoxic drugs (such as vincristine, hydroxyurea) may help if there is eosinophilia or evidence of recent necrotic damage in the endomyocardial biopsy. Chronic restrictive cardiomyopathy requires diuretic and anticoagulant therapy.

SPECIFIC HEART MUSCLE DISEASE

The WHO Task Force on the definition and classification of heart muscle disease has confined the term 'cardiomyopathy' to conditions of unknown cause. 'Specific heart muscle diseases' are either of known cause or associated with systemic disease. The former terms 'primary' and 'secondary' cardiomyopathy respectively are now obsolete. A summary of specific heart muscle disease classification is given in Table 4.6. The list is enormous and only the more important will be briefly described.

The pathophysiological effects of the various specific heart muscle diseases vary widely, but in general terms the functional defects are analogous to those of the cardiomyopathies—dilated, hypertrophic and restrictive (Table 4.7). For specific heart muscle disease the functional classification is a guide only—there are many exceptions. Most conditions display the same fault as dilated cardiomyopathy. A condition appearing in more than one

Table 4.7

SPECIFIC HEART MUSCLE DISEASES CLASSIFIED BY MAIN PATHOPHYSIOLOGICAL ABNORMALITY

Dilated	*Hypertrophic*	*Restrictive*
Myocarditis	Friedreich's ataxia	Carcinoid syndrome
Sarcoidosis	Noonan's syndrome	Methysergide toxicity
Haemochromatosis	Lentiginosis	Sarcoidosis
Haemosiderosis	Acromegaly	Amyloidosis
Connective tissue disorders (especially scleroderma)	Pompe's disease	Malignant infiltration
		Glycogen storage disease
Progressive muscular dystrophies		Scleroderma
Dystrophia myotonica		
Myocardial toxins cobalt toxicity anthracycline drugs (Adriamycin, daunorubicin)		
Beriberi		
Amyloidosis		

category may show either or both functional defects in a given individual. Thus amyloid infiltration combines failure of systolic contraction with the indistensibility of the 'restrictive' ventricle.

Infective Disorders

Virus myocarditis

Definition

This is inflammation of the myocardium, sometimes with vasculitis, caused by virus invasion of the myocyte.

Background

Viruses are the commonest cause of acute myocarditis in the United Kingdom. Coxsackie group B is the usual aetiological agent but many viruses may be responsible. Transient electrocardiographic changes may be observed during the course of many viral illnesses, such as influenza, respiratory infection, measles, poliomyelitis, without clinical signs of cardiac involvement. Conversely, myocarditis may progress rapidly to death in severe heart failure. Progression from virus myocarditis to dilated cardiomyopathy is suspected but not proven.

Symptoms and signs

Malaise, fever, skeletal myalgia, dyspnoea, palpitations and chest pain are common. Tachycardia is disproportionate to fever or evidence of heart failure.

Investigation and management

Virus complement fixation titres are often unhelpful. Endomyocardial biopsy may indicate the use of steroids and immunosuppressive drugs if the inflammatory process is active. Most patients make a spontaneous and complete recovery.

Diphtheria

Acute myocarditis complicates diphtheria in one quarter of subjects. Cardiac damage is due to the release by the bacillus of exotoxin that inhibits protein synthesis. Cardiac dilatation and severe congestive cardiac failure appear at the end of the first week, often progressing to heart block and cardiogenic shock. Diphtheritic myocarditis is fatal in most infants and in one-quarter of adults. Antitoxin and penicillin should be given as early as possible. Supportive measures include drug therapy of cardiac failure and transvenous pacing. Residual electrocardiographic abnormalities are common in survivors but chronic myocardial damage is rare.

Trypanosomiasis (Chagas' disease)

Chagas' disease is caused by the protozoon *Trypanosoma cruzi* and is the commonest form of heart disease in South America. It is transmitted to humans by infected reduviid bugs which acquire the organism from infected animals. After human inoculation the protozoa multiply and disseminate throughout the body. *Acute* trypanosomiasis occurs in a minority of cases, usually young children, as a febrile illness with myocarditis. After an average latent period of 20 years an immune-mediated *chronic* trypanosomiasis appears. Cardiac dilatation, progressive heart failure, ventricular arrhythmias, emboli and heart block are common. Clinical and epidemiological evidence of chronic Chagas' disease is confirmed by the complement fixation (Machado–Guerreiro) test. Death due to cardiac failure and ventricular arrhythmias is common.

Endocrine and Metabolic Disorders

Diabetes mellitus

Heart muscle disease in diabetes mellitus may develop as a result of:

(i) Atheromatous coronary artery disease, which is common and more severe in diabetics.
(ii) Myocardial microvascular disease, similar to and often coexisting with, diabetic retinopathy, neuropathy and renal disease.

Abnormal left ventricular function is detectable in the absence of significant atheromatous coronary artery disease. The combined vascular lesions may account for the higher incidence of heart failure in diabetics when compared with the non-diabetic population.

Thyroid disorders

Thyroid hormone affects the level of general tissue metabolism and oxygen consumption, and acts directly on the myocardium. The effects of hyperthyroidism and hypothyroidism are summarised in Table 4.8.

In *hyperthyroidism* the complications of heart failure and atrial fibrillation may be due solely to thyroxine excess but usually

Table 4.8
CARDIOVASCULAR EFFECTS OF THYROID DISORDERS

	Hyperthyroidism	*Hypothyroidism*
General tissue metabolism and O_2 consumption	Increased	Decreased
Cardiac output	Increased	Decreased
Cardiac rhythm	Sinus tachycardia Atrial fibrillation	Sinus bradycardia Low voltage ECG
Myocardial contractility	Increased	Decreased
Heart size	Increase in hypertrophy and heart failure	Increase often due to pericardial effusion
Specific myocardial lesions	None. Focal leucocytic infiltration and fibrosis reported in thyroid hormone abuse	None, but mucoid infiltration and interstitial oedema occur

imply the aggravation of underlying heart disease. Rapid control of tachyarrhythmias is best achieved by beta-adrenoceptor blockade with propranolol. Atrial fibrillation is relatively unresponsive to digoxin in untreated hyperthyroidism but is readily cardioverted by DC shock to sinus rhythm once the disease is controlled. Conventional therapy is used for heart failure. Radioiodine is the preferred specific treatment for patients with thyrotoxic heart disease.

Hypothyroidism and the associated type III hyperlipidaemia probably predispose to atheromatous coronary artery disease. Thyroid replacement reverses the cardiovascular abnormalities but may provoke the symptoms of underlying coronary artery disease.

Acromegaly

Cardiac enlargement and marked hypertrophy of the left ventricle are invariable. Asymmetrical hypertrophy of the interventricular septum may occur, similar to the structural defect in hypertrophic cardiomyopathy. Hypertension is common and 25% of patients develop cardiac failure. Myocardial hypertrophy reflects generalised organomegaly due to growth hormone excess, increased cardiac work and the effect of hypertension. Cardiovascular complications of acromegaly are often the cause of death.

Haemochromatosis

Haemochromatosis is a chronic disease due to excessive deposition of iron in the liver and other tissues including the heart. The disease may be *genetic* due to an inborn error of the regulation of iron absorption, or *acquired* due to the administration of iron in the tissues but with no resultant tissue damage.

Heart involvement presents as a dilated cardiomyopathy often associated with slate-grey skin, diabetes mellitus and gonadal atrophy. The serum iron level is raised (> 30 mol/l) with a reduction in total iron-binding capacity and elevated transferrin saturation. Myocardial iron deposits are demonstrated by endomyocardial biopsy. The iron may be mobilised by repeated phlebotomy and partial reversal of the cardiac lesion has been described.

Table 4.9

CARDIOVASCULAR INVOLVEMENT IN JOINT AND CONNECTIVE TISSUE DISEASES

(principal manifestations are shown in italics)

Condition (% cardiac involvement)	*Pathology*	*Myocardium*	*Pericardium*	*Endocardium*	*Other*
Polyarteritis nodosa (80%)	Necrotising arteritis	*Myocardial infarction* Congestive failure	*Acute pericarditis*	—	*Coronary arteritis* Superventricular tachycardia Hypertension Cardiac involvement is second commonest cause of death after renal disease

Systemic lupus erythematosus (60%)	Fibrinoid necrosis of small arteries, arterioles and capillaries	*Myocarditis* Congestive failure Conduction defects	*Fibrinoid pericarditis*	Libman-Sachs endocarditis with mitral valve vegetations. Rare	Aortic regurgitation Hypertension
Scleroderma (50%)	Fibrosis	Conduction defects Arrhythmias Dilatation and congestive failure	Acute pericarditis *Chronic fibrotic pericarditis*	—	Systemic hypertension Pulmonary hypertension Cor pulmonale
Rheumatoid arthritis (50%)	Vasculitis Granulomata	Non-specific and granulomatous inflammation	*Pericarditis* *Pericardial effusion* especially in nodular rheumatoid arthritis	*Valvulitis* of aortic > mitral valve. Clinical evidence rare	Coronary arteritis
Ankylosing spondylitis (4%)	Chronic inflammatory cell infiltrate	Dilatation and congestive failure Conduction defects	Pericarditis	—	*Aortitis* *Aortic regurgitation* in cases exceeding 15 years duration

Beriberi

Beriberi is due to thiamine deficiency. In eastern countries primary deficiency is associated with a diet of polished rice. In the West deficiency is secondary to a low intake, usually in chronic alcoholics. Polyneuropathy (dry beriberi) or congestive cardiac failure (wet beriberi) are the typical features. Thiamine deficiency results in the accumulation of lactate and pyruvate which reduce peripheral vascular resistance, increase venous return and in the early stage cardiac output is high. Congestive cardiac failure and a fall in cardiac output develop later. Parenteral and oral thiamine may produce rapid resolution of the cardiac and neurological abnormalities.

Kwashiorkor

Protein energy malnutrition may result in cardiac dilatation and severe congestive cardiac failure with pulmonary and systemic emboli. Arrhythmias and heart block accompany atrophy of the conducting system. Dietary correction and rest are required.

Glycogen storage disease

Absence of the enzyme alpha-glucosidase is an autosomal recessive disorder resulting in the accumulation of normal glycogen in cardiac and skeletal muscle. Specific heart muscle disease is most characteristic of type II glycogenesis (Pompe's disease) and resembles hypertrophic cardiomyopathy with massive thickening of the left ventricular myocardium. There is no treatment and death is usual in the first year of life.

Collagen vascular disease

The heart is involved in a variety of collagen vascular disease. The findings are summarised in Table 4.9.

Amyloidosis

Amyloid is an abnormal fibrillar protein which may be found in almost any organ. The main protein types are composed of immunoglobulin light chains (AL), non-immunoglobulin protein (AA) and a unique type found in senile cardiac amyloid (ASc_1).

The main clinical forms are summarised in Table 4.10. Amyloidosis is not clinically apparent unless there is extensive disease. Cardiac amyloidosis is a disease of the elderly and usually presents with heart failure. Macroglossia occurs in one-quarter of immunocyte-related amyloidosis. Signs include a small volume pulse, low blood pressure and raised jugular venous pressure. The following are useful investigations:

(i) *ECG*: low voltage tracing, conduction disturbances.
(ii) *Two-dimensional echocardiography*: small and immobile ventricles, thick right ventricular wall, characteristic 'glittering' echoes from the myocardium.
(iii) *Cardiac catheter*: diastolic pressures are unequally increased in both ventricles, higher in the left ventricle than the right.
(iv) *Endomyocardial biopsy*: electron microscopy is most specific for amyloid detection.

Colchicine is effective in familial Mediterranean fever, but no specific treatment exists in other forms of amyloidosis.

Table 4.10
MAJOR CLINICAL TYPES OF AMYLOIDOSIS

Type	*Major protein*	*Usual site of deposition*	*Cardiac involvement*
Primary and immunocyte dyscrasia (for example, myeloma)	AL	Systemic, especially heart and tongue, or organ specific	Very common
Secondary (chronic infection, inflammation, malignancy)	AA	Systemic	Unusual
Familial, including Mediterranean fever	Various	Heart or nerve or kidney	Common
Senile	ASc_1	Heart	Very common

Table 4.11

CARDIAC ABNORMALITIES IN HEREDOFAMILIAL NEUROMYOPATHIC DISORDERS

	Duchenne muscular dystrophy	*Dystrophia myotonica*	*Friedreich's ataxia*
Definition	Primary degenerative myopathy	Systemic disorder including myotonia, facial myopathy, cataracts, frontal balding, gonadal atrophy, dementia	Progressive spinocerebellar degeneration
Inheritance	X-linked recessive	Autosomal dominant	Autosomal recessive
Frequency of cardiac involvement	Half	Three-quarters	Half
Clinical features	Progressive heart failure; sudden death	Progressive heart failure; Stoke–Adams attacks; sudden death	Arrhythmias, angina pectoris, congestive heart failure, sudden death
ECG	Sinus tachycardia, tall R waves in right chest leads and deep Q waves in left are specific. Also found in unaffected female carriers	Sinus bradycardia, tachy-brady syndrome, atrioventricular and bundle branch blocks	Sinus tachycardia LV hypertrophy S–T/T wave changes
Pathology	Posterobasal scarring of left ventricle may correlate with specific ECG abnormality. Medial hypertrophy at intramural coronary arteries	Often normal. Specialised conducting system may be specifically affected	Left ventricular hypertrophy Intimal proliferation of coronary arteries

Sarcoidosis

Sarcoidosis is a systemic granulomatous disease which may affect the heart. Myocardial sarcoidosis occurs in about 20% of cases studied at autopsy, but is clinically apparent only when massive infiltration has occurred. It presents with ventricular arrhythmias, atrioventricular conduction defects, congestive cardiac failure and sudden death. The condition is underdiagnosed partly because patients with infiltration of the heart extensive enough to cause cardiac dysfunction rarely have evidence of dysfunction of another organ system. The presence of characteristic non-caseating epithelial cell granulomas in lymph node and myocardial biopsies substantiates the diagnosis. Sudden death is the commonest mode of death in patients with cardiac dysfunction, and may affect young adults. Corticosteroid therapy causes healing of myocardial sarcoid granulomas and replacement by fibrous tissue, but whether steroids alter the natural history of myocardial sarcoidosis remains uncertain.

Neurological and Neuromuscular Disorders

Cardiac abnormalities are an important cause of death in three heredofamilial myopathic, myotonic and neurological conditions: Duchenne's progressive muscular dystrophy, dystrophia myotonica, and Friedreich's ataxia. The principal features are summarised in Table 4.11.

FURTHER READING

Benotti J.R., Grossman W., Cohn P.F. (1980). The clinical profile of restrictive cardiomyopathy. *Circulation*; **61**, 1206.

Demakis, J.G., Rahimtoola, S.H. (1971). Peripartum cardiomyopathy. *Circulation*; **44,** 964.

Editorial (1986). Natural history of dilated cardiomyopathy. *Lancet*; **i**, 248.

Fleming H.A. (1974). Sarcoid heart disease. *Br Heart J*; **36**, 54.

Goodwin J.F. (1985). Mechanisms in cardiomyopathies. *J Mol Cell Cardiol*; **17**, 5.

Goodwiun J. E. and Oakley C.M. (1972). The cardiomyopathies. *Br Heart J*; **34**, 545.

Olsen E.G.J. (1985). The problem of viral heart disease. How often do we miss it? *Post grad Med J*; **61**, 479.

Report of the WHO/ISFC Task Force on the Definition and Classification of Cardiomyopathies (1980). *Br Heart J*; **44**, 672.

Unverferth (1985). Etiologic factors, pathogenesis and prognosis of dilated cardiomyopathy. *J Lab Clin Med* **106**, 349.

Wigle E.D., Sasson Z., Henderson M.A., Ruddy T.D., Fullop J., Rakowski H., Williams W.G. (1985). Hypertrophic cardiomyopathy. The importance of the site and extent of hypertrophy. *Prog Cardiovasc Dis*; **28**, 1.

Chapter Five

Congenital Heart Disease

Definition

Congenital heart disease has been defined as an abnormality of cardiocirculatory structure or function existing at birth.

Background

It is widely quoted that six to eight in every 1000 children born alive has a cardiovascular malformation. This is an underestimate of the total incidence because it fails to include the two commonest structural abnormalities.

(i) Congenital non-stenotic bicuspid aortic valve.
(ii) The valve leaflet abnormality of mitral valve prolapse, and the frequent occurrence of
(iii) Patent ductus arteriosus in preterm births.
(iv) Congenital heart disease in stillbirths.

Extracardiac anomalies are present in 25% of infants with significant congenital heart disease. These anomalies are often multiple and increase mortality. The highest mortality occurs in the neonatal period but survival after 1 year of age carries a fairly good prognosis. Reasons for increased longevity include improved invasive and non-invasive diagnosis, improved anaesthesia, advances in interventional catheter techniques and surgical management, and a clearer understanding of cardiac anatomy. About three per 1000 babies undergo surgery for congenital heart disease in the first year of life, 50% presenting within the first 4 weeks. Patients with congenital heart disease are increasingly encountered in adolescent or adult life as the natural survivors of mild or compensated lesions, or more commonly as the surgical survivors of palliative or 'corrective' procedures.

Incidence

Table 5.1 shows the incidence of congenital cardiac defects. Ventricular septal defect is the commonest clinically apparent abnormality. Bicuspid aortic valve is the commonest anomaly found at autopsy. Eight lesions make up 80% of cases. The remaining 20% include complex and rare abnormalities.

Table 5.1

FREQUENCY OF CONGENITAL HEART DEFECTS

	Per 1000 live births	*Percentage*
Ventricular septal defect	2·0	30
Atrial septal defect	0·7	10
Patent ductus arteriosus	0·7	10
Pulmonary stenosis	0·5	7
Coarctation of the aorta	0·5	7
Aortic stenosis	0·4	6
Tetralogy of Fallot	0·4	6
Transposition of the great arteries	0·3	4
Other	1·5	20
Total	7	100

The overall sex incidence of congenital heart disease is equal but some lesions show a preponderance:

(i) Commoner in males:
  (a) aortic valvular stenosis;
  (b) coarctation of the aorta;
  (c) tetralogy of Fallot.

(ii) Commoner in females:
  (a) atrial septal defect;
  (b) patent ductus arteriosus.

Aetiology

No cause is known for the great majority of congenital cardiovascular abnormalities, which fall into one of three groups;

Table 5.2
ENVIRONMENTAL CAUSES OF CONGENITAL HEART DISEASE

Syndrome	Major clinical features Cardiac	Non-cardiac
Rubella	Patent ductus arteriosus Pulmonary valve stenosis Pulmonary artery stenosis Atrial septal defect	Deafness Cataracts Microcephaly
Alcohol	Ventricular septal defect	Microcephaly Micrognathia Microphthalmia Low birth weight
Thalidomide	Various	Limb deformities
Maternal lupus erythematosus and phenylketonuria	Congenital complete heart block	
Maternal insulin-dependent diabetes	Various	

(i) *Multifactorial disorders*: 90% of lesions are of unknown cause and probably result from the interaction of several genetic and environmental factors. Table 5.2 shows the environmental factors recognised to disturb normal cardiovascular development.

(ii) *Single gene disorders*: eight lesions are known to be caused by single gene mutations, accounting for only 5% of all congenital heart disease (Table 5.3). Transmission is by mendelian inheritance. The gene mutation disrupts the function of a single protein essential for normal development of the heart and other involved systems.

(iii) *Chromosomal disorders*: chromosomal disorders account for about 5% of cases of congenital heart disease. The two commonest disorders are Down's syndrome (trisomy 21) and Turner's syndrome (XO) (Table 5.4). Much rarer are trisomy 13, trisomy 18 and cri-du-chat syndrome (short arm deletion of chromosome 5) in which ventricular septal defect is the usual cardiac anomaly.

Table 5.3

SINGLE GENE DISORDERS IN CONGENITAL HEART DISEASE

		Major clinical features	
Syndrome	*Transmission*	*Cardiac*	*Non-cardiac*
Noonan	Autosomal dominant	PS ASD HOCM	Short stature Webbed neck Skeletal, genitourinary abnormalities
LEOPARD	Autosomal dominant	*L*entigines, *E*CG conduction defects, *O*cular hypertelorism, *P*ulmonary valve stenosis, *A*bnormal genitals, *R*etardation of growth, *D*eafness	
Kartagener	Autosomal recessive	Situs inversus with dextrocardia	Sinusitis Bronchiectasis

Holt–Oram	Autosomal dominant	ASD Heart block	Upper limb deformities
Familial ASD with prolonged atrioventricular conduction	Autosomal dominant	Syndrome as named	None
Ellis–Van Creveld	Autosomal recessive	Single atrium Various	Small stature Bilateral polydactyly Shortened extremities
Familial supravalvar aortic stenosis	Autosomal dominant	Pulmonary and systemic arterial stenoses	*Normal* facies and mental development (see fetal hypercalcaemia syndrome)
Familial primary pulmonary hypertension	Autosomal dominant	Abnormal small pulmonary vasculature	None

PS = pulmonary stenosis ASD = atrial septal defect HOCM = hypertrophic cardiomyopathy

Table 5.4

CHROMOSOMAL DISORDERS IN CONGENITAL HEART DISEASE

Syndrome	*Major clinical features* Cardiac	Non-cardiac
Down's (trisomy 21)	Endocardial cushion defect, ASD, VSD, tetralogy of Fallot	Mongol faces, mental retardation, hyperextensile joints, hypotonia
Turner's (XO)	Coarctation of the aorta	Female, short stature, webbed neck

ASD = atrial septal defect VSD = ventricular septal defect

INHERITANCE AND RECURRENCE RISK

Genetic counselling of a family in which congenital heart disease has occurred requires knowledge of the mode of inheritance and recurrence risk of the condition (the risk of transmitting the condition to future offspring).

Multifactorial Disorders

Most common congenital heart disorders for which there is no known cause may run in families. A polygenic hypothesis of inheritance, determined by a number of genes of small effect, has been supported by family studies. For the common congenital lesions (see Table 5.1) 2·5–5·0% of siblings or offspring of an affected parent also have heart defects, a two- to five-fold increase in risk. The defect may be the same or similar within families. Since the recurrence risk is low if one parent is free of congenital heart disease such families are rarely discouraged from having further children.

Single Gene Disorders

Single gene disorders (see Table 5.3) are transmitted by mendelian inheritance. The principal features of autosomal dominant and recessive disorders are summarised in Table 5.5. The gene

Table 5.5
CHARACTERISTICS OF AUTOSOMAL INHERITANCE

	Dominant	*Recessive*
Clinical expression	Heterozygotes	Homozygotes only
Sexes affected	Both equally	Both equally
Parents	One affected*	Clinically normal
Offspring	Normal and affected offspring in equal proportions (one in two recurrence risk)	Offspring unaffected; only siblings are affected

*Unless the disorder arose as a new mutation.

responsible for an autosomal disorder is located on one of the 22 autosomes.

Chromosomal Disorders

Chromosomal disorders are present in 0.5% of live births (one in 200). Most occur as new mutations so the recurrence risk is low. The commonest chromosomal defect causing heart disease is trisomy 21 (Down's syndrome, mongolism); it occurs in one in 600 neonates half of whom have congenital heart defects. Maternal age is the main risk factor increasing from one in 1200 between 20 and 29 years to one in 80 between 40 and 44 years. If a couple has had one offspring with Down's syndrome the recurrence risk is 2% (one in 50) irrespective of maternal age.

CLASSIFICATION OF CONGENITAL HEART DISEASE

A preoccupation with conflicting classifications has long dogged the history and confused the student of congenital heart disease. Three commonly used systems are:

(i) Functional
  (a) communications between systemic and pulmonary circulations, for example, ASD, VSD, patent ductus arteriosus;

(b) obstructive lesions, for example, aortic stenosis, aortic coarctation, pulmonary stenosis;
(c) displacement of structures, for example, transposition of the great vessels, dextrocardia.

(ii) Anatomical: sequential chamber analysis (see Further reading section, p. 160).
(iii) Clinical: this is shown in Table 5.6.

The morphological description of simple and complex malformations by sequential chamber analysis has clarified scientific communication by its logic and consistency, but may be difficult for the student at the bedside. The definition of congenital lesions as discrete entities becomes inadequate when describing the rarer complex malformations. Functional classifications are flawed if

Table 5.6
CLASSIFICATION OF CONGENITAL HEART DISEASE

Acyanotic
Normal pulmonary blood flow
  Pulmonary stenosis
  Bicuspid aortic valve
  Coarctation of the aorta
  Heart muscle/endocardial diseases

Increased pulmonary blood flow
  Ventricular septal defect
  Atrial septal defect
  Patent ductus arteriosus
  Anomalous pulmonary venous drainage

Cyanotic
Decreased pulmonary blood flow
  Tetralogy of Fallot
  Pulmonary stenosis with VSD
  Pulmonary atresia with VSD
  Tricuspid atresia
  Ebstein's anomaly

Increased pulmonary blood flow
  Transposition of the great vessels
  Common mixing situations (common atrium, univentricular hearts, truncus arteriosus)

the dynamic nature of congenital heart lesions is forgotten: a subtle abnormality at birth may be clinically obvious later in life; a ventricular septal defect may close spontaneously; the development of pulmonary arterial hypertension may convert an acyanotic lesion with increased pulmonary blood flow to a cyanotic lesion with reduced pulmonary blood flow. No classification is perfect. The scheme favoured for the purposes of this book is shown in Table 5.6. It has the virtue of simplicity and easy clinical use. Congenital heart lesions are divided into acyanotic and cyanotic categories, then subdivided according to pulmonary blood flow. Prudent use of the scheme with the chest X-ray, electrocardiogram and echocardiogram provides a useful framework for clinical diagnosis.

CLINICAL APPLICATION

Cyanosis

Central cyanosis occurs when the concentration of reduced haemoglobin in the circulation is more than 5 g/dl. The clinical detection of cyanosis depends on both the haemoglobin concentration (g/dl) and the oxygen saturation (%). Central cyanosis in congenital heart disease is caused by the entry of venous blood into the systemic circulation without passing through the lungs (intracardiac or extracardiac right-to-left shunt). Blood passing through the lungs is fully oxygenated so inhalation of 100% oxygen will not improve the patient's colour. If central cyanosis is due to pulmonary disease the inhalation of oxygen will improve or abolish cyanosis.

Differential cyanosis is present when the upper part of the body is pink and the lower part of the body blue. It occurs most commonly in patients with patent ductus arteriosus and severe pulmonary arterial hypertension.

Pulmonary Blood Flow

The chest X-ray is used to decide whether blood flow through the lungs is normal, increased or reduced (Table 5.7).

Table 5.7

PULMONARY PLETHORA AND OLIGAEMIA

	X-ray sign	*Explanation of sign*
Increased pulmonary blood flow (pulmonary plethora)	Increased pulmonary vascular markings	Acyanotic lesions: left-to-right shunt Cyanotic lesions: transposition of great vessels; common mixing situations
Decreased pulmonary blood flow (pulmonary oligaemia)	Decreased pulmonary vascular markings	Obstruction to pulmonary blood flow *plus* a defect allowing right-to-left shunt

ACYANOTIC LESIONS WITH NORMAL PULMONARY BLOOD FLOW

Pulmonary Stenosis

Background

Pulmonary stenosis may occur at several levels.

(i) *Valvar*: a common defect in which the pulmonary valve is 'domed' with a central orifice and fused commissures; obstruction may be mild to critical.
(ii) *Infundibular*: isolated stenosis is rare; secondary pulmonary infundibular stenosis is common as part of right ventricular hypertrophy.
(iii) *Supravalvar*: rare, associated with hypercalcaemia in infancy; peripheral pulmonary artery stenosis is associated with maternal rubella and thalidomide ingestion.

Symptoms

Mild or moderate pulmonary stenosis is asymptomatic. Effort breathlessness, angina pectoris and heart failure may accompany severe stenosis.

Physical signs

These are summarised in Table 5.8.

Table 5.8
PHYSICAL SIGNS OF PULMONARY STENOSIS

Sign	*Explanation of sign*
Large 'a' wave in jugular venous pressure	Right atrium empties into a hypertrophied right ventricle
Parasternal heave	Right ventricular hypertrophy
Soft, delayed second heart sound	Prolonged right ventricular systole
Loud, harsh midsystolic murmur in second left interspace	Long murmur with a late peak correlates with severity of stenosis; ejection click precedes murmur if cusps are mobile
Cyanosis	Seen late in severe stenosis; right atrial pressure rises allowing right-to-left shunting across a patent foramen ovale

Investigations

(i) *Chest X-ray*: the heart size is usually normal, pulmonary vascular markings are normal, not reduced; poststenotic dilatation of the pulmonary artery is marked.

(ii) *ECG*: right ventricular hypertrophy is present, the height of R waves in leads V_1 and V_4R being proportional to the severity of stenosis. Precordial T-wave inversion indicates severe hypertrophy. Right atrial enlargement is common.

(iii) *M-mode echocardiogram*: the pulmonary valve echogram has an exaggerated 'a' wave. Atrial contraction may open the pulmonary valve just before the onset of ventricular systole.

(iv) *Cardiac catheter*: right ventricular pressure is increased and pulmonary artery pressure is normal or low. The pressure gradient is proportional to the severity of stenosis. Right ventricular angiography defines the anatomy of the lesion.

Treatment

If the pressure gradient exceeds 60 mmHg the stenosis is relieved by surgical valvotomy. Percutaneous balloon valvuloplasty is an effective and increasingly popular alternative.

Aortic Stenosis

Aortic stenosis is discussed in Chapter 8. Congenital aortic stenosis may occur in three sites.

(i) *Valvar*: the commonest congenital cardiac anomaly, a *bicuspid aortic valve* occurs in about 1% of the population. It is usually non-stenotic but mild, moderate or severe obstruction may be present. A bicuspid valve is the usual substrate of isolated calcific aortic stenosis in adult life.

(ii) *Subvalvar*: in *discrete subvalvar aortic stenosis* a fibromuscular diaphragm obstructs the left ventricular outflow tract and involves the anteroseptal leaflet of the mitral valve. Less frequently there is a tubular stenosis of the subvalvar region.

(iii) *Supravalvar*: *supravalvar aortic stenosis* may be associated with a syndrome of 'elfin' facies, pulmonary arterial stenosis, hypercalcaemia and mental retardation.

Coarctation of the Aorta

See Hypertension, Chapter 12, page 340.

Heart Muscle Disease

See specific heart muscle disease, Chapter 4.

ACYANOTIC LESIONS WITH INCREASED PULMONARY BLOOD FLOW

Ventricular Septal Defect (VSD)

Background

Isolated VSD is the commonest congenital cardiac lesion seen in childhood after bicuspid aortic valve; 70% of defects subsequently undergo spontaneous closure. Defects in the membranous part of the interventricular septum are commonest but occur also in the muscular and subarterial sites. Muscular defects may be multiple. When the membranous septum is defective the aorta may override the right ventricle by up to 50% of its orifice area, and aortic regurgitation may result from prolapse of an inadequately supported right coronary cusp.

Pathophysiology

Small VSDs restrict flow from the high pressure left ventricle to the low pressure right ventricle allowing only a small increase in pulmonary flow. Larger defects are progressively less restrictive allowing a pulmonary blood flow which is up to five times systemic flow, and pulmonary artery pressure may increase to systemic levels. Severe pulmonary arterial hypertension may result in shunt reversal and cyanosis (Eisenmenger's syndrome). This usually results from progressive pulmonary vascular disease secondary to high pulmonary blood flow but may rarely occur if the high pulmonary vascular resistance at birth fails to fall.

Clinical features

The symptoms and signs of VSD depend on its size. The clinical features are summarised in Table 5.9.

Investigations

Echocardiography

In small defects the echocardiogram is normal. Large defects may be visualised directly. Left atrial and biventricular dilatation occurs if the left-to-right shunt is large. Flow across the defect is detected by Doppler echocardiography and may be visualised by Doppler colour-flow imaging which is particularly useful in small or multiple lesions.

Cardiac catheterisation

Intracardiac pressures are normal in small defects. Larger defects result in elevated right ventricular pressure, and very large defects

Table 5.9

CLINICAL FEATURES OF VENTRICULAR SEPTAL DEFECT

	Small VSD (Maladie de Roger)	*Large VSD*
Symptoms	None	Heart failure and failure to thrive in infancy
Signs		
Precordial heave	Absent	Present due to biventricular hypertrophy
Second heart sound	Normal	Split
Murmur	Loud, pansystolic, thrill at left sternal edge	Same, *plus* S3 and mitral diastolic rumble due to high volume flow
Cyanosis	Never	May occur if pulmonary arterial hypertension develops
ECG	Normal	Left or biventricular hypertrophy; right atrial hypertrophy; right bundle branch block
Chest X-ray	Normal	Biventricular enlargement; increased pulmonary vascular markings

S3 = third heart sound

allow equalisation of right and left ventricular pressures. The left-to-right shunt causes a stepup in oxygen saturation at ventricular level. If pulmonary arterial hypertension has developed mixed shunting with systemic oxygen desaturation occurs. Angiography shows the site and number of defects.

Treatment

Small defects require no treatment. Large symptomatic defects are closed surgically in infancy. Surgery is not indicated when severe pulmonary hypertension and mixed shunting has developed. Antibiotic prophylaxis against infective endocarditis is mandatory for any surgical procedure whatever the size of the defect.

Atrial Septal Defect (ASD)

Background

ASD is the commonest congenital heart lesion encountered in adults after bicuspid aortic valve. Lesions are classified according to their anatomy.

(i) *Ostium secundum ASD* (90%): a defect in the floor of the fossa ovalis.

(ii) *Ostium primum ASD*: a *partial atrioventricular canal defect* due to defective fusion of the septum primum and endocardial cushions allowing communication between right and left atrium. There is usually a cleft in the mitral valve. When the upper part of the interventricular septum is also deficient a *complete atrioventricular canal defect* (complete endocardial cushion defect) is present allowing communication between all four cardiac chambers.

(iii) *Sinus venosus defect*: a defect high on the atrial septum adjacent to the orifice of the superior vena cava, associated with partial anomalous drainage of the right lung into the vena cava.

ASD is usually isolated but is not uncommonly associated with pulmonary stenosis, VSD or anomalous pulmonary venous drainage. ASD may be essential to survival in some lesions, for example, tricuspid atresia, complete transposition of the great vessels. This section describes only isolated ASD.

Pathophysiology

Pressures in the right and left atria are equal. Blood flows from left atrium to right atrium because of the greater compliance (easier distensibility) of the thinner-walled right ventricle. Pulmonary blood flow commonly exceeds systemic flow by up to five times, yet pulmonary artery pressure is little raised because pulmonary vascular resistance falls. Rarely pulmonary vascular resistance rises leading eventually to shunt reversal and cyanosis (Eisenmenger's syndrome).

Symptoms

ASD is usually asymptomatic and is discovered on routine examination. Effort breathlessness, paroxysmal atrial tachyarrhythmias or atrial fibrillation may develop in adult life, especially if mitral regurgitation complicates an ostium primum defect.

Physical signs

These are shown in Table 5.10.

Table 5.10
PHYSICAL SIGNS OF ATRIAL SEPTAL DEFECT

Sign	*Explanation of sign*
'v' wave > 'a' wave in jugular venous pressure (reversal of normal)	Maximum left-to-right shunting during late ventricular systole and early diastole
Parasternal impulse	Large shunts, due to right ventricular dilatation
Second heart sound widely split; 'fixed' on respiration	Prolonged right ventricular systole delays pulmonary valve closure; ASD equilibrates effect of respiratory pressure variations
Pulmonary midsystolic murmur	High flow across pulmonary valve
Tricuspid mid-diastolic rumble	Large shunts; high flow across tricuspid valve
Apical pansystolic murmur	Ostium primum defects. Mitral regurgitation due to cleft mitral valve

Investigations

(i) *Chest X-ray*: depending on shunt size the right atrium, right ventricle and pulmonary artery shadows are enlarged. The lung fields show increased vascular markings.

(ii) *ECG*: right bundle branch block is almost invariable. The frontal plane QRS axis is helpful in distinguishing several lesions characterised by the physical signs of atrial septal defect (Table 5.11).

(iii) *Echocardiogram*: with large left to right shunts M-mode echocardiography indicates right ventricular volume overload—increased right ventricular diastolic dimension and reversed septal motion. On two-dimensional imaging in the 'four-chamber' view the atrial septal defect may be directly visualised. Flow across the defect is visualised by Doppler colour flow imaging.

(iv) *Cardiac catheterisation*: a stepup in oxygen saturation is present at atrial level. The catheter passes easily across the defect to the left atrium. Left ventricular angiography is normal in ostium secundum defects. In primum defects the abnormal mitral valve position elongates the left ventricular outflow tract causing a characteristic 'gooseneck' deformity on left ventricular angiography. Regurgitation through the cleft mitral valve may also be seen.

Table 5.11

SIGNS OF ATRIAL SEPTAL DEFECT (ASD) RELATED TO ECG AND CYANOSIS

ECG	*Acyanotic*	*Cyanotic*
Right axis deviation	Secundum ASD	Total anomalous pulmonary venous drainage
Left axis deviation	Primum ASD	Common atrium

Treatment

If the shunt is significant (pulmonary: systemic flow ratio = 2:1 or more) an ostium secundum or sinus venosus defect is closed by direct suture or a patch. Operative mortality is about 1%. Surgical correction of ostium primum lesions is more difficult depending on the extent of the endocardial cushion defect. Patch closure of the defect and mitral valve repair are often complicated by traumatic complete heart block owing to the proximity of conducting tissue. Operative mortality may reach 5%.

Patent Ductus Arteriosus

Background

In the normal fetus the ductus arteriosus, part of the sixth aortic arch, connects the junction of the main and left pulmonary arteries to the descending aorta just distal to the origin of the left subclavian artery. The main bulk of right ventricular output passes through the ductus arteriosus, bypassing the high resistance pulmonary circulation, and down the descending aorta to be reoxygenated in the placenta. At birth there is a sudden fall in pulmonary vascular resistance and a rise in systemic vascular resistance. The ductus arteriosus begins to constrict under the influence of increased oxygen saturation and vasoactive substances—possibly the inhibition of prostaglandin synthesis. In the full-term fetus ductal closure is complete by 1 week, with permanent obliteration by subsequent fibrosis. Closure is often delayed in premature neonates in whom higher circulating levels of prostaglandin are found, in rubella syndrome babies and in those born at high altitude. Patent ductus arteriosus is commoner in females.

Pathophysiology

The normal postnatal changes in vascular resistance allow a left-to-right shunt through a patent ductus arteriosus. The magnitude of the shunt then depends on the size of the ductus which usually is partly constricted or, more rarely, widely patent.

Clinical features

These depend on the size of the left-to-right shunt (Table 5.12).

Table 5.12

CLINICAL FEATURES OF PATENT DUCTUS ARTERIOSUS

	Small shunt	*Large shunt*
Symptoms	None	Heart failure, especially in premature infants. Failure to thrive. Respiratory infections
Signs		
Pulse volume	Normal	Bounding, wide pulse pressure
Murmur	Continuous or 'machinery' murmur at upper left sternal edge	
ECG	Normal	Left ventricular hypertrophy
Chest X-ray	Normal	Left atrial and left ventricular enlargement
Cardiac catheter	Catheter passes from pulmonary artery to aorta through ductus. Oxygen saturation stepup in pulmonary artery indicates presence and magnitude of left-to-right shunt	

Natural history

Most patients with a large shunt are detected and treated in infancy. Those surviving into childhood and adult life with a large shunt are prone to heart failure, infective endocarditis (endarteritis) in the ductus, and progressive pulmonary arterial hypertension. The latter may result in shunt reversal (Eisenmenger's syndrome) with differential cyanosis.

Differential diagnosis

Patent ductus arteriosus is the commonest cause of a continuous parasternal murmur in an acyanotic child, but rarer lesions need consideration (Table 5.13). Most are confirmed by angiography.

Treatment

Surgical ligation or division of any isolated patent ductus arterio-

Table 5.13

DIFFERENTIAL DIAGNOSIS OF A CONTINUOUS MURMUR IN AN ACYANOTIC CHILD

Lesion	*Cause of murmur*
Patent ductus arteriosus	Communication between aorta and pulmonary artery via ductus
VSD plus aortic regurgitation	Aortic cusp prolapse
Ruptured sinus of Valsalva	Sinus of Valsalva aneurysm ruptures into right atrium or ventricle
Aortopulmonary window	Direct communication between ascending aorta and main pulmonary artery
Coronary arteriovenous fistula	Fistula between coronary artery and right side of heart
Congenital pulmonary incompetence	Congenital absence of pulmonary valve
Aorto-left ventricular tunnel	Sinus of Valsalva to left ventricle communication

sus is indicated to prevent infective endocarditis and the development of pulmonary vascular disease. Prior cardiac catheterisation is preferable to exclude existing pulmonary arterial hypertension with right-to-left shunting, or the presence of additional congenital lesions. In some infants pharmacological closure may be achieved using prostaglandin synthetase inhibitors (aspirin, indomethacin).

CYANOTIC LESIONS WITH DECREASED PULMONARY BLOOD FLOW

Fallot's Tetralogy

Background

This is the most common congenital heart lesion causing cyanosis after 1 year of age. The four components are:

(i) Ventricular septal defect (VSD).
(ii) Right ventricular outflow tract (RVOT) obstruction due to pulmonary infundibular stenosis.
(iii) Overriding of the interventricular septum by the aorta.
(iv) Right ventricular hypertrophy.

The primary abnormality is an anterior deviation of the infundibular septum which divides the aortic and pulmonary trunks. The anatomical consequence of this anterior deviation is to produce a VSD, an overriding aorta and infundibular stenosis. Right ventricular hypertrophy develops in response to increased pressure work.

The degree of anterior deviation of the infundibular septum is of fundamental importance. The more anterior the deviation the larger is the size of the aorta at the expense of the pulmonary artery, and the greater is the RVOT obstruction. Extreme anterior deviation causes pulmonary atresia with a VSD, in which the right ventricle is blind-ended. The severity of RVOT obstruction also depends on hypertrophy of the infundibular walls. Initially mild RVOT obstruction often becomes increasingly severe as hypertrophy progresses. One-quarter of patients have additional pulmonary valvar stenosis.

The VSD is large and non-restrictive to blood flow; it is high on the septum just below the aortic valve. The aorta straddles or overrides the VSD to a varying degree. When the override exceeds one-half the aortic diameter the condition is defined as double outlet right ventricle.

Clinical features

The severity of the RVOT obstruction determines the size of the right-to-left shunt through the VSD and hence the clinical presentation (Table 5.14). Exercise increases the degree of cyanosis and children often 'squat' to decrease the right-to-left shunt. Cyanotic 'spells' of extreme right-to-left shunting are due to pulmonary infundibular spasm and may be fatal. They are relieved by propranolol, oxygen administration and correction of acidosis.

Investigations

(i) *Chest X-ray*: the heart is of normal size and 'boot'-shaped

Table 5.14

CLINICAL FEATURES OF FALLOT'S TETRALOGY

	Severe RVOT obstruction	*Mild RVOT obstruction*
Symptoms	Dyspnoea	Often asymptomatic with systolic murmur
	Squatting Cyanotic 'spells'	Heart failure by age 3 months due to large left-to-right shunt via VSD 'Spells' may occur
Signs	Cyanosis at rest before age 1 year	Acyanotic initially but few remain so
	Finger-clubbing	Soft, late pulmonary second sound
	Right ventricular heave Single (aortic) second heart sound	Loud midsystolic murmur (loudness inversely proportional to severity of RVOT obstruction)
	Midsystolic murmur in 2nd, 3rd left interspace	
	Aortic ejection click (large diameter aorta)	

due to right ventricular hypertrophy and a small pulmonary artery. The lung fields are oligaemic. The aortic arch is right-sided in 25% of patients.

(ii) *ECG*: when RVOT obstruction is mild there is biventricular hypertrophy at first progressing to right ventricular hypertrophy as the obstruction increases.

(iii) *Echocardiogram*: discontinuity between the aorta and the interventricular septum and a large aortic root are present.

(iv) *Cardiac catheterisation*: oxygen saturation is normal in the left atrium and reduced in the left ventricle and aorta. Left and right ventricular pressures are equal (systemic level) while pulmonary artery pressure beyond the obstruction is low. Cineangiography using 'situp' views demonstrates the anatomy of the RVOT and pulmonary arteries.

Treatment

Surgical management may be palliative or corrective. 'Total correction' is now ultimately performed in almost all cases.

Palliative

These procedures reduce hypoxaemia and increase pulmonary blood flow. This may encourage development of the pulmonary artery and left heart chambers prior to eventual corrective surgery. Palliation is indicated for severe cyanosis in the early months of life, and involves the creation of a surgical systemic–pulmonary anastomosis (Table 5.15). The most commonly constructed shunt is now the modified Blalock Taussig. Alternatively, the RVOT obstruction may be relieved leaving the VSD (Brock procedure).

Table 5.15
PALLIATIVE OPERATIONS FOR FALLOT'S TETRALOGY

Operation	*Shunt*
Blalock–Taussig	Right subclavian artery to right pulmonary artery
Modified Blalock–Taussig	As above, using a 'Gore-Tex' tube
Waterston	Direct anastomosis, back of aorta to front of right pulmonary artery
Potts	Direct aortopulmonary trunk anastomosis

Corrective

Total correction under cardiopulmonary bypass is indicated for children over 1 year of age, or in infancy as a primary procedure if the pulmonary arteries are well developed. The operation involves relief of RVOT obstruction and closure of the VSD. Overall operative mortality is about 10%.

Tricuspid Atresia

Anatomy

Anatomically described as 'univentricular heart with absent right atrioventricular connexion', tricuspid atresia is the commonest variety of univentricular heart. The essential features are:

(i) A normal or enlarged ventricle of left ventricular morphology with only a rudimentary right ventricle.
(ii) Absent tricuspid valve.

Most patients also have:

(iii) Pulmonary stenosis.
(iv) Normally related aorta and pulmonary artery.

Pathophysiology

Systemic venous return passes from the right atrium across an interatrial communication to the left atrium. Here it mixes with oxygenated blood from the lungs then passes on through the mitral valve into the ventricular chamber. Pulmonary stenosis frustrates the entry of blood into the pulmonary artery, increasing cyanosis. If pulmonary stenosis is mild or absent cyanosis may be clinically undetectable, but arterial desaturation is always present.

Clinical features

Most patients are cyanotic at birth and fail to thrive. The jugular venous pulse shows a large 'a' wave and there is a pulmonary midsystolic murmur. Clinical features vary greatly depending on the effective pulmonary blood flow and the presence of associated anomalies.

Investigations

(i) *ECG*: almost pathognomonic, this shows right atrial hypertrophy, left axis deviation and left ventricular hypertrophy.

(ii) *Chest X-ray*: the heart size is usually increased. Pulmonary vascular markings are decreased.

(iii) *Echocardiography*: demonstrates a large left ventricle, a diminutive or absent right ventricular chamber and absence of the tricuspid valve.

(iv) *Cardiac catheterisation*: oxygen saturations indicate a right-to-left shunt at atrial level. Angiography confirms the type of pulmonary stenosis and the relationship between the great vessels.

Treatment

Balloon atrial septostomy and palliative systemic–pulmonary surgical shunts improve symptoms and diminish cyanosis. 'Corrective' surgery involves connection of the right atrium to the pulmonary artery using a prosthetic conduit (Fontan procedure).

Ebstein's Anomaly

Anatomy

The tricuspid valve is displaced downwards into the right ventricle due to anomalous attachment of its leaflets. The part of the ventricle above the valve becomes part of the right atrium ('atrialised') which is thin-walled and often massively dilated. An atrial septal defect is usually present. The part of the ventricle below the valve is small but hypertrophied. The anatomy is subject to much variation and 20% of patients have coexistent cardiac anomalies.

Incidence

The malformation is rare, accounting for 1% of congenital heart disease.

Pathophysiology

The dilated, poorly contractile right atrium and the small subvalvar right ventricle result in reduced pulmonary blood flow. Raised right atrial pressure causes right-to-left shunting across a patent foramen ovale or atrial septal defect in 80% of patients. Tricuspid incompetence is usual.

Symptoms

Cyanosis, effort breathlessness or right heart failure occur. Adults with a mild version (forme fruste) of Ebstein's anomaly may be asymptomatic. Paroxysmal supraventricular tachycardia is common.

Signs

Cyanosis, low volume pulses, prominent 'a' or 'v' waves in the jugular venous pulse, a split first heart sound (delayed tricuspid valve closure) and a scratchy diastolic murmur are characteristic. If the tricuspid valve is incompetent a pansystolic murmur is present.

Investigations

(i) *Chest X-ray*: massive cardiomegaly and reduced pulmonary vascular markings are usual.

(ii) *ECG*: giant right atrial P waves, a long P–R interval and right bundle branch block occur frequently. A common alternative is type B Wolff–Parkinson–White syndrome, simulating the appearance of left bundle branch block.

(iii) *Echocardiography*: M-mode tracings show prominent tricuspid valve echoes and reversed septal motion; two-dimensional images demonstrate the abnormal position of the tricuspid valve and the dilated right atrium.

(iv) *Cardiac catheterisation*: pressure is raised in the right atrium but low in the right ventricle and pulmonary artery. Oxygen saturations indicate a right-to-left shunt. Characteristic recordings are obtained by withdrawing an electrode catheter from right ventricle to right atrium. Right ventricular electrograms arise from the 'atrialised' portion of the right ventricle while recording right atrial pressure waveforms. Further withdrawal to the true right atrium records atrial electrograms and atrial pressure waveforms together.

Treatment

Improved pulmonary blood flow can be achieved by closure of the atrial septal defect and repair or replacement of the incompetent tricuspid valve. The results are variable with a hospital mortality of up to 30%.

CYANOTIC LESIONS WITH INCREASED PULMONARY BLOOD FLOW

Transposition of the Great Arteries

Background

Sequential chamber analysis

The anatomy of many complex congenital cardiac malformations is best understood by sequential chamber analysis. This describes the position, morphology and connections of the heart chambers and great arteries. In the normal heart a right-sided right atrium connects with a morphologically right ventricle which in turn connects with a pulmonary artery, and a left-sided left atrium connects with a morphologically left ventricle and thence an aorta. Identification is made in practice using radiographic methods. If a plain chest X-ray shows that the liver is right-sided it can be inferred that the inferior vena cava and the right atrium are right-sided (situs solitus = usual position). If the liver is left-sided the right atrium will be left-sided (situs inversus). The morphology of the ventricle is decided by angiography. Thus, in the normal heart there is *situs solitus* of the atria with *concordant atrioventricular* and *ventriculoarterial connections.* If a morphologically right atrium connects with a morphologically left ventricle, or a left atrium with a right ventricle, there is *atrioventricular discordance.* Similarly, if a right ventricle connects with an aorta, or a left ventricle with a pulmonary artery there is *ventriculoarterial discordance.*

Anatomy of transposition of the great arteries (TGA)

This is summarised in Table 5.16. TGA is anatomically defined as ventriculoarterial discordance. TGA may be:

Table 5.16

ANATOMY OF TRANSPOSITION OF THE GREAT ARTERIES

	Physiologically complete transposition	*Physiologically corrected transposition*
Atrial situs	Solitus	Solitus
Atrioventricular connection	Concordant	Discordant
Ventriculoarterial connection	Discordant	Discordant
Course of the circulation	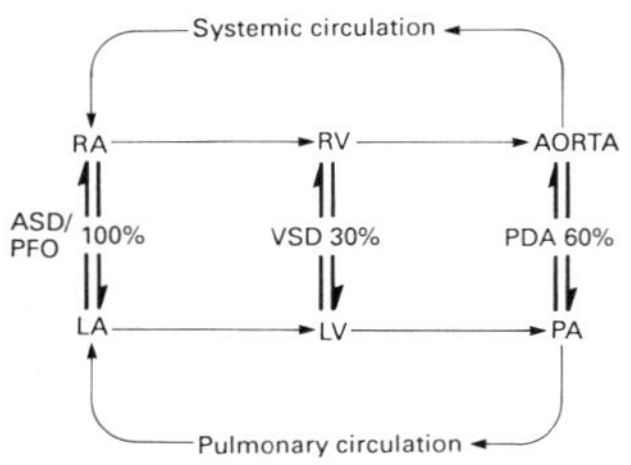 Systemic circulation; RA → RV → AORTA; ASD/PFO 100%; VSD 30%; PDA 60%; LA → LV → PA; Pulmonary circulation	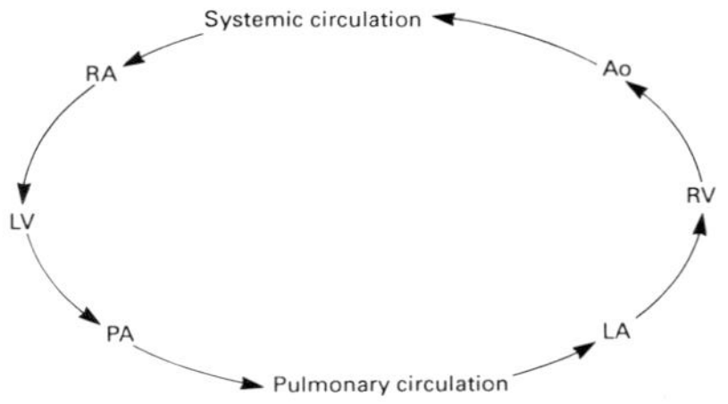 Systemic circulation → RA → LV → PA → Pulmonary circulation → LA → RV → Ao → Systemic circulation

RA = right atrium, RV = right ventricle, LA = left atrium, LV = left ventricle, PA = pulmonary artery
ASD = atrial septal defect, PFO = patent foramen ovale VSD = ventricular septal defect
PDA = patent ductus arteriosus. Percentages indicate the incidence of the communication between the systemic and pulmonary circulation

(i) *Physiologically complete*: systemic venous return passes to the aorta, and pulmonary venous return passes to the pulmonary artery. This results in two separate circulations. For survival there must be some communication between the circulations; this may occur at atrial or ventricular level, or through a patent ductus arteriosus. The shunt must be bidirectional or one circulation would drain the other, so the net volume exchange per unit time between the two circulations is equal. The magnitude of the shunt is affected by the number of communications and by the coexistence of other lesions, for example, pulmonary stenosis.

(ii) *Physiologically corrected*: 'correction' occurs because there is additional atrioventricular discordance. Systemic venous return passes to the lungs. Cyanosis or abnormal pulmonary blood flow are not features of corrected transposition.

Complete Transposition

Complete transposition of the great arteries is the commonest congenital heart lesion causing cyanosis in the newborn. Without treatment 30% of patients die in the first week, 50% in the first month and 90% in the first year of life.

Clinical features

Cyanosis is often marked and is the main presenting feature. If there is a large ventricular septal defect or patent ductus arteriosus congestive cardiac failure may predominate. Cyanosis may then be less easy to detect clinically but arterial oxygen desaturation, not reversed by giving 100% oxygen, will always be present.

Physical signs

Apart from cyanosis the physical signs are largely dependent on which associated lesions are present. Ventricular overload due to a large ventricular septal defect or patent ductus arteriosus will cause a prominent precordial heave and will be accompanied by the appropriate murmurs on auscultation.

Investigations

(i) *Chest X-ray*: the heart may have an 'egg-on-its-side' shape and the lung fields show increased vascular marking. Neither finding is invariable and the chest X-ray can be normal.

(ii) *ECG*: right ventricular hypertrophy and right axis deviation are usual. Biventricular hypertrophy accompanies a large shunt.

(iii) *Echocardiogram*: two-dimensional echocardiography demonstrates the abnormal relationship of the great arteries and may identify associated defects.

(iv) *Cardiac catheterisation*: the catheter passes from the right ventricle to the aorta. Pressure is higher in the right ventricle than the left ventricle. Oxygen saturations show bidirectional shunting at the level of the communication between the two circulations. The origins of the great arteries are displayed by angiography.

Treatment

Palliative

Palliative treatment at the time of cardiac catheterisation consists of passing an inflatable balloon catheter through the foramen ovale from the right to the left atrium. The balloon is jerked back tearing the atrial septum (Rashkind procedure) to allow increased shunting at atrial level.

Corrective

Corrective surgery aims at rerouting systemic and pulmonary venous return to the appropriate ventricle by making an intra-atrial baffle made of Dacron (Mustard's operation) or an atrial wall flap (Senning's operation). More recently a direct switch operation between the aorta and pulmonary artery has been used (Jatene operation) but surgical mortality can be high.

Corrected Transposition

Physiologically corrected transposition as an isolated anomaly causes no functional disturbance and is asymptomatic. Three clinical clues to its presence are:

(i) A loud single aortic second heart sound—the aorta lies anterior to the pulmonary artery.
(ii) A high incidence of complete atrioventricular block.
(iii) A high incidence of arrhythmias.

The commonest associated lesions are ventricular septal defect, pulmonary stenosis and tricuspid incompetence.

Double Outlet Right Ventricle (DORV)

By definition DORV is present when the pulmonary artery and more than half of the aorta arise from the right ventricle. It is usually associated with situs solitus and atrioventricular concordance. A ventricular septal defect is almost invariably present. Echocardiography and cardiac catheterisation are the most useful diagnostic procedures. Balloon septostomy provides early palliation. Total surgical correction involves the use of a baffle which directs blood from the left ventricle to the aorta.

SPECIAL SITUATIONS IN CONGENITAL HEART DISEASE

Chronic Cyanosis

Adolescents and adults with unrelieved cyanosis due to congenital heart disease may develop important extracardiac complications (Table 5.17). The most common lesion producing cyanosis in the adult population is Fallot's tetralogy. Other causes include Eisenmenger's syndrome and complex cyanotic congenital defects which have not been diagnosed in childhood. The incidence of the latter is low in developed communities.

Infective Endocarditis

Infective endocarditis may occur in association with many con-

Table 5.17

EXTRACARDIAC COMPLICATIONS OF CENTRAL CYANOSIS IN CONGENITAL HEART DISEASE

Complication	*Mechanism of complication*	*Management*
Clubbing of digits	Increased capillaries, connective tissue, and atrioventricular aneurysm formation in distal phalanges	Regression with correction of cyanotic lesion
Polycythaemia (Hb > 19 g/dl)	Chronic hypoxaemia	Venesection to Hb 17 g/dl Volume replacement, for example, dextran is mandatory
Cerebral thrombosis	Hypoxaemia	Heparin in acute stage. Consider antiplatelet agent long-term
Cerebral abscess	Hypoxaemia; infected embolism	Differentiate from thrombosis by brain scan; conventional management; often fatal
Haemoptysis	Pulmonary vascular obstruction Ruptured bronchial collateral vessels	Conservative. Correct clotting disorders Fresh blood transfusion
Gout	Increased red cell turnover Impaired renal function	Conventional for acute attack Allopurinol prophylaxis
Renal impairment	Polycythaemia, hypovolaemia X-ray contrast media	Volume replacement, 'loop' diuretics, dialysis
Impaired growth	Hypoxaemia, metabolic disorders	Correction of cyanotic lesion

genital cardiac lesions. Antibiotic prophylaxis to reduce the risk should always be considered. Table 5.18 shows lesions which present a high risk and those in which the risk is so low that antibiotic prophylaxis is unnecessary.

Table 5.18

RELATIVE RISK OF INFECTIVE ENDOCARDITIS IN CONGENITAL HEART DISEASE

High risk: antibiotic prophylaxis required	*Low risk: antibiotic prophylaxis not required*
Left-to-right shunts, uncorrected or residual after surgery	Pulmonary valve stenosis
Left-sided valvular heart disease	Surgically closed atrial or ventricular septal defect without coexisting left-sided lesion (for example, mitral or aortic valve disease)
Prosthetic valve or conduit implanted	Surgically closed ductus arteriosus
Fallot's tetralogy	

Eisenmenger's Syndrome

Definition

This is pulmonary hypertension at systemic level due to high pulmonary vascular resistance in which reversal of a left-to-right shunt has occurred across a pulmonary–systemic communication.

Eisenmenger's original description applied to patients with severe pulmonary hypertension and shunt reversal across a ventricular septal defect (Eisenmenger's complex). The definition was extended by Paul Wood to include shunts at any level—ventricular, great arterial or atrial.

Background

Elevated pulmonary artery pressure occurs in many congenital cardiac lesions as a result of increased pulmonary blood flow and/or resistance. Initially the increase in resistance may be due to increased vascular tone but progressive obliterative changes in the pulmonary vascular bed lead to fixed pulmonary arterial hypertension. Patients at high risk of developing Eisenmenger's syndrome early in life are those with a large ventricular septal defect, complete transposition of the great arteries, double outlet right ventricle and Down's syndrome. In atrial septal defect the syndrome tends to develop later in life.

Clinical features

The common *symptoms* are effort breathlessness, effort syncope, angina pectoris, haemoptysis which may be massive (pulmonary apoplexy) and fatal, right heart failure and arrhythmias. The physical *signs* of pulmonary hypertension are discussed in Chapter 8 (p. 217).

Management

Fixed pulmonary hypertension with a predominant right-to-left shunt contraindicates surgery for the underlying defect. Heart–lung transplantation is appropriate in some patients. Pregnancy is totally contraindicated. Major hazards are listed in Table 5.19.

Table 5.19
POTENTIALLY FATAL HAZARDS IN EISENMENGER'S SYNDROME

Pregnancy
General anaesthesia
Oral contraceptives
Minor surgery
Trauma
Haemorrhage
High altitude

PREGNANCY IN WOMEN WITH CONGENITAL HEART DISEASE

Maternal and fetal risk is low in most acyanotic lesions with normal pulmonary vascular resistance. Risks are increased by pulmonary arterial hypertension and pregnancy is completely contraindicated in Eisenmenger's syndrome. Congenital heart

Table 5.20

RISKS OF PREGNANCY IN WOMEN WITH CONGENITAL HEART DISEASE

Lesion	*Maternal risk*	*Potential hazards*
Secundum ASD	Low	Atrial arrhythmias Paradoxical embolism
Patent ductus arteriosus	Low	Infective endocarditis
Pulmonary valvular stenosis	Low	Rare, even with significant obstruction
Ventricular septal defect	Low	Infective endocarditis Heart failure in large VSD
Fallot's tetralogy	High (fetal and maternal)	Hypoxia; infective endocarditis Surgical correction allows subsequent low risk pregnancy
Eisenmenger's syndrome	Very high	Up to 70% maternal mortality
Bicuspid non-stenotic aortic valve	Low	Infective endocarditis
Aortic valvular stenosis	Low to moderate	Infective endocarditis Syncope, angina and heart failure with significant obstruction
Coarctation of aorta	Low to moderate	Infective endocarditis, heart failure, aortic dissection, cerebral haemorrhage
Congenital heart block	Low	Peripartum Stokes–Adams attacks. Consider temporary pacemaker to cover delivery

lesions with the highest prevalence in women of childbearing age relative maternal risk and potential hazards are summarised in Table 5.20.

FURTHER READING

Allan L.D. (1986). Examining the foetal heart. *British Journal of Obstetrics and Gynaecology*, **92,** 305.

Becker A.E. and Anderson R.H. (1981). *The Pathology of Congenital Heart Disease*. London: Butterworth.

Dickinson D.F., Arnold R. and Wilkinson J.L. (1981). Congenital heart disease among 160, 480 liveborn children in Liverpool, 1960–1969: Implications for surgical treatment. *British Heart Journal*, **46,** 55.

Engle M.A. (1976). Reviews: cyanotic congenital heart disease. *American Journal of Cardiology*, **37,** 283.

Perloff J.K. (1970). *The Clinical Recognition of Congenital Heart Disease*. Philadelphia: W.B. Saunders.

Roberts W.C. (1979). *Congenital Heart Disease in Adults*. Philadelphia: Davis.

Rudolph A.M. (1970). The changes in the circulation after birth: their importance in congenital heart disease. *Circulation*, **41,** 343.

Shinebourne E.A. and Anderson R.H. (1980). *Current Paediatric Cardiology*. Oxford: Oxford University Press.

Somerville J. (1979). Congenital heart disease—changes in form and function. *British Heart Journal*, **41,** 1.

Chapter Six

Ischaemic Heart Disease

Definitions

Ischaemic heart disease

This is heart muscle disease caused by deficiency or cessation of its blood supply.

Coronary artery disease/coronary heart disease

This implies the presence of atherosclerotic lesions in the coronary arteries resulting in three main clinical manifestations—angina pectoris, myocardial infarction or sudden death.

Arteriosclerosis

This is caused by fibrous or myxofibrous lesions of the intima with no lipid infiltration or necrosis, commonly observed in large stenotic arteries and in diabetics.

Atherosclerosis

This is a form of arteriosclerosis made unique by its high lipid content.

Background

Coronary artery disease is often asymptomatic, but presents clinically in one of three ways:

(i) Angina pectoris.
(ii) Acute myocardial infarction.
(ii) Sudden cardiac death.

The mechanisms responsible for their development have attracted intensive research. Final answers are not available but much evidence supports the hypotheses summarised in this chapter. Acute coronary artery thrombosis and coronary arterial spasm, proposed earlier this century and later discarded, are now known to be important. It is agreed, however, that the substrate of coronary artery disease in the majority of patients is the atherosclerotic plaque.

Pathogenesis of the atherosclerotic plaque

Arterial lesions leading to the fully developed atheroma plaque begin in childhood and early adult life, long before symptoms of ischaemic heart disease present.

The early lesion

Figure 6.1 summarises the main factors thought to be involved in the formation of the developed atheroma plaque.

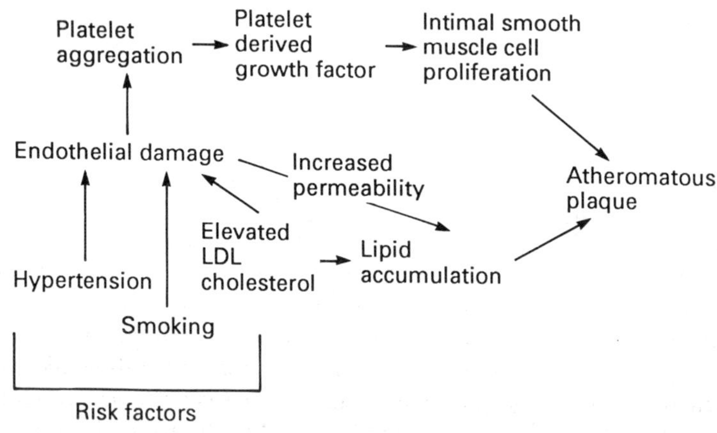

Fig. 6.1. Early development of the atheromatous plaque

Experimental work suggests that minimal endothelial damage and raised low density lipoprotein (LDL)–cholesterol levels are required to initiate a progressive plaque. Endothelial damage may occur at sites of disordered blood flow such as arterial bifurcations and curves. Elevated LDL–cholesterol levels also induce injury to the endothelium which is further damaged by the effects of arterial hypertension and cigarette smoking. Blood platelets aggregate on the injured vascular endothelium and are activated to release a platelet-derived growth factor which stimulates the proliferation of the intimal smooth muscle cells. Smooth muscle cell proliferation may also be stimulated by raised LDL levels. The increased permeability of damaged endothelium allows the accumulation of cholesterol rich LDL within the lesion. The major components of advanced atherosclerotic plaque are:

(i) A necrotic core of cholesterol and cell debris.
(ii) A fibrous cap of proliferated smooth muscle cells, collagen and lipid.

Both components are hazardous—the fibrous cap may fracture and ulcerate exposing the thrombogenic core substances.

The advanced lesion

The advanced lesion (Fig. 6.2) produces clinical effects because it is a space-occupying lesion causing stenosis and because it has thrombogenic qualities related to plaque fracture. Some advanced lesions progress slowly by the mechanisms described above causing angina pectoris, and may result in vessel occlusion. Myocardial infarction is not inevitable if an adequate collateral circulation has developed. However, unstable angina, myocardial infarction and sudden death usually follow rapid progression of the lesion by plaque fracture and acute thrombus formation. The events precipitating fracture of the plaque possibly include haemorrhage into the lesion, wall shear stresses of blood flow and mechanical torsion of the artery during cardiac contraction. Plaque fracture exposes collagen and the thrombogenic core which attract blood platelets to aggregate over the lesion. Collagen interacts with platelet membrane phospholipase A_2 releasing arachidonic acid which is converted by cyclo-oxygenase enzyme to thromboxane A_2 (TXA_2). TXA_2 promotes the mechanism in two ways. It stimulates circulating platelets to adhere and aggregate; it is also a potent vasoconstrictor which may induce local spasm in the remaining normal arterial circumference.

Coronary blood flow is acutely reduced, again favouring platelet aggregation. In the vessel wall, however, arachidonic acid

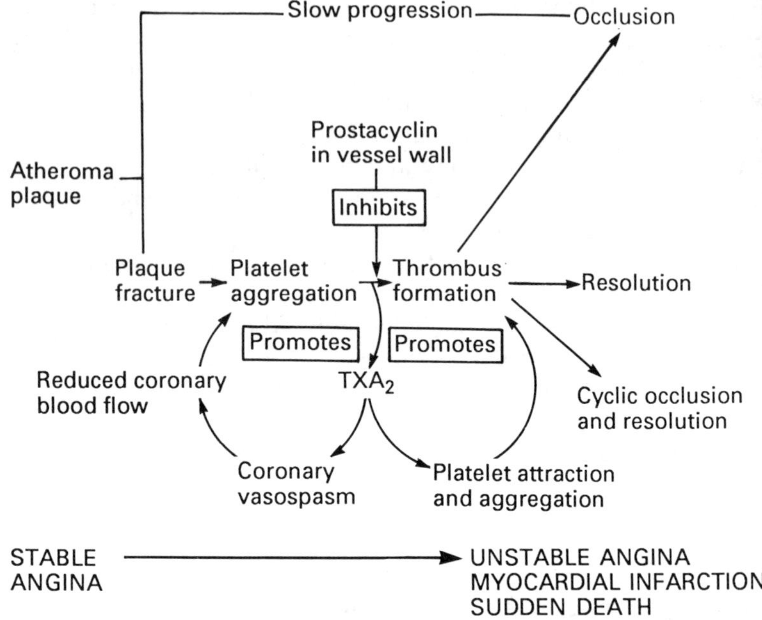

Fig. 6.2. Mechanisms of slow and rapid progression of the developed atheroma plaque

is converted by cyclo-oxygenase not to TXA_2 but to prostacyclin, a powerful antiaggregatory and vasodilator substance. The arachidonic acid pathway may therefore exert a dynamic balance between the effects of TXA_2 and prostacyclin, and resolution of the developing thrombus is possible.

Pathology of clinical ischaemic heart disease

The pathological processes described unify the clinical syndromes of ischaemic heart disease.

Stable angina pectoris

This results mainly from the space-occupying effect of the slowly progressing atheromatous lesion. During exercise the increased myocardial demand for oxygen (blood) cannot be met by increased supply because of the stenosis, and myocardial ischaemia develops.

Acute myocardial infarction

Angiographic and pathological studies have shown atherosclerosis with total thrombotic occlusion of the infarct-related coronary artery in up to 90% of cases. Sudden and prolonged occlusion is the mechanism leading to regional transmural myocardial infarction.

Unstable angina pectoris

Short-term cyclical occlusion and resolution of thrombus over the fractured plaque with associated coronary vasospasm have been demonstrated experimentally and angiographically and may explain intermittent rest angina.

Sudden cardiac death

Between one-third and two-thirds of patients dying within 6 hours of the onset of symptoms of ischaemic heart disease have an acute lesion in which plaque rupture and thrombosis lead to acute arterial occlusion and presumably to fatal ventricular fibrillation. However, a substantial proportion of patients show no recent thrombus, and studies from Seattle demonstrate that many patients resuscitated from 'sudden cardiac death' have no subsequent evidence of myocardial infarction. Chronic myocardial ischaemia is postulated but the mechanisms triggering ventricular fibrillation in these patients is unknown.

CHRONIC ISCHAEMIC HEART DISEASE

This is most commonly due to atherosclerotic obstruction of the coronary arteries. Myocardial ischaemia without atherosclerosis occurs in aortic valve disease, hypertrophic cardiomyopathy, and syphilitic coronary ostial stenosis causing typical angina pectoris. Angina pectoris and rarely myocardial infarction may occur in the presence of angiographically normal coronary arteries; the cause is unknown although coronary artery spasm and embolism have been implicated.

The presenting symptom of chronic ischaemic heart disease is usually angina pectoris although congestive cardiac failure or cardiac arrhythmias may predominate. Electrocardiographic monitoring has shown that the majority of angina patients commonly develop asymptomatic ischaemic episodes—ST segment and T wave changes in the absence of chest pain suggesting that myocardial ischaemia must reach a given severity before pain is produced. 'Silent myocardial ischaemia' is also common in diabetics due to autonomic denervation.

Angina Pectoris

Background

The word angina is derived from the Greek 'agkhone' which means strangling, and was first used by William Heberden in his lecture on angina pectoris to the Royal College of Physicians in 1768. He also noted that the sensation was accompanied by fear of death (angor animi); his description of angina pectoris is still regarded as complete and accurate.

How the symptom is produced is uncertain. Metabolic products of ischaemia appear to stimulate the sensory end-plates of cardiac sympathetic nerves, neural impulses passing via the sympathetic ganglia (C7–T4), spinal ganglia, spinal cord and thalamus to the cerebral cortex. The sensation is then 'referred' to the corresponding peripheral dermatomes which may include those of the neck and medial aspect of the arm.

Pathophysiology

Myocardial ischaemia and hence angina pectoris result from an imbalance between myocardial oxygen demand and supply. The principal factors involved are shown in Table 6.1.

An increase in heart rate, the force and velocity of contraction or left ventricular wall tension increase the demand of the myocardium for oxygen (blood). This must be met by an adequate oxygen supply which depends upon the aortic perfusion pressure and an adequate coronary arterial circulation. During ventricular systole the myocardial compressive forces on the intramyocardial vessels is high, so a large proportion of coronary blood flow to the left ventricle occurs during diastole. Systolic compression is much greater in the subendocardial region of the myocardium which is consequently more susceptible to ischaemia.

Table 6.1

MAIN FACTORS DETERMINING MYOCARDIAL OXYGEN DEMAND AND SUPPLY

Oxygen demand	*Oxygen supply*
Heart rate	Patent coronary arteries
Myocardial contractility	Aortic diastolic pressure
Left ventricular wall tension ventricular volume systolic pressure	Coronary vascular tone Collateral blood flow

The coronary arterial system consists of conductive vessels (the large epicardial arteries) and resistance vessels (the small intramural arteries) which are capable of dilatation or constriction. During maximal exercise coronary blood flow increases five-fold due to dilatation, mainly in the resistance vessels. Drugs such as glyceryl trinitrate and calcium antagonists dilate the large epicardial conductance vessels, including collateral vessels and those with atherosclerotic stenoses, increasing blood flow and o_2 supply to normal and ischaemic myocardium. Conversely, coronary arterial spasm reduces myocardial oxygen supply, and may occur in both normal and atherosclerotic epicardial arteries. Since atherosclerotic plaques are often eccentric, severe transient obstruction may be produced by spasm in the overlying healthy vessel wall. Myocardial ischaemia can thus result from a transient primary reduction in myocardial oxygen supply in the absence of any increase in oxygen demand.

In summary, myocardial ischaemia may occur as a result of:

(i) Fixed, stenotic atherosclerotic lesions.
(ii) Reversible coronary artery spasm.
(iii) Transient platelet aggregation.

The clinical consequences may be angina pectoris, cardiac arrhythmias, electrocardiographic changes and depressed left ventricular function. Persistent obstruction results in myocardial necrosis.

Characteristics of angina pectoris

Angina pectoris is a symptom not a diagnosis. It is identified from the clinical history. Its characteristics are well known (Table 6.2)

Table 6.2
CHARACTERISTICS OF ANGINA PECTORIS

Quality
Pressure, weight, gripping
Breathlessness with constriction
Gradual increase then gradual waning

Location
Typically retrosternal, between neck and epigastrium
Radiation across chest; to medial aspect of either arm; jaw, teeth; back
May occur exclusively in a site of radiation

Duration
Lasts 0·5–15 min (may be longer in unstable angina)

Precipitating factors
Physical exercise
Mental stress
Sexual intercourse
Worse after eating, walking in wind or cold

Relieving factors
Relief within 1–5 min
Cessation of activity
Glyceryl trinitrate

but should be sought carefully because the differential diagnosis of chest pain is a challenging one. The five cardinal features of angina pain are its quality, location, duration and the factors precipitating or relieving it. The history also affords important clues to a variable component due to coronary arterial spasm. These include marked day-to-day variability in effort tolerance, sensitivity to cold, relief by eructation, the occurrence of pain at rest and sensitivity to emotional stress especially in a patient already receiving beta-adrenergic blocking drugs.

Physical examination in chronic stable angina

Examination is often entirely normal. The aims of a general and cardiovascular examination are:

General

(i) Exclude factors exacerbating angina:

- (a) *reduced oxygen supply*:
  anaemia
  hypoxia (obstructive airways disease, pulmonary infection);
- (b) *increased oxygen demand*:
  tachycardia;
  hypertension;
  anxiety, stress;
  inappropriate lifestyle;
  hyperthyroidism;
  phaeochromocytoma;
  acid–base disturbance (for example, diabetic ketoacidosis).

(ii) Identify risk factors:
- (a) xanthomata, premature arcus cornealis;
- (b) hypertensive retinopathy;
- (c) nicotine stained fingers;
- (d) obesity.

Cardiovascular

(i) Identify non-atherosclerotic causes of angina:
- (a) aortic valve disease;
- (b) hypertrophic cardiomyopathy;
- (c) pulmonary arterial hypertension.

(ii) Signs of ischaemic heart disease:
- (a) third heart sound;
- (b) loud fourth heart sound;
- (c) palpable 'a' wave at apex;
- (d) precordial 'bulge' due to dyskinetic left ventricle or aneurysm;
- (e) mitral regurgitation due to papillary muscle dysfunction;
- (f) diastolic murmur across left anterior descending coronary artery stenosis (rare).

Differential diagnosis

A careful history of chest pain is mandatory; laboratory tests are no substitute. Pain may be difficult to describe, especially for patients of limited literacy, and gestures should be observed.

Table 6.3

CAUSES OF CHEST PAIN RESEMBLING ANGINA PECTORIS

Cardiovascular
Pericarditis
Mitral valve prolapse
Aortic dissection
Thoracic aortic aneurysm
Non-cardiac
Oesophageal motility of disorder
Gastro-oesophageal acid reflux
Chest wall pain
Peptic ulcer
Biliary disease
Thoracic outlet syndrome
Hyperventilation syndrome
Psychogenic (Da Costa's syndrome)

Clenching of the fist over the chest is a reliable indicator of angina pectoris.

Non-anginal chest pain may arise in thoracic, abdominal or chest wall structures, and may be psychogenic (Table 6.3). Some discriminating features are summarised below:

(i) *Quality*: stabbing or pricking pains and tenderness are rarely cardiac. 'Sharp' may be synonymous with 'severe' for some patients.

(ii) *Location*: rarely cardiac are pains localised to the left nipple, costochondral joints or ribs and pointed to by the patient. Predominant back pain may suggest a thoracic or dissecting aneurysm.

(iii) *Duration*: pain which is momentary or lasts less than 30 s is often musculoskeletal. Prolonged pain, greater than 15 min, may or may not be ischaemic.

(iv) *Precipitating factors*: pain at rest or during mental stress may often be ischaemic. Postural variability occurs in pericarditis and oesophageal reflux. Induction by vomiting or swallowing is found in oesophageal disease. Thoracic outlet pain may radiate to the medial aspect of the arms especially with arm movement, but is not related to walking.

(v) *Relieving factors*: glyceryl trinitrate may alleviate oesophageal spasm, and beta-adrenergic blockers ameliorate the atypical chest pain of prolapsing mitral valve syndrome. Chest pain due to pericarditis is relieved by leaning forward. Food, antacids and milk relieve peptic ulcer pain.

Investigation of chronic ischaemic heart disease

Background

The usual questions which need to be answered and the tests which are useful (+) or indispensable (+ +) in routine practice are summarised in Table 6.4.

Coronary angiography demonstrates the pathological anatomy of the coronary arterial tree. It is the final arbiter in detecting the presence and severity of atheromatous disease and in the evaluation of the patient for surgical coronary artery bypass grafting (CABG) or percutaneous transluminal coronary angioplasty (PTCA). However, it is an expensive, invasive procedure with a small but definite mortality and morbidity which is unsuitable for serial observations. Furthermore it does not assess the functional effects of impaired coronary blood flow. Exercise stress testing, radionuclide studies and echocardiography are commonly used to provide diagnostic, functional and prognostic data in patients with ischaemic heart disease (see Chapter 3).

Laboratory investigations

(i) *Biochemical screening* identifies potentially treatable risk factors such as hyperlipidaemia and hyperglycaemia. A non-fasting sample is satisfactory for the estimation of total cholesterol but the full evaluation of hyperlipoproteinaemia requires a fasting sample. Concentrations of plasma cholesterol and low density lipoprotein may fall by 60% early in acute myocardial infarction and fluctuations persist for 6 weeks; stable levels should be obtained after 2–3 months.

Hypercholesterolaemia is an unequivocal risk factor for coronary artery disease, but evidence linking serum triglycerides is inconclusive. High density lipoproteins (HDL) have been inversely associated with coronary artery disease risk. Unfortunately, there is little evidence

Table 6.4

INVESTIGATIONS IN CHRONIC ISCHAEMIC HEART DISEASE

Aim of investigation	*Exercise stress testing*	*Radionuclide studies*	*Two-dimensional echocardiography*	*Cardiac catheter*
Diagnosis of the presence of CAD	+	+ (TS)		+ +
Assess severity of myocardial ischaemia	+ +	+ (TS)		
Assess left ventricular function	+	+ (RA)	+	+ +
Efficacy of drug therapy	+			
Preoperative assessment for CABG and PTCA	+	+ (TS/RA)	+	+ +
Postoperative assessment of CABG and PTCA	+	+ (TS/RA)	+	+ +
Prediction of future coronary events and survival	+			

TS = Thallium scintigraphy
RA = Radionuclide angiography
CAD = Coronary artery disease
CABG = Coronary artery bypass grafting
PTCA = Percutaneous transluminal coronary angioplasty

that the reduction of elevated lipid levels confers any significant benefit once symptomatic ischaemic heart disease is present.

(ii) *Exercise stress testing* is valuable in provoking symptoms and assessing effort tolerance. Heart rate and blood pressure response to exercise must be measured in addition to morphological ECG changes and cardiac arrhythmias. A strongly positive exercise stress test (low exercise tolerance due to angina, marked S–T segment depression, failure to rise or a fall in systolic blood pressure) indicates the possible presence of life-threatening coronary artery lesions—left main coronary artery stenosis or triple vessel disease—and the need for coronary angiography.

(iii) *Radionuclide studies*: thallium scintigraphy identifies areas of reversible myocardial ischaemia induced by exercise stress testing. Radionuclide angiography using technetium 99^{m} provides non-invasive evaluation of left ventricular function. Their use is limited by availability but they may increase the sensitivity and specificity of conventional stress testing to the presence and severity of coronary artery lesions.

(iv) *Two-dimensional echocardiography* is widely available and provides reliable qualitative and semiquantitative data on overall left ventricular function and regional left ventricular wall motion abnormalities due to myocardial ischaemia and infarction. M-mode echocardiography is unsuitable for assessing the ischaemic left ventricle because the small area sampled may be unrepresentative of the whole chamber.

(v) *Cardiac catheterisation*: coronary angiography is performed by selective catheterisation of the left and right coronary ostia using special preformed catheters. It demonstrates the site and severity of obstructive lesions. The left ventriculogram visualises overall ventricular function, regional wall motion abnormalities due to ischaemia, infarction or aneurysm formation and the presence of mitral regurgitation. The usual indications for coronary angiography are shown in Table 6.5.

Table 6.5

INDICATIONS FOR CORONARY ANGIOGRAPHY

Angina refractory to medical treatment
Angina with a strongly positive exercise test
Unstable angina
Postinfarction angina
Prinzmetal's variant angina
Assessment of life-threatening ventricular arrhythmias in ischaemic heart disease
Preoperative assessment of postinfarction ventricular septal defect and acute mitral regurgitation
Preoperative assessment in valvular heart disease
Assessment of suspected cardiomyopathy

Treatment of angina pectoris

This may be broadly considered as:

(i) Medical management:
  (a) control of 'risk factors' (see Chapter 14);
  (b) control of factors exacerbating angina pectoris;
  (c) drug therapy (nitrates, beta-adrenergic blocking agents, calcium antagonists).

(ii) Coronary artery bypass surgery.

(iii) Percutaneous transluminal coronary angioplasty.

Drug therapy

Most patients with moderate to severe angina pectoris will benefit from 'triple therapy' with nitrates, beta-adrenergic blocking agents and calcium antagonists because in many respects their modes of action are complementary. These drug classes are discussed in Chapter 11; their specific use in angina pectoris is discussed here.

Nitrates Nitrates have beneficial effects on both myocardial oxygen demand and supply (Fig. 6.3). There are several formulations the use of which depends on the desired duration of action and patient preference.

(i) *Sublingual nitrates*: glyceryl trinitrate (nitroglycerin)

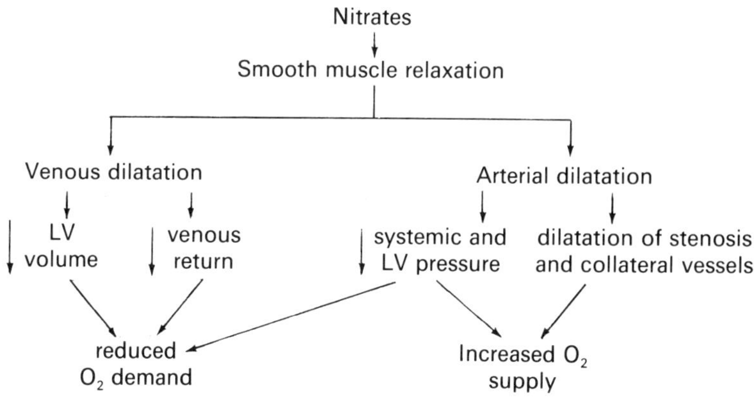

Fig. 6.3. Beneficial effects of nitrates in angina pectoris. Venous dilatation is the principal effect

500 μg abolishes the acute attack within 1–3 min and is protective for up to 20 min. It should also be used just prior to exertion known to produce symptoms. Nitrate headache may be prevented by using part of a tablet or by discarding it once the exertion is completed. Tablets deteriorate in light and moisture so must be kept in a cool, dark bottle and renewed every 2 months. An aerosol spray form is an effective, stable but expensive alternative. Chewable sublingual isosorbide dinitrate is also effective.

(ii) *Oral nitrates* increase exercise tolerance and reduce the frequency of attacks for up to 12 h. Isosorbide dinitrate (ISDN) undergoes extensive first-pass metabolism in the liver, producing the active mononitrate metabolite (ISMN). ISDN is commenced at 10 mg t.d.s. and increased to the limit of tolerable side-effects. ISMN may have a narrower dose range.

(iii) *Topical nitrates*: glyceryl trinitrate patches deliver the drug transdermally, and have superseded ointments. Although designed to act for 24 hours the drug levels have probably become ineffective before the next patch is due. Since continuous nitrate levels may induce tachyphylaxis the resulting 'pulsed' administration is possibly advantageous.

(iv) *Buccal nitroglycerin* in tablet form is placed between the gum and the cheek. It is effective for up to 6 h by mucosal absorption.

Beta-adrenergic blocking agents These drugs (see page 332) all reduce myocardial oxygen demand by reducing heart rate, myocardial contractility and systolic pressure. Although they increase ventricular volume, which increases oxygen demand, this is outweighed by the beneficial effects and may also be counteracted by the simultaneous use of nitrates. They are extremely effective in controlling angina of effort, and since their introduction 20 years ago they have improved the prognosis of ischaemic heart disease. However, abrupt withdrawal of beta-adrenergic blocking agents may induce sudden clinical deterioration and the drugs should be tailed off gradually when indicated.

Calcium antagonists Reduced myocardial contractility and dilatation of vascular smooth muscle result in a reduction of myocardial oxygen demand. Dilatation of both systemic and coronary arteries occurs, so that they are the drugs of first choice in Prinzmetal's variant angina and in patients whose history suggests a component of coronary artery spasm (see page 314).

A strategy for drug therapy in angina pectoris

Sublingual nitrates are the drugs of choice for the immediate relief of angina and must be supplied to all affected patients. A combination of beta-adrenergic blocking agents and long-acting nitrates increases exercise tolerance in most patients with chronic stable angina. Ineffectively low doses are often prescribed. Nitrate dosage should be increased progressively to obtain maximum benefit until the limit of tolerated side-effects is reached; nitrate headache often diminishes or disappears shortly after commencing treatment. Beta-adrenergic blockade should achieve a resting heart rate of 50–60 beats/min and should blunt the rate increase on moderate exercise to 10–15 beats/min. This usually requires 240–320 mg propranolol/day or its equivalent for another beta-adrenergic blocker. Calcium antagonists often provide further benefit and should be added at an early stage, especially when coronary artery spasm is likely. The use of such 'triple therapy' satisfactorily controls angina in many patients. Angina can be described as refractory only when full doses of all three drug classes have been tried.

Coronary artery bypass surgery

Background The procedure was introduced in 1964. Autologous saphenous vein is anastomosed proximally to the aorta and distally to the diseased coronary artery beyond the stenosis. Blood flow is restored to previously ischaemic myocardium. The left internal mammary artery may be used instead of saphenous vein. The procedure is performed under cardiopulmonary bypass and moderate hypothermia (24°C–32°C).

Several factors affect the operative mortality, including sex, age, left ventricular function and the number of grafts. The operative risk for patients under 65 years of age with good left ventricular function is about 2% for men and 5% for women.

Relief of angina

About 90% of patients remain free of angina one year after surgery, and 50% are asymptomatic for 10 years. Recurrence of angina is caused by graft occlusion and progression of atherosclerosis in the native coronary arteries.

Improved prognosis

Patients with significant stenosis of the left main coronary artery, or with disease in all three main coronary artery trunks (right, left anterior descending and left circumflex coronary arteries) have a better 5 year survival rate following bypass surgery than with medical treatment. The prognosis in patients with poor left ventricular function is also improved by operation.

Percutaneous transluminal coronary angioplasty

A steerable guide wire is passed down the coronary artery and past the stenotic lesion. A balloon catheter is passed over the wire and the balloon positioned adjacent to the stenosis. The balloon is inflated and dilates the stenosis by rupture of the atherosclerotic plaque and stretching of the elastic media. The procedure is indicated in patients with angina pectoris who would otherwise be candidates for bypass surgery, and who have a lesion suitable for angioplasty. Ideally the stenosis is proximal, discrete and concentric. Success rates may be as high as 90%. At the present time approximately 15% of patients are suitable but indications are widening rapidly as experience accumulates.

Unstable Angina Pectoris

Definition

(i) Increased frequency, severity or duration of angina.
(ii) Angina of recent onset.
(iii) Angina at rest or on minimal exertion.

Background

Unstable angina was previously called crescendo angina, preinfarction angina, intermediate coronary syndrome or acute coronary insufficiency. In fact, most patients with unstable angina do not develop infarction in the short term if they are stabilised promptly by medical treatment in hospital. However, the mortality and the incidence of infarction are approximately 15–20% after 1 year of followup and investigation by arteriography is required shortly after symptoms have stabilised in order to plan treatment.

Acute myocardial infarction is often preceded by a period of unstable angina. The converse is not true—unstable angina infrequently proceeds directly to acute infarction (less than 10%).

Investigations

(i) *The ECG* invariably shows transient depression or elevation of the S–T segment, often with T wave inversion, associated with pain or in isolation (silent myocardial ischaemia). Pathological Q waves do not develop.
(ii) *Cardiac enzymes* are not elevated since, by definition, this implies myocardial infarction.
(iii) *Coronary angiography* may show normal coronary arteries (5%) or one, two or three vessel coronary artery disease. The left anterior descending artery is the most com-

monly affected. The extent of disease is no different to that found in stable angina, but the morphology of the atherosclerotic lesion may suggest plaque fracture and thrombosis. Coronary artery spasm has been demonstrated during spontaneous episodes of pain.

Management

Patients with unstable angina must be admitted to hospital, preferably to a cardiac intensive care unit. Management consists of three phases: medical stabilisation, investigation by coronary arteriography, and definitive management.

Medical stabilisation

(i) Bedrest, reassurance, sedation.
(ii) Exclusion of factors exacerbating angina (see page 00).
(iii) Nitrates (often intravenously), beta-adrenergic blockade and calcium antagonists in optimal dosage to prevent angina.
(iv) Aspirin (324 mg/day orally) has been shown to result in a 50% reduction in mortality and acute non-fatal myocardial infarction.

Angina pectoris is abolished by these measures within 48 h in 95% of patients. Coronary angiography should be performed, preferably during the same hospital admission, to identify those patients suitable for coronary artery bypass grafting or angioplasty.

When medical treatment fails intra-aortic balloon counterpulsation is commenced prior to urgent coronary angiography and surgery or angioplasty.

Variant Angina Pectoris

Definition

Angina pectoris at rest, not precipitated by increased myocardial oxygen demand, and accompanied by S–T segment elevation in the electrocardiogram.

Background

Prinzmetal described variant angina in 1959. It is caused by reversible spasm in a large epicardial coronary artery, often associated with a severe proximal atherosclerotic stenosis. Maseri has shown, however, that spasm may occur in normal coronary arteries and in all grades of atherosclerotic disease. Variant angina may be associated with ventricular tachycardia, ventricular fibrillation and sudden death.

Diagnosis

(i) *ECG*: marked transient S–T segment elevation during spontaneous pain establishes the diagnosis. A 12-lead ECG or ambulatory ECG monitoring using a suitable low-frequency recorder are used.

(ii) *Coronary angiography*: localised discrete spasm is demonstrated during spontaneous pain or on provocation with ergometrine 500 μg intravenously in divided doses.

Management

Management is directed at the relief of coronary artery spasm which causes myocardial ischaemia by reduction of myocardial oxygen supply. Nitrates and calcium antagonists are extremely effective in abolishing and preventing coronary artery spasm. Non-selective beta-adrenergic antagonists may worsen symptoms by allowing unopposed alpha-adrenergic mediated vasoconstriction.

Prognosis

Sudden death occurs in 15% of patients with variant angina but is less likely in those with angiographically normal coronary arteries. Coronary artery bypass grafting is contraindicated in patients with pure spasm, but is helpful in those with associated severe atherosclerotic stenosis.

Angina with Angiographically Normal Coronary Arteries

About 20% of patients investigated for angina-like chest pain have normal coronary angiograms; 20% of these patients have positive exercise stress tests and a very small proportion show myocardial lactate production (ischaemia) on exercise. Because the cause is unknown the name 'syndrome X' has been given. Treatment with antianginal drugs is often unsatisfactory. The prognosis is excellent.

ACUTE MYOCARDIAL INFARCTION (AMI)

Definition

Myocardial necrosis due to cessation or interruption of the blood supply.

Epidemiology

This is discussed in Chapter 14.

Pathology

The pathophysiology of atherosclerosis and coronary thrombosis are discussed on page 182. Myocardial infarction results almost invariably from atherosclerotic occlusion of a coronary artery. Histological changes cannot be recognised for up to 8 h following the occlusion; thereafter, two patterns of distribution are seen:

(i) *Regional infarction*: a specific wedge of myocardium related to the area of supply of a major artery (Table 6.6). Infarction proceeds from the endocardial to the

Table 6.6
SITE OF MYOCARDIAL INFARCTION RELATED TO ARTERIAL SUPPLY

Occluded artery	*Site of left ventricular infarct*
Left anterior descending	Anterior/apical interventricular septum
Left circumflex	Lateral/inferoposterior
Right	Inferoposterior, inferior interventricular septum, posteromedial papillary muscle

epicardial surface resulting in subendocardial or transmural infarction.

(ii) *Diffuse infarction*: occurs in widespread atherosclerosis, in diabetics and as an extension of regional infarction with cardiogenic shock. Diffuse subendocardial necrosis may complicate severe left ventricular hypertrophy with or without atherosclerotic coronary artery disease. Other non-atherosclerotic causes of myocardial infarction are relatively rare (Table 6.7).

Table 6.7

NON-ATHEROSCLEROTIC CAUSES OF MYOCARDIAL INFARCTION

Congenital coronary artery anomalies
Non-atheromatous coronary artery disease
arteritis
spasm
trauma
Coronary artery embolism
Aortic stenosis
Polycythaemia vera, hypercoagulability
Myocardial infarction with normal coronary arteries

Pathophysiology

Ischaemic damage to the myocardium causes impairment of:

(i) *Left ventricular systolic pump function*: reduced cardiac output, stroke volume, blood pressure and myocardial contractility.

(ii) *Left ventricular diastolic function*: stiffening (reduced compliance) of the myocardium, raised ventricular diastolic pressure, pulmonary venous congestion.

Impairment of function is related to the extent of damage. Clinical heart failure and cardiogenic shock result from loss of more than 25% and 40% of the left ventricular myocardium respectively.

Symptoms

(i) *Prodomal symptoms*: unstable angina pectoris, non-specific chest discomfort or excessive fatigue occur in up to 50% of patients. Precipitating factors, for example, severe exertional or emotional stress, are rare.

(ii) *Chest pain*: the quality and location resembles angina pectoris. Severity may be mild to intolerable. Its duration usually exceeds 30 min and glyceryl trinitrate fails to provide relief.

(iii) *Other symptoms*: these are common in the elderly. Left ventricular failure, syncope, severe fatigue, sweating and vomiting may predominate over or replace chest pain.

(iv) *'Silent' myocardial infarction*: recognised only on routine ECG or postmortem examination. Infarction may be truly silent, especially in diabetics, or the patient may forget an atypical symptom. About one-fifth of myocardial infarctions are clinically unrecognised.

Differential diagnosis

Unstable angina pectoris, pulmonary embolism, acute aortic dissection, acute pericarditis, pleurisy and Bornholm disease may simulate the chest pain of acute myocardial infarction.

Physical signs

(i) *General appearance*: normal to pale, sweating, anxious, fearful. Fever within 12 hours.

(ii) *Cardiovascular*:

(a) Pulse: rapid, thready. Bradycardia is frequent in inferior myocardial infarction.

(b) Blood pressure: often elevated initially, later falling below preinfarction levels. Early hypotension usually signifies extensive infarction.

(c) Palpation: systolic bulging may be felt over the left precordium due to a left ventricular wall motion abnormality. Fourth and third heart sounds may be palpable if extensive myocardial damage has occurred.

(d) Heart sounds: a fourth heart sound is almost invariable; a third sound accompanies extensive myocardial damage.

(e) Pericardial friction: indicates extensive transmural damage. It is usually very transient, occurring between the 2nd and 4th days. Rubs are audible in at least 20% of patients.

(iii) *Lungs*: Crepitations or frank pulmonary oedema occur if sufficient left ventricular dysfunction is present. Often the chest is clear.

(iv) *New cardiac murmurs*: usually indicate the development of a mechanical complication of myocardial infarction.

Diagnosis

Electrocardiography

Morphology A definitive diagnosis of myocardial infarction depends on QRS complex abnormalities:

(i) Localised and inappropriate reduction in R wave amplitude.

(ii) An abnormal Q wave:
   (a) duration greater than 40 ms;
   (b) depth greater than one quarter of the size of the succeeding R wave.

Sequential changes A typical sequence of changes occurs.

(i) *Hours*: the ECG may appear within normal limits during the first few hours of infarction. ST segment elevation—the current of injury to the myocardial cell membrane—is the earliest change. It represents ischaemia rather than infarction and may resolve completely without QRS changes or enzyme evidence of infarction (see variant angina pectoris, page 179). ‘Reciprocal’ ST segment depression may occur in leads opposite the infarct.

(ii) *Days*: reduced R wave voltage and pathological Q waves reflect loss of viable myocardium. ST segment elevation diminishes; T wave inversion appears.

(iii) *Weeks*: S–T segments revert to normal; deep symmetrical T wave inversion is common; reduced or absent R waves and pathological Q waves persist.

(iv) *Months*: QRS abnormalities are usually permanent.

Their regression indicates scar shrinkage. Persistent ST elevation suggests left ventricular aneurysm formation.

Regional location of infarction

The site of a regional myocardial infarction is predicted by the ECG leads showing the primary QRST abnormalities (Table 6.8).

Table 6.8
LOCATION OF MYOCARDIAL INFARCTION

Region of infarct	*ECG leads*
Extensive anterior	V_1–V_6, I, aVL
Anteroseptal	V_1, V_2, V_3
Anterolateral	V_4, V_5, V_6, I, aVL
High lateral	aVL
Inferior	II, III, aVF
Inferolateral	II, III, aVF, V_5, V_6
True posterior	Tall R and T waves in V1 and V2

(i) *Transmural or subendocardial infarction*: infarction of the full thickness of myocardium from endocardium to epicardium is termed 'transmural' infarction. R waves are lost completely, leaving QS complexes. Substantial but less than full thickness infarction causes reduction in R-wave amplitude with pathological Q waves. Infarction of the subendocardial zone alone causes deep symmetrical T wave inversion without QRS changes. It should be noted that a clear electrocardiographic differentiation between transmural and subendocardial infarction has not been substantiated by some pathological studies, although abnormal Q waves usually indicate more extensive infarction. It may be more accurate merely to distinguish between 'Q-wave infarcts' and 'non-Q-wave infarcts' unless there is pathological confirmation of the thickness of infarction. There is no difference in the incidence of complications or prognosis of patients with or without abnormal Q waves.

Table 6.9

TIME COURSE OF SERUM ENZYME ACTIVITY IN ACUTE MYOCARDIAL INFARCTION

	Rise begins	*Peak level*	*Normalises*
CK	6–8 h	24 h	3–4 days
AsAT	8–12 h	8–36 h	3–4 days
LDH	24–48 h	3–6 days	8–14 days
MB-CK	4–6 h	18–24 h	36–48 h
LDH_1	8–12 h	3 days	10–14 days

CK: creatine kinase; AsAT: aspartate aminotransferase; LDH: lactic dehydrogenase

(ii) *Cardiac enzymes*: three enzymes released into the circulation by myocardial cell death are usually measured: creatine kinase (CK), aspartate aminotransferase (AsAT) formerly called glutamic oxaloacetic transaminase (GOT), and lactic dehydrogenase (LDH). The activity of each has a different time course (Table 6.9). Elevation of these enzymes is a sensitive but non-specific test for acute myocardial infarction (Table 6.10), and specificity is improved by measuring the myocardial isoenzymes of CK (MB-CK) or LDH (LDH_1). MB-CK is the most sensitive and specific—in 15% of patients with acute myocardial infarction MB-CK is elevated despite normal total CK levels.

(iii) *Other investigations* are rarely required but may provide useful confirmatory evidence:

(a) Radionuclide scanning: technetium pyrophosphate 'hot spot' or thallium scintigraphy 'cold spot'.

(b) Elevated ESR, WBC (12 000–15 000) and blood glucose.

General management of acute myocardial infarction

Background

Half of all deaths presumed due to myocardial infarction occur within 2 h of the onset of symptoms; many deaths are instan-

Table 6.10

CAUSES OF A FALSE-POSITIVE CARDIAC ENZYME RISE

CK	*AsAT*	*LDH*
Skeletal muscle disease/injury	Liver disease/congestion	Liver disease/congestion
Intramuscular injection	Skeletal muscle-disease/injury	Haemolysis
Vigorous exercise	Intramuscular injection	Megaloblastic anaemia
Diabetes mellitus	Pulmonary embolus	Leukaemia
Pulmonary embolus	Shock	Renal disease
	Pericarditis	Neoplasm
		Pulmonary embolus
		Shock
		Myocarditis

CK = creative kinase; AsAT = aspartate aminotransferase; LDH = lactic dehydrogenase taneous, and 90% of deaths due to AMI are caused by ventricular fibrillation. The incidence of ventricular fibrillation falls dramatically during the first 6 h after the onset of infarction—60% of episodes occur within 4 h and 80% within 12 h. Since the average delay between the onset of symptoms and admission to a coronary care unit is about 4 h the period of maximum risk has already passed. Reduction in mortality during the high, prehospital risk period has been achieved using public education in cardiopulmonary resuscitation (Seattle Heartwatch programme) and coronary ambulances (Belfast, Brighton).

Home or hospital care?

Three United Kingdom studies suggest that hospital admission offers no clear advantage to patients who have survived the early hours of infarction and have no pain, arrhythmias or heart failure. Such patients have clearly selected themselves as a low risk group.

Cardiac intensive care unit (CICU) or general ward?

Ventricular fibrillation occurs in about 10% of patients admitted to hospital with acute myocardial infarction. Immediate recognition and electrical defibrillation on CICUs has reduced the mortality from primary ventricular fibrillation almost to zero, and the overall hospital mortality of acute myocardial infarction from 25% to 15%. A definitive comparison of CICU versus general ward care is lacking but it is almost universally accepted that patients with early definite or suspected acute myocardial infarction do better in a CICU than a general ward. By contrast CICUs have made little impact on heart failure and cardiogenic shock which account almost entirely for the 15% hospital mortality from acute myocardial infarction.

General management of uncomplicated acute myocardial infarction

Early acute myocardial infarction is uncomplicated in one-half of patients admitted to hospital. Fewest complications occur in young patients and first infarcts. General measures include:

(i) *Pain relief*: the first priority; diamorphine 2.5–5 mg incre-

Table 6.11
INDICATIONS FOR FULL ANTICOAGULATION IN ACUTE MYOCARDIAL INFARCTION

Congestive cardiac failure
Prolonged immobilisation
Cardiogenic shock
Sustained atrial fibrillation
Current venous thrombosis
Current or previous venous or systemic embolism
Long-term anticoagulant treatment

ments every 10 min to a maximum of 25 mg. Opiate narcosis is reversed with naloxone 0.4 mg intravenously.

(ii) *Reassurance*: rehabilitation commences with reassurance and explanation at the time of admission.

(iii) *Oxygen*: 2–4 l/min at 100% humidified oxygen by mask or nasal prongs counters hypoxaemia (cardiac failure, opiates).

(iv) *Anticoagulants*: low dose (5000 units subcutaneously every 12 h) helps prevent venous thromboembolism. Full dose anticoagulation is required for increased thromboembolic risk (Table 6.11).

(v) *Hypertension*: often responds promptly to pain relief, sedation and nitrates. Persistent hypertension and tachycardia accompany sympathetic overactivity or left ventricular failure. Severe persistent hypertension without heart failure responds to labetalol 10 mg intravenously over 5 min repeated at 10 min intervals to a maximum of 100 mg.

(vi) *Mobilisation*: prolonged bedrest increases the risk of venous thromboembolism. If there are no complications gentle mobilisation is started on the second or third day.

Limitation of myocardial infarct size

Myocardial pump failure causes the majority of hospital deaths from acute myocardial infarction and is related to necrosis of a critical mass of myocardium. Infarct size is the major predictor of acute and long-term prognosis. Reduction of infarct size has been attempted by:

(i) *Drug treatment* to reduce myocardial oxygen demand (beta-blockers, vasodilators, etc.). No certain benefit has been clinically demonstrated, and the hypothesis that an ischaemic but viable 'border zone' is present and can be preserved is losing credibility.

(ii) *Reperfusion of the occluded artery* by:

(a) coronary artery bypass grafting cannot usually be achieved in time to prevent myocardial necrosis. Similar delays apply to emergency coronary balloon angioplasty which also has a high incidence of complications in acute myocardial infarction when used alone or in combination with intravenous coronary thrombolysis.

(b) coronary thrombolysis: most cases of acute myocardial infarction are caused by intra-coronary thrombus formation secondary to plaque disruption. Large scale clinical trials published since 1986 demonstrate that intravenous thrombolytic agents given early in acute infarction reduce infarct size, preserve left ventricular function and achieve a highly significant reduction in mortality. Accordingly, thrombolytic therapy, in the absence of contraindications, is the treatment of choice for acute myocardial infarction.

Coronary thrombolysis

Several thrombolytic agents have been evaluated for the immediate treatment of acute myocardial infarction. These include Streptokinase, recombinant tissue-type plasminogen activator (rt-PA), anisoylated plasminogen-streptokinase activator complex (APSAC, anistreplase) and urokinase. In early 1989 there is no definitive evidence that any one agent is significantly better than another in achieving the major aims of mortality reduction and myocardial preservation, but intensive study of newer agents and combinations is in progress. The largest thrombolytic trial performed, by the International Studies of Infarct Survival (ISIS) group, demonstrates the powerful effect of treatment with a combination of Streptokinase and aspirin (see Further Reading) in more than 17,000 patients. The current choice of patients for

Table 6.12

INCLUSION AND EXCLUSION CRITERIA FOR THROMBOLYSIS IN PATIENTS WITH ACUTE MYOCARDIAL INFARCTION

Inclusion

Myocardial ischaemic pain for at least 30 minutes
ECG: 2 mm S–T segment elevation in at least 2 leads, limb or precordial

Exclusion

Symptom duration greater than 6 hours (up to 24 hours if pain recurrent)
Age above 75 years
Systolic BP sustained at or above 200 mmHg
Bleeding diathesis
Cerebrovascular accident within 3 months
Active peptic ulcer
Gastrointestinal haemorrhage within 6 months
Current menstruation or pregnancy
Aortic dissection or acute pericarditis not excluded
Major surgery/trauma/cardiac massage within 6 weeks
Proliferative diabetic retinopathy
Concurrent serious or lifethreatening illness
Streptokinase or anistreplase in past 6 months: allergy (use alternative agent e.g. rTPA)

Table 6.13

THROMBOLYTIC TREATMENT REGIME IN PATIENTS WITH ACUTE MYOCARDIAL INFARCTION

ASPIRIN :	300 mg orally at presentation, then 300 mg daily indefinitely
STREPTOKINASE :	1,500,000 units intravenously over 1 hour in 100 ml 0.9% saline

thrombolytic therapy (Table 12) and the treatment regime (Table 13) in the Liverpool Cardiac Intensive Care Unit is based on the results of recent trials.

Complications of acute myocardial infarction

(i) Arrhythmias.
(ii) Conduction disturbances.
(iii) Left ventricular failure.
(iv) Cardiogenic shock.
(v) Right ventricular infarction.
(vi) Mechanical complications:
  (a) interventricular septal rupture;
  (b) acute mitral regurgitation;
  (c) left ventricular free wall rupture;
  (d) left ventricular aneurysm.
(vii) Embolism.
(viii) Dressler's syndrome.

Arrhythmias

Some disorder of cardiac rhythm is almost invariable. Important arrhythmias and their in-hospital incidence are:

(i) *Ventricular fibrillation* (10%): *primary* ventricular fibrillation occurs suddenly early in uncomplicated infarction. The prognosis after defibrillation is excellent; *secondary* ventricular fibrillation terminates a complicated infarction with myocardial pump failure.

  Treatment is by DC shock with 200–400 joules. Ventricular fibrillation is often initiated by R-on-T ventricular ectopic beats, but few such ectopics result in fibrillation. The concept of 'warning arrhythmias' (frequent or coupled ventricular ectopics, brief self-limiting ventricular tachycardia) is discredited and their treatment is inappropriate. Ventricular fibrillation is recurrent in 15% of patients initially resuscitated and lignocaine infusion is the preventive management of choice.

(ii) *Ventricular tachycardia* (20%): defined as three or more consecutive ventricular ectopics, rate greater than 120 beats/min. Haemodynamic deterioration or degeneration to ventricular fibrillation are common. If poorly tolerated immediate DC cardioversion is mandatory. Lignocaine is the drug of choice if the arrhythmias are

Table 6.14
USE OF HAEMODYNAMIC MONITORING IN SINUS TACHYCARDIA FOLLOWING ACUTE MYOCARDIAL INFARCTION

Cause	*PCWP*	*Treatment*
Pain, anxiety	N	Analgesia, sedation
Sympathetic overactivity	N	Beta-blockade
Left ventricular failure	↑	Diuretics, vasodilators
Hypovolaemia	↓	Restore blood volume

N = normal; ↑ = above normal; ↓ = below normal; PCWP = pulmonary capillary wedge pressure

well tolerated; procainamide, disopyramide and amiodarone are alternatives.

(iii) *Accelerated idioventricular rhythm* (15%): defined as three or more consecutive ventricular ectopics at a rate of 60–120 beats/min. It is usually a benign escape rhythm due to underlying bradycardia and enhanced automaticity of Purkinje cells. Treatment is that of the bradycardia.

(iv) *Sinus bradycardia* (25%): common in inferior infarction. Atropine or temporary cardiac pacing are indicated if hypotension results.

(v) *Sinus tachycardia* (30%): usually due to pain and anxiety but sympathetic overactivity, left ventricular failure or hypovolaemia may be responsible. Persistent sinus tachycardia increases myocardial oxygen demand. Pulmonary capillary wedge pressure (PCWP) measurement by Swan–Ganz catheter may be needed to determine the cause and appropriate treatment (Table 6.14).

(vi) *Atrial fibrillation* (15%) is associated with left ventricular failure, pericarditis and atrial infarction. Usually transient or paroxysmal it predicts increased mortality. Digoxin, propranolol or verapamil are helpful. Amiodarone infusion is often effective.

(vii) *Paroxysmal atrial/junctional rhythm* (1–2%): left ventricular failure and digoxin toxicity must be excluded.

Conduction disturbances

(i) *Complete heart block*: complete heart block develops in 5–10% of patients with acute myocardial infarction. In

Table 6.15
CHARACTERISTICS OF COMPLETE HEART BLOCK (CHB) IN ACUTE MYOCARDIAL INFARCTION

	Inferior infarction	*Anterior infarction*
Incidence	10%	5%
Myocardial damage	Mild/moderate	Severe
Mortality	25%	50–80%
Defect preceding CHB	1° atrioventricular block, 2° Type I (Wenckebach)	RBBB, (LBBB less often)
Site of block	Atrioventricular node/His bundle	Bilateral bundle branch block
QRS complexes	Usually narrow	Wide
Asystolic periods	Rare	Common
Temporary pacing	Only for symptomatic bradycardia	Always

RBBB: right bundle branch block; LBBB: left bundle branch block

90% of people the nutrient artery of the atrioventricular node arises from the right coronary artery; in 10% it arises from the left circumflex coronary artery. Occlusion of either vessel results in inferior infarction and may cause atrioventricular block with only limited myocardial damage. Conversely, the bundle branches are supplied by the left anterior descending artery, and massive damage to the interventricular septum is required to cause complete heart block during anterior infarction. The development and prognosis of complete heart block thus differs between inferior and anterior infarction (Table 6.15). Complete heart block and some intraventricular conduction defects predispose to sudden ventricular asystole and temporary pacemaker insertion may be indicated (Table 6.16). Complete heart block in acute myocardial infarction usually resolves within 2–3 weeks and permanent pacing is almost never needed. Neither temporary nor permanent pacing affects the poor long-term prognosis which depends principally on the extent of myocardial damage.

(ii) *First degree and type I second degree block*: occur in 10% of infarcts. The site of block is above or within the atrioventricular node and progression to complete heart block is uncommon. Survival is not affected.

Table 6.16

INDICATIONS FOR TEMPORARY PACING IN ACUTE MYOCARDIAL INFARCTION

Sinus bradycardia (symptomatic, unresponsive to atropine)
Mobitz type II 2° atrioventricular block
Complete heart block
New bilateral bundle branch defects
  RBBB + LAFB
  RBBB + LPFB
  Alternating RBBB and LBBB
  LBBB with 1° A–V block

RBBB = right bundle branch block; LBBB = left bundle branch block; LA(P)FB = left anterior (posterior) fascicular block; 1° atrioventricular block = first degree atrioventricular block

(iii) *Type II second degree block*: occurs in only 1% of infarcts, usually anterior, and often progresses to complete heart block. The site of block is distal to the His bundle.

Left ventricular failure

Pulmonary venous congestion or frank pulmonary oedema on the chest X-ray provide the earliest diagnosis of left ventricular failure—breathlessness and crepitations are late signs. Radiographic signs are, however, slow to clear after effective diuretic and/or vasodilator treatment. The use of intravenous diuretics and vasodilators is discussed in Chapter 11. In patients who fail to respond promptly the measurement of pulmonary capillary wedge pressure (PCWP) using a Swan–Ganz catheter is valuable in the titration of intravenous vasodilators and inotropic agents. Forrester *et al.* have used haemodynamic monitoring to identify subsets of patients as a guide to treatment and prognosis (Table 6.17). Some overlap between subsets is inevitable in practice.

Cardiogenic shock

Definition (United States National Heart, Lung and Blood Institute)

(i) Systolic blood pressure less than 90 mmHg, or 60 mmHg below the previous basal level.

Table 6.17

HAEMODYNAMIC SUBSETS IN ACUTE MYOCARDIAL INFARCTION (AFTER FORRESTER)

Subset	*Cardiac index (litres/min/m²)*	*PCWP (mmHg)*	*Treatment*	*Mortality (%)*
I No failure	> 2·2	< 18	None	2
II Pulmonary congestion	> 2·2	> 18	Normal blood pressure: diuretics Elevated blood pressure: vasodilators	10
III Peripheral hypoperfusion	< 2·2	< 18	Elevated heart rate: volume expansion Depressed heart rate: pacing	22
IV Congestion and hypoperfusion	< 2·2	> 18	Depressed blood pressure: inotropes Normal blood pressure: vasodilators	55

(ii) Evidence of reduced blood flow as shown by all of the following:
   (a) urine output less than 20 ml/h, usually with a low sodium content;
   (b) impaired mental function;
   (c) peripheral vasoconstriction with cold, clammy skin.

Management None is consistently effective. Useful measures include:

(i) Analgesia, oxygenation, prompt treatment of arrhythmias, correction of electrolyte and acid–base imbalance.
(ii) Urinary catheter to monitor urine flow.
(iii) Haemodynamic monitoring using a Swan–Ganz catheter and intra-arterial pressure monitoring to control volume depletion, inotropic or vasodilator drugs as required.
(iv) Intra-aortic balloon counterpulsation to reduce afterload and improve coronary arterial perfusion. This is useful only in the short-term and does not alter the prognosis unless there is a surgically correctable lesion, such as ventricular septal rupture or acute mitral regurgitation.

Prognosis Necrosis of about 40% of the left ventricular myocardium has occurred. Mortality is approximately 80% at 1 month.

Right ventricular infarction

Diagnosis Right ventricular failure (raised JVP and hepatic engorgement) without radiographic or clinical signs of pulmonary congestion.

Clinical features Usually associated with inferior myocardial infarction. Swan–Ganz monitoring shows elevated right atrial and right ventricular diastolic pressures with a normal or modestly elevated PCWP. Arterial hypotension is common.

Management Inotropic drugs and fluid loading are required. Misdiagnosis of right ventricular infarction as a manifestation of left ventricular failure is hazardous since diuretics and vasodilators cause haemodynamic deterioration. The condition is probably underdiagnosed.

Mechanical complications of acute myocardial infarction

Rupture of the interventricular septum This presents during the first week after infarction as sudden haemodynamic deterioration accompanied by a new pansystolic murmur maximal at the lower left sternal edge. The size of the defect determines the magnitude of the left to right shunt and hence the clinical severity. The shunt is readily detected by demonstrating a 'stepup' in oxygen saturation in the right ventricle and pulmonary artery on Swan–Ganz catheterisation.

Anterior infarcts are responsible slightly more often than inferior. Recent results favour prompt surgical repair after acute haemodynamic stabilisation.

Rupture of papillary muscles This may be partial or complete. Complete rupture causes sudden severe mitral regurgitation and gross pulmonary oedema which is usually fatal. Partial rupture with acute mitral regurgitation presents as haemodynamic deterioration with a new pansystolic murmur. Clinical distinction from ventricular septal rupture is often impossible but is easily made by Swan–Ganz catheterisation; the PCW pressure waveform shows massive 'v' waves and there is no 'stepup' in oxygen saturation. In severe acute mitral regurgitation aortic balloon counterpulsation controls gross left heart failure prior to emergency mitral valve replacement.

Left ventricular free wall rupture This accounts for 10% of hospital deaths from acute myocardial infarction. It is most common in the first week and in elderly, female hypertensive patients with large infarction. Immediate death from cardiac tamponade is usual.

Left ventricular aneurysm This develops in up to 15% of patients surviving myocardial infarction. The diagnosis is suggested by a palpable left precordial systolic 'bulging', persistent S–T segment elevation on the ECG and a localised deformity of the radiographic heart shadow.

It is confirmed by two-dimensional echocardiography and left ventricular angiography. Left ventricular aneurysms are often asymptomatic and rupture is rare, although mural thrombus in the sac may cause systemic embolism. Surgical excision is indicated for intractable left ventricular failure or persistent ventricular tachyarrhythmias.

Embolism

Systemic embolism Left ventricular thrombus develops over an acute infarct in just under one-half of patients, and often resolves spontaneously. Clinically recognisable systemic emboli occur in under 5% of patients and prophylactic oral anticoagulation is not generally advocated.

Venous thrombosis and embolism Early mobilisation and low dose anticoagulation has reduced the incidence of death from pulmonary embolism to a rarity.

Dressler's syndrome

Local pericarditis occurs in 50% of patients during the first week of infarction. It is easily confused with Dressler's (post-myocardial infarction) syndrome—pericarditis, pleurisy and pneumonitis—which appears 1–6 weeks after infarction and has an autoimmune mechanism. The pain and fever are usually controlled with non-steroidal anti-inflammatory drugs.

Following myocardial infarction

The management of convalescence from myocardial infarction is often woefully neglected. Consideration must be given to:

(i) *Explanation and reassurance* throughout the admission are essential to successful rehabilitation. Anxiety, depression, loss of confidence, marital problems, sexual dysfunction and inappropriate fear of death become serious, permanent problems unless sympathetic counselling is given from the outset.

(ii) *Exercise*: guarded increase in normal activity is advised, including daily walks of 1·6–3·2 km (1–2 miles) by 4–6 weeks after infarction. Isometric exercise and any activity causing angina or undue breathlessness is avoided. Sexual activity may resume when the patient is capable of climbing one or two flights of stairs normally.

(iii) *Employment*: 85% of uncomplicated infarct survivors return to work by 3 months. Ability to work prior to infarction is obviously an important factor in subsequent employment. Cardiac rehabilitation programmes can favourably influence the rate of return to work. Special regulations may apply; heavy goods (HGV) and public service (PSV) licences are almost invariably withdrawn. Private licence driving, in the absence of symptoms, may recommence at eight weeks.

(iv) *Risk factor modification*: ex-smokers have half the subsequent mortality of those who continue to smoke after infarction. There is no consistent evidence that reduction of elevated blood pressure or lipid levels is useful. Reduction of stress, attainment of optimal weight and a 'healthy lifestyle' are generally advocated.

(v) *Secondary prevention*: see Chapter 14.

(vi) *Postinfarct assessment*: the concept of 'risk stratification' attempts to identify patients at increased risk of further infarction or premature death. At 6–8 weeks after infarction a poor prognosis is indicated by:
   (a) poor exercise tolerance or electrocardiographic evidence of myocardial ischaemia or exercise stress testing;
   (b) frequent or repetitive ventricular ectopic activity on 24 h ambulatory electrocardiographic monitoring.

Whether medical or surgical treatment improves the prognosis in such patients is not yet known. Cardiac catheterisation and angiography is best reserved for patients with significant postinfarction angina.

Prognosis

Many factors determine the prognosis following acute myocardial infarction. The most important are the state of left ventricular function and the severity of atherosclerosis in the coronary vessels supplying the remaining viable myocardium. Overall, the mortality in the first year following myocardial infarction, including hospital mortality, is 20%. Thereafter mortality is 5% per year and between 5 and 11 years there is no excess risk if the patient remains asymptomatic.

FURTHER READING

Campbell R.W.F., Murray A., Julian D.G. (1981). Ventricular arrhythmias in first 12 hours of acute myocardial infarction: Natural history study. *Br. Heart J.*, **46,** 351.

Chesebro J.H., Holmes D.R., Mock M.B., Gersh B.J., Fuster V. (1988). Thrombolysis in acute myocardial infarction. *Cardiology Clinics*, **6,** 1.

Christie L.G., Conti C.R. (1981). Systematic approach to evaluation of angina-like chest pain: Pathophysiology and clinical testing with emphasis on objective documentation of myocarfdial ischaemia. *Am. Heart J.*, **102,** 897.

Cohn P.F. (1987). Silent myocardial ischaemia: present status. *Mod. Con. Cardiovasc. Dis.*, **56,** 1.

Cooper I.C., Signy M., Webb-Peploe M.M., Coltart D.J. (1987). Coronary angioplasty. *Postgrad. Med. J.*, **63,** 327.

Davies M.J. (1981). Pathological view of sudden cardiac death. *Br Heart J.*, **45,** 88.

Dawber T.D. (1980). *The Framingham Study*. Harvard University Press, Cambridge, Mass. and London.

Feldman R.L. (1987). A review of medical therapy for coronary artery spasm. *Circulation*, **75,** V-96.

Forfar J.C., Irving J.B., Miller H.C., Kitchin A.H., Wheatley D.J. (1980). The management of ventricular septal rupture following myocardial infarction. *J. Med.*, **47,** 205.

Forrester J.S., Diamond G., Chatterjee K. and Swan H.J.C. (1976). Medical therapy of acute myocardial infarction by application of haemodynamic subsets. *N. Engl. J. Med.*, **295,** 1404.

ISIS-2 Collaborative Group (1988). Randomized trial of intravenous streptokinase, oral aspirin, both, or neither among 17,187 cases of suspected myocardial infarction. *Lancet*, **2,** 349.

Nellen M., Naurer B., Goodwin J.F. (1973). Value of physical examination in acute myocardial infarction. *Br. Heart J.*, **35,** 777.

Norris R.M., Caughey D.E., Mercer C.J., Scott P.J. (1974). Prognosis after myocardial infarction—six years follow-up. *Br. Heart J.*, **36,** 786.

Smitherman T.C. (1986). Unstable angina pectoris: the first half century: natural history, pathophysiology and treatment. *Am. J. Med. Sci.*, **292,** 395.

Varnauskas E. (1986). Lessons learned from the three randomised coronary by-pass surgery trials. *Cardiology*, **73,** 204.

Chapter 7

Structure and Functions of the Heart and Circulation

The primary function of the heart is to deliver oxygenated blood to the peripheral tissues according to their metabolic needs. The adult heart weighs 250–350 g and pumps a cardiac output of 5 litres/min at rest which can increase to 30 litres/min during exercise. Intracardiac and intravascular pressures are maintained within narrow limits during normal function.

The circulation is the transport system for oxygen, nutrients, waste products of cellular metabolism, hormones and body defences. It serves to regulate body heat.

EMBRYOLOGY

The heart begins to form at the end of the 3rd week. Heart-forming cells in the cephalic portion of the embryo collect into solid strands across the midline and down each side which acquire a lumen forming contractile *endocardial tubes*. As the embryo folds the two tubes fuse into a single endocardial tube. Differentiation of surrounding mesoderm results in a tube consisting of three layers—endocardium, myocardium and pericardium. During the fourth week, at the 5 mm embryo stage, rapid growth of the heart tube leads to longitudinal bending into a *cardiac loop* with cephalic and caudal limbs. Grooves appear in the heart tube as it bends demarcating the primitive heart chambers (Fig. 7.1).

Between 4 and 8 weeks the following changes occur to form a definitive heart with four chambers and four valves.

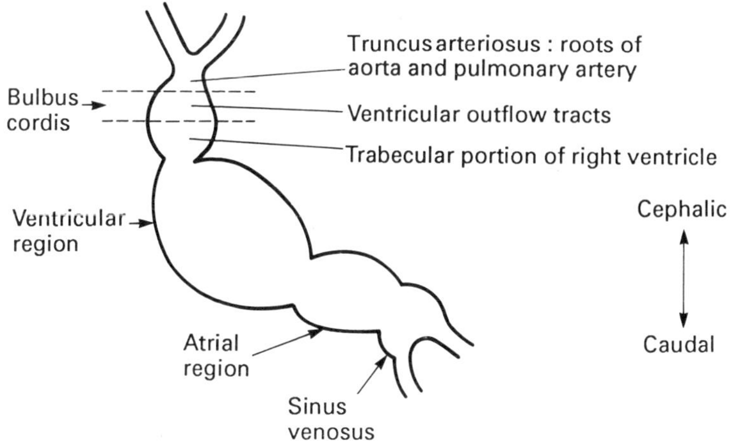

Fig. 7.1. Diagrammatic representation of the cardiac loop

Septation of the Atria and Atrioventricular Canal

The division of the common atrial region into a right and left side begins with the formation of the *septum primum* which grows down from the atrial roof towards the atrioventricular canal. At the same time anterior and posterior thickenings, the *endocardial cushions*, develop in the canal and eventually fuse forming the right and left atrioventricular canals. The gap between the septum primum and the fusing endocardial cushions is the *ostium primum*. Further growth of the septum primum and endocardial cushions closes the ostium primum but before this is complete the septum primum develops a hole in its upper part, the *ostium secundum*. During the 7th week the *septum secundum* grows down from the roof of the right atrium to overlap the ostium secundum. The residual gap between the two atria is termed the *foramen ovale* through which blood flows from right to left during fetal life.

Abnormal development of the atrial septum

Normally the septum primum and septum secundum fuse. In one-quarter of adult hearts a catheter can be passed from right atrium to left atrium through a *patent foramen ovale*, although no shunting of blood occurs because the higher left atrial pressure keeps the overlapping edges of the foramen ovale together.

Abnormal development of either atrial septum may result in a persistent opening between the two atria, an *ostium secundum atrial septal defect*. Complete failure of septal development results in the condition of *common atrium*.

Abnormal development of the atrioventricular canal

Normally the endocardial cushions:

(i) Fuse to form the right and left atrioventricular canals in which develop the tricuspid and mitral valves respectively.
(ii) Help form the upper (membranous) part of the interventricular septum.
(iii) Help close the ostium primum.

Total failure of fusion thus results in a *common atrioventricular canal* containing abnormal valve leaflets. Partial failure of fusion may result in an *ostium primum atrial septal defect* usually associated with a cleft in the anterior mitral valve leaflet.

Septation of the Ventricles

The interventricular septum has an upper membranous part, below the aortic root, which is formed partly from endocardial cushion tissue and a lower muscular part which develops from the floor of the bulboventricular region.

Defects in the membranous part of the interventricular septum are seen frequently as isolated lesions. Defects in the muscular part are less common and may be multiple. Complete absence of the interventricular septum is usually associated with transposition of the aorta and pulmonary artery.

Development of the Great Arterial Trunks and Semilunar Valves

During the 5th–7th weeks ridges of tissue develop to form a septum which divides the cephalic part of the truncus forming the aortic and pulmonary trunks. Rotation of the septum locates the pulmonary trunk anterior and to the right of the aorta. Secondary ridges of tissue in the roots of the aorta and pulmonary artery develop into the semilunar valves.

Anomalous development of the septum between the aortic and pulmonary trunks may result in *tetralogy of Fallot* or *transposition of the great vessels*. Fusion of the semilunar valve cusps commonly results in *stenosis of the aortic or pulmonary valves*.

FUNCTIONAL ANATOMY

The circulation is a closed system comprising two major divisions, the pulmonary circulation and the systemic circulation. The two divisions are hydraulic circuits connected in series. Unidirectional flow is ensured by normal function of the cardiac valves. Each division consists of a pump, a distributing system, an exchange system and a collecting system (Table 7.1).

Table 7.1

PULMONARY AND SYSTEMIC CIRCULATIONS

	Pulmonary circulation	*Systemic circulation*
Pump	Right ventricle	Left ventricle
Distributing system	Pulmonary arteries	Aorta, arterial branches
Exchange system	Capillaries	Capillaries
Collecting system	Pulmonary veins	Systemic veins, venae cavae
Operating pressure (systolic pressure)	Low (25 mmHg)	High (120 mmHg)
Blood volume	15%	85%
Pump wall thickness	2 mm	10 mm
Resistance to flow	Low	High

The Heart

The heart lies in the mediastinum related anteriorly to the

sternum, posteriorly to the oesophagus and descending aorta between the fourth and ninth vertebrae, and laterally to the lungs which envelop it except for the cardiac notch in the upper lobe of the left lung, an important window for echocardiography. The right heart lies anterior and to the right of the left heart so that the atrial and ventricular septa lie at 45° to the median plane. The pericardium is a strong, stiff sac which surrounds the heart and is attached to the aorta, venae cavae and pulmonary vessels and diaphragm. The inner visceral pericardium is intimately attached to the surface of the heart and reflects back to form the outer parietal pericardium. The resulting sac normally contains about 50 ml of fluid. Functions of the pericardium include anatomical fixation of the heart, and its protection from surrounding structures. However, clinical cardiac function is unaffected by surgical removal or congenital absence of the pericardium.

Cardiac chambers

The atria

The atria are thin-walled structures which act as reservoirs of blood and 'priming pumps' for the ventricles.

The *right atrium* receives systemic venous return from the superior vena cava, the inferior vena cava and the coronary sinus. Its smooth-walled cavity is separated from the trabeculated right atrial appendage by the crista terminalis. The *left atrium* receives pulmonary venous return from the pulmonary veins and has a trabeculated appendage. Posteriorly it is separated from the pericardial space by the oblique sinus of the pericardium. For this reason an echo-free space is not seen behind the left atrium in the detection of a pericardial effusion by echocardiography; a retrocardiac pleural effusion often produces an echo-free space behind the left atrium. In normal sinus rhythm there are three components to atrial function:

(i) Atrial systole enhances ventricular filling by about 25%, the increased stretch of the ventricular myocardial fibres resulting in a greater force of contraction (Starling's law).
(ii) Facilitation of venous return by maintenance of a low filling pressure.

(iii) Atrial systole assists in the closure of the mitral and tricuspid valves. After atrial systole pressure in the atria falls more rapidly than in the ventricles, helping the valves to close with the onset of ventricular systole.

The ventricles

The ventricles are the main pump elements of the circulation. The cavity of the *right ventricle* is trabeculated and its septal surface displays a prominent band of muscle, the trabecula septomarginalis. The right ventricular outflow tract is a muscular tube terminating at the pulmonary valve. The right ventricle contains the tricuspid valve and its three papillary muscles (anterior, posterior and medial). The tricuspid valve is not in fibrous continuity with the pulmonary valve, being separated from it by the crista supraventricularis.

The *left ventricle* is finely trabeculated and contains the mitral valve with its two papillary muscles (anterior and posterior). The mitral and aortic valves are in fibrous continuity so the outflow tract of the left ventricle is formed by the interventricular septum and the anterior cusp of the mitral valve. There is no infundibulum.

The ventricles receive blood from the atria at approximately zero (that is, atmospheric) pressure. The muscle mass of each ventricle is proportional to the pressure work done and so the ratio of peak systolic pressure developed in each ventricle is similar to the ratio of their wall thickness at approximately 5:1 (see Table 7.1).

The Circulation

The systemic circulation is a high resistance circuit. The aorta is predominantly an elastic structure with smaller proportions of smooth muscle and fibrous tissue. Towards the periphery the arterial vessel walls became thinner and smooth muscle predominates. Pulsatile flow from the heart is converted to continuous flow at the periphery by distension of the aorta and arterial branches during ventricular systole, elastic recoil of the arteries during ventricular diastole and frictional resistance of the arterioles. In the distributing system blood velocity is high while frictional resistance and pressure drop are small. Peripheral resistance is determined principally at the arterioles and is reflected in the sharp fall in pressure between the arterioles and the capillaries. The total cross-sectional area of the capillaries is extremely high so blood flow is slow allowing full exchange of diffusable substances between blood and the tissues across the single-celled (1 μm) capillary wall.

The collecting system of venules, veins and venae cavae contains 60% of the blood volume. As the central veins are approached the vessel walls of the system contain increasing amounts of fibrous tissue and smooth muscle, total cross-sectional area decreases and blood velocity increases. The capacity of the venous system is capable of wide variation. Since the total blood volume is constant the venous pool allows for redistribution of blood under changing physiological conditions.

The *pulmonary circulation* operates in a similar manner to the systemic circulation but is a low volume, low pressure, low resistance circuit comprising shorter, thinner vessels.

Myocardial cell

The contractile mechanism of cardiac and skeletal muscle is similar. However, important structural and functional differences exist (Table 7.2).

Structure and function of the sarcomere

The resting sarcomere is between 2·0 and 2·2 μm in length from Z line to Z line. Thin *actin* filaments attached to the Z line interdigitate with thick *myosin* filaments producing the familiar banded appearance on electron microscopy (Fig. 7.2). The essential process of contraction and relaxation is thought to occur in the following way. When the cell is depolarised a sudden rise in the intracellular concentration of free Ca^{2+} ions activates the proteins of the actin and myosin filaments and the *crossbridges* between them. Repetitive attachment and detachment of the crossbridges pulls the thin actin strands along the thick myosin strands, pulling the Z lines towards each other and causing contraction of the myofibril. Relaxation ensues when free Ca^{2+} is pumped out of direct contact with the myofibrils by the cell membranes. The protein strands are thereby deactivated and recoil to their resting length. In the intact heart this produces a

Table 7.2

DIFFERENCES BETWEEN CARDIAC AND SKELETAL MUSCLE

Cardiac muscle	*Skeletal muscle*
Functional syncytium of branched, interconnecting fibres	Discrete fibres
Indefinite, repetitive contraction	Limited repetitive or sustained 'tetanic' contraction
All-or-none-response to depolarisation	Graded response
Action potential has plateau phase during which extracellular Ca^{2+} enters cell via 'slow calcium' channels	Action potential has no plateau phase. Contraction is independent of extracellular Ca^{2+}
No oxygen debt	Capable of anaerobic metabolism and oxygen debt
Numerous mitochondria	Fewer mitochondria

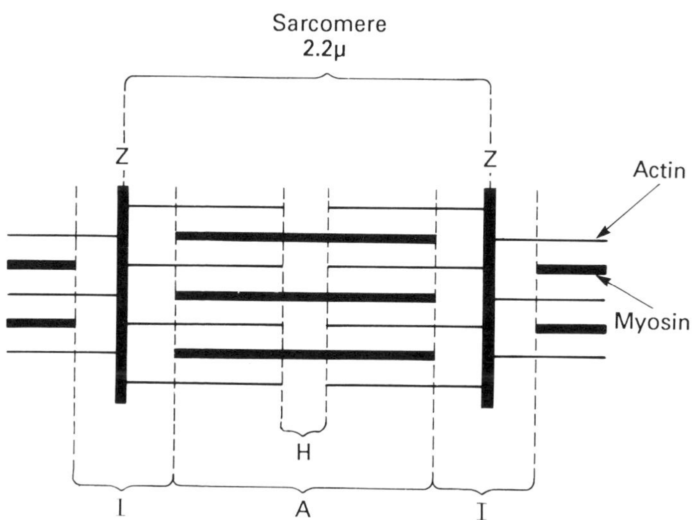

Fig. 7.2. The sarcomere showing overlapping filaments of thin actin and thick myosin

small negative pressure in the ventricles which may assist their diastolic filling.

It is now necessary to consider in more detail the structure of the sarcomere. Four proteins are involved in the contraction process—actin, myosin, tropomyosin, and troponin complex. Troponin complex itself comprises three proteins—troponin C which binds calcium, troponin I which inhibits interaction between actin and myosin, and troponin T which attaches the troponin complex to tropomyosin. Tropomyosin and troponin complex exert a regulatory effect on the fundamental actin–myosin reaction during excitation–contraction coupling.

Each thin actin filament consists of two chains of actin molecules wound round each other in a helix. In the groove of the helix lies a tropomyosin strand. Attached to every sixth actin molecule is a troponin complex. These composite filaments are arranged in groups of six around one thick myosin filament. The myosin filament is made up of myosin molecules in helical arrangement and each myosin molecule has a protruding *head* which forms a crossbridge with an active site on the actin strand. The myosin head contains the enzyme myofibrillar ATP-ase which reduces ATP to provide energy for the interaction of crossbridges.

Excitation–contraction coupling

Free calcium ions (Ca^{2+}) are the link between excitation and contraction. Their delivery to initiate contraction and subsequent removal during relaxation depends on special structural features of the myocardial cell—the transverse (T) tubules of the sarcolemma and the sarcoplasmic reticulum.

The *sarcolemma* is the membrane which surrounds the myocardial cell. The *T-tubules* are invaginations of sarcolemma from the cell surface which pass down to each Z line of each myofibril. Within the myocardial cells is an extensive *sarcoplasmic reticulum*, a tubing system permeating the whole cell, which acts as an intracellular store of Ca^{2+}. Dilatations of the sarcoplasmic reticulum, the lateral cysternae, are located near the Z lines and are in close contact with the T-tubules.

The T-tubules allow rapid transmission of electrical depolarisation from the outside of the cell to its interior, releasing previously bound Ca^{2+} from storage sites in the sarcoplasmic reticulum and lateral cisternae into the cytoplasm. The release of this so called 'activator Ca^{2+}' initiates the contraction process by combining with troponin C which releases the inhibitor troponin I and moves tropomyosin out of the way so that actin molecules can form a crossbridge with the myosin heads. The number of crossbridges activated simultaneously determines the resultant force of contraction, and this number is related to the intracellular Ca^{2+} concentration.

Summary of the excitation–contraction mechanism

Precise details of the entire mechanism are not known with certainty but the following is a probable sequence of events.

(i) The cardiac impulse begins with a spontaneous discharge from the sinoatrial node which passes through the atrial myocardium, through the atrioventricular node, bundle of His, bundle branches and Purkinje fibres to the ventricular myocardium. The sum of the action potentials affecting each cell in the atrial and ventricular myocardium is recorded at the body surface as the electrocardiogram.

(ii) Depolarisation of the myocardial cell membrane (excitation) results from a sequence of changes in selective permeability to Na^+, Ca^{2+} and K^+. This sequence of voltage changes is the action potential. The resting membrane potential is -80 mV. During the first, rapid phase of the action potential Na^+ floods into the cell through 'fast channels' carrying positive charge. When the voltage has reached -40 mV the membrane allows the ingress of extracellular Ca^{2+} through 'slow channels'.

(iii) Deplorisation of the cell membrane (sarcolemma and T-tubules) and the entry into the cytoplasm of extracellular Ca^{2+} triggers the release of previously bound Ca^{2+} from the sarcoplasmic reticulum and cisternae. If the cytoplasmic concentration of Ca^{2+} is insufficient contraction will not be triggered.

(iv) The combination of activator Ca^{2+} and troponin complex removes the inhibitory effect of tropomyosin allowing the interaction of myosin heads with corresponding sites on the actin filaments–crossbridge formation.

(v) The crossbridges act as a 'rachet' mechanism, pulling the actin and myosin strands over each other and resulting in contraction of the myofibril.

(vi) After the plateau phase of the action potential intracellular Ca^{2+} is pumped out of the cell or is rebound to the sarcoplasmic reticulum, crossbridges are deactivated and the myofibril relaxes.

Energy supply

Free fatty acids, glucose and lactate are the major substrates for myocardial metabolism. Oxygen is consumed in the mitochondria to generate adenosine triphosphate (ATP) most of which reacts with creatine to form creatine phosphate. Energy is transported in this form throughout the cell. ATP is regenerated and its energy released by the enzyme ATPase at sites where energy is required. More than 80% of myocardial energy supply is required for contraction.

Myocardial function

The principal factors affecting myocardial function are preload, afterload and myocardial contractility. Their significance in pathological states is discussed in Chapters 8 and 10.

Preload

Preload is the extent to which the myocardium is stretched prior to the next ventricular contraction. Starling's law implies that, within physiological limits, the force of myocardial contraction depends on the initial length of the myocardial fibres—the greater the length the more forceful the contraction. The Frank–Starling curve relates stroke volume (the volume of blood ejected from the ventricle during one ventricular systole) to end diastolic volume. End diastolic volume is determined by venous return and the 'pump-priming' or 'booster effect' of atrial systole. As end diastolic volume increases, stroke volume increases until over-stretching occurs. At this point the Frank–Starling curve becomes flat. Further increases in end diastolic volume do not produce an increase in stroke volume. In clinical practice it is more usual to measure end diastolic pressure. The pulmonary wedge pressure, or indirect left atrial pressure, serves as an indication of left ventricular end diastolic pressure under many circumstances.

Afterload

Afterload is the ventricular wall tension during ventricular ejection. It is determined by the impedance imposed by the peripheral vascular resistance. Left ventricular afterload is increased by pathological forces opposing ejection such as aortic valvular stenosis and systemic arterial hypertension.

Myocardial contractility

During constant preload and afterload the force and velocity of contraction depend on the state of myocardial contractility. A precise definition of contractility is difficult—it has humorously been described as the 'myocardial nick'. Myocardial contractility is increased by sympathetic stimulation, inotropic drugs and increased heart rate. It is decreased by hypoxia, beta-adrenergic blocking drugs, many antiarrhythmic drugs and by intrinsic myocardial disease. The Frank–Starling curve is shifted upwards and to the left by increased contractility, and downwards and to the right by decreased contractility.

Pressure and volume changes during the cardiac cycle

The cardiac cycle (Fig. 7.3) is often described in terms of the pressure and volume changes occurring in the left ventricle: I: isovolumetric contraction period; II: systolic ejection period; III: isovolumetric relaxation period; IV: filling phase.

Isovolumetric contraction period

With the onset of left ventricular contraction the mitral valve closes producing the first heart sound. Intraventricular pressure rises rapidly but since the aortic valve is not yet open the volume of the ventricle remains unchanged.

Systolic ejection period

As soon as left ventricular pressure exceeds aortic pressure the

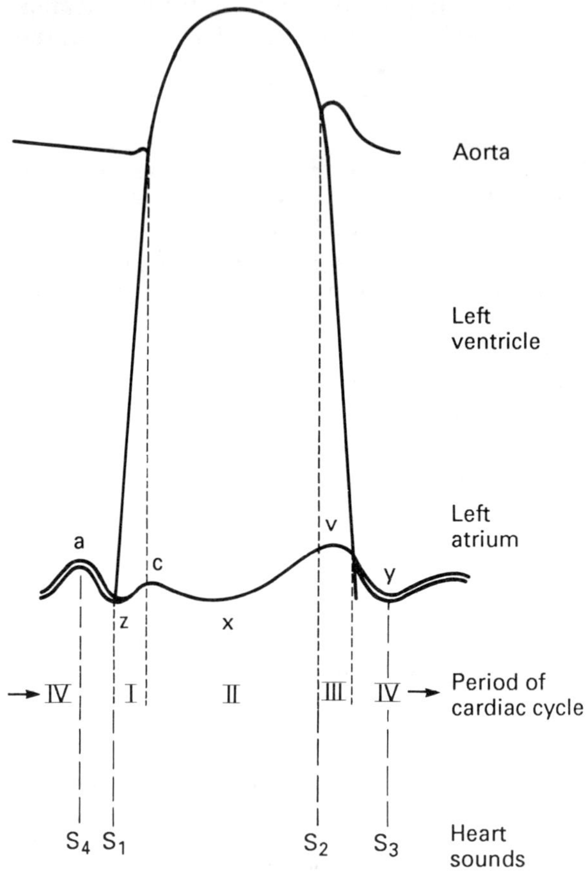

Fig. 7.3. The cardiac cycle; ... period of the cardiac cycle designated by Roman numerals (see text); --- timing of heart sounds

aortic valve opens and blood is ejected rapidly into the aorta. As ventricular systole proceeds the rate of ejection falls until the end of systole when ejection ceases. The quantity of blood delivered into the aorta during this period is the *stroke volume*, and the ventricle is left more than half empty. The stroke volume divided by the initial ventricular volume is called the *ejection fraction*, which is one of the most commonly used indices of ventricular function.

Isovolumetric relaxation period

Shortly after ejection ceases pressure in the ventricle falls below that in the aorta and the aortic valve closes generating the second heart sound. The dicrotic notch is seen on the aortic pressure tracing at this time. As diastole begins left ventricular pressure falls rapidly but its volume remains the same because the aortic and mitral valves are shut.

Filling phase

When left ventricular pressure falls below left atrial pressure the mitral valve opens and rapid passive filling of the ventricle occurs. This may generate a third heart sound. As the ventricle fills flow from the atrium diminishes and pressures in the atrium and ventricle equilibrate. Echocardiography has shown that the mitral valve closes during this period of diastole. In late diastole, however, atrial systole sharply reopens the mitral valve causing rapid active filling of the ventricle. A fourth heart sound may occur at this time. Shortly after the end of atrial systole the cycle is ready to begin again.

The atrial pressure tracing

The left atrial pressure tracing (see Fig. 7.3) shows three positive waves designated a, c and v each followed by a descent designated z, x and y respectively. These represent the following events:

- 'a': atrial systole
- 'z': atrial relaxation
- 'c': mitral valve cusps bulge into the left atrium during the isovolumetric contraction period
- 'x': mitral ring descends as the ventricular volume falls during the systolic ejection period
- 'v': left atrial pressure rises with increasing pulmonary venous return during ventricular systole when the mitral valve is shut. The rise in pressure ceases as the mitral valve opens, and the peak of the 'v' wave occurs at this point
- 'y': blood flows from the atrium to the ventricle during this time.

The right heart

The same events occur in the right atrium and right ventricle except that:

(i) The pressures are lower.
(ii) The events occur slightly later so that the tricuspid first heart sound follows the mitral first heart sound and the pulmonary second heart sound follows the aortic second heart sound. The timing of the second heart sounds are further affected by respiration. The negative intrathoracic pressure during inspiration enhances systemic venous return to the right side of the heart and decreases pulmonary venous return to the left side of the heart. As a result right ventricular systole takes slightly longer while left ventricular systole is slightly shorter. Thus pulmonary valve closure is relatively later and aortic valve closure relatively earlier resulting in increased 'splitting' of the second heart sound on auscultation during inspiration. Setting aside these transient small variations the stroke volume of the right and left ventricles are equal.

The atrial pressure waves described are derived from direct intra-atrial pressure recordings. Clinical inspection of the jugular venous pressure waveform reveals only the 'a' and 'v' waves and the 'x' and 'y' descents.

FURTHER READING

Berne R.M., Levy M.N. (1981). *Cardiovascular physiology*, ed. 4. C.V. Mosby, St. Louis.

Shepherd J.T., Vanhoutte P.M. (1979). *The human cardiovascular system, facts and concepts*. Raven Press, New York.

Chapter 8

Valvular Heart Disease

Background

Valvular heart disease in adults affects predominantly the mitral and aortic valves. In rheumatic heart disease the mitral valve is affected in almost all patients, the aortic valve in 35% and the tricuspid valve in less than 15%. The decline in rheumatic fever in developed countries means that rheumatic disease may not now be the commonest aetiology of valvular lesions, and degenerative conditions of the mitral and aortic valves are increasingly recognised. The clinical assessment of valvular heart disease requires consideration of the underlying cause and its pathophysiology.

Natural history of valvular heart disease

The most important goal in the evaluation of valvular heart disease is to decide the proper timing of surgery. The natural history of a valvular lesion, upon which the decision is based, depends principally on its aetiology and pathophysiology. In particular an understanding of left ventricular overload is central to the course and management of aortic and mitral valve disease.

Pathophysiology of left ventricular overload

See Table 8.1. Left-sided valvular lesions may increase the work of the left ventricle because of:

(i) Pressure overload.
(ii) Volume overload.
(iii) A combination of both.

Table 8.1

THE EFFECT OF LEFT VENTRICULAR LOADING CONDITIONS AND PHYSIOLOGICAL STATE IN VALVULAR HEART DISEASE

	LV overload	*LV work*	*Adaptive process*	*Vasodilatation*	*Isotonic exercise* $CO\uparrow PVR\downarrow HR\uparrow$	*Isometric exercise* $CO\uparrow PVR\uparrow HR\rightarrow$
Aortic stenosis	Pressure	+ + +	Hypertrophy	DANGER! Hypotension	↑gradient	↑gradient
Aortic regurgitation	Volume	+ +	Dilatation and hypertrophy	↓leak	↓leak	↑leak
Mitral regurgitation	Volume	+	Mainly dilatation	↓leak	↑leak	↑leak

LV = left ventricle, CO = cardiac output, PVR = peripheral vascular resistance, HR = heart rate, ↑ = increased, ↓decreased, → = unchanged.

The severity of valvular gradients and regurgitation varies with the physiological state of the patient. An increase in cardiac output requires a rise in the pressure gradient across a stenotic valve. A decrease in peripheral vascular resistance reduces the amount of aortic and mitral regurgitation and vasodilator drugs make it easier for the left ventricle to eject its stroke volume forwards. In addition, tachycardia decreases aortic regurgitation by shortening ventricular diastole—isotonic exercise is thus well-tolerated.

Pressure overload

The greatest burden on the left ventricle is imposed by the pure pressure overload of aortic stenosis. When aortic stenosis is severe (aortic valve orifice area 0·5 cm^2) the left ventricle must work as hard to overcome the obstruction as it does to maintain peripheral blood pressure. The left ventricle adapts to chronic pressure overload by concentric hypertrophy, the volume of the ventricle being normal or reduced.

Volume overload

Aortic and mitral regurgitation impose a volume overload on the left ventricle. In diastole, normal filling of the ventricle is augmented by the regurgitant volume of blood from the aorta or left atrium respectively. In aortic regurgitation the increased volume of blood must then be ejected wholly into a high pressure chamber, the aorta. In mitral regurgitation part of the increased volume is ejected into a low pressure chamber, the left atrium. The energy cost to the ventricle of aortic regurgitation is therefore less than that of aortic stenosis but more than that of mitral regurgitation. The left ventricle adapts to chronic volume overload by dilatation, the enlarged chamber allowing ejection of a very large total stroke volume.

Chronic effects of left ventricular overload

Ventricular hypertrophy and dilatation may compensate for severe chronic pressure or volume overload for some years but not indefinitely. Left ventricular performance is eventually impaired, at first without irreversible myocardial depression. Finally, myocardial damage is permanent and irreversible. In aortic stenosis the onset of symptoms carries a short life expectancy of 2–5 years and early valve replacement is required. Chronic volume overload is tolerated longer; in aortic regurgitation the average life expectancy is 9 years after the onset of symptoms of left ventricular failure and the natural history of mitral regurgitation is even more gradual.

Implications for management

Severe preoperative left ventricular depression in aortic stenosis is often reversible after aortic valve replacement has relieved the pressure overload. In aortic regurgitation left ventricular function may improve after valve replacement but heart failure continues if surgery has been delayed too long. In mitral regurgitation the 'low pressure leak' (left ventricle to left atrium) can mask deteriorating left ventricular function which may appear well preserved on angiography even when irreversible damage has developed. Mitral valve replacement unmasks the left ventricular damage and the patient has persistent left ventricular failure despite a technically successful operation. Therefore, the primary aim in the assessment and management of valvular heart disease is to decide the proper timing of operation. Surgery must not be delayed so long that the patient is left with irreversible heart failure despite a satisfactory operation. Yet surgery should not be too early because artificial valves may cause embolic or infective complications, and may develop mechanical malfunction. No certain method is yet available which will accurately determine the proper timing of operation in the individual patient. The place of surgery is currently decided by the severity of patient's symptoms and the natural history of the lesion. Serial non-invasive investigations and cardiac catheterisation help to confirm the decision.

MITRAL STENOSIS

Background

Rheumatic heart disease is by far the commonest cause of mitral stenosis, though a history of rheumatic fever is obtained in only 50% of cases; 25% of all patients with rheumatic heart disease have pure mitral stenosis, two-thirds of whom are female. Non-rheumatic causes of mitral stenosis are all rare (Table 8.2); of more importance are conditions which mimic mitral stenosis (Table 8.3). In parallel with rheumatic fever, mitral stenosis is commoner and more rapidly progressive in developing countries.

Pathology

Rheumatic fever causes fusion of the mitral valve cusps, commissures and chordae tendinae resulting in a funnel-shaped

Table 8.2

NON-RHEUMATIC CAUSES OF MITRAL STENOSIS

Congenital
Associated with left heart malformations
Parachute mitral valve (single papillary muscle)

Acquired
Systemic lupus erythematosus (Libman–Sachs endocarditis)
Eosinophilic endocarditis
Obstruction by infective vegetations
Calcified mitral valve ring
Lutembacher's syndrome (chance association of rheumatic mitral stenosis and atrial septal defect)

Table 8.3

CONDITIONS WHICH MAY MIMIC MITRAL STENOSIS

Condition	*Mechanism*
Pure mitral regurgitation	Increased mitral diastolic flow
Ventricular septal defect	Increased mitral diastolic flow
Austin–Flint murmur	Mid-diastolic murmur in moderate–severe aortic regurgitation due to early partial closure of mitral leaflets
Left atrial myxoma	Can mimic all signs of mitral stenosis. Tumour 'plop' simulates opening snap
Tricuspid stenosis	Analogous to mitral stenosis
Atrial septal defect (ostium secundum type)	Increased tricuspid diastolic flow
Cor triatriatum	Left atrium divided into upper and lower chambers by a diaphragm left by failure of reabsorption of common pulmonary vein. Small communicating orifice causes mid-diastolic murmur
Carey-Coombs murmur	Variable, high pitched mid-diastolic murmur due to active mitral valvulitis during acute rheumatic fever

narrowing of the mitral orifice. Calcification of the cusps and valve ring is common. The left atrium is dilated, with mural thrombus usually developing on the free wall. Chronic elevation of left atrial pressure may cause thickening of the pulmonary vessels and multiple small haemorrhages lead to haemosiderosis with subsequent nodular bone formation in the lungs.

Pathophysiology

The normal mitral valve has a cross sectional area of 5 cm^2. Ventricular filling is impaired when the orifice is reduced to 2 cm^2 and a transvalvular pressure gradient develops on exercise. At 1 cm^2, regarded as critical mitral stenosis, a pressure gradient of about 20 mmHg is required to maintain a normal cardiac output at rest. The elevated left atrial pressure causes a passive rise in pulmonary venous and pulmonary capillary pressures resulting in breathlessness on exertion. If pulmonary capillary pressure rises rapidly to exceed 25 mmHg, usually with exertion or the onset of artrial fibrillation, pulmonary oedema develops. If the pressure rise is gradual the slow exudation of fluid causes thickening of the capillary–alveolar wall and much higher pressures are tolerated without the development of severe pulmonary oedema. In severe mitral stenosis the chronic elevation of left atrial pressures leads to active constriction of the pulmonary arterioles. This protects the lungs from pulmonary oedema during a sudden rise in right ventricular pressure on exercise, but causes a disproportionate elevation of pulmonary artery pressure with eventual right ventricular failure and functional tricuspid regurgitation. The process is usually reversed by mitral valve surgery, but in extreme cases structural changes in the pulmonary arterioles result in irreversible pulmonary hypertension.

Symptoms

Mitral stenosis may present with any of the following symptoms.

(i) *Effort intolerance* due to gradually increasing breathlessness is the usual presentation. Orthopnoea and paroxysmal nocturnal dyspnoea may develop abruptly with the onset of atrial fibrillation and in pregnancy. *Fatigue*, due to a low resting cardiac output and its failure to rise on exercise, is characteristic of more severe mitral stenosis.

(ii) *Recurrent chest infection* often accompanied by increased dyspnoea and pulmonary oedema.
(iii) *Haemoptysis* due to pulmonary oedema, pulmonary infarction, chest infection or the rupture of a dilated bronchial vein (pulmonary apoplexy).
(iv) *Pulmonary oedema* and right heart failure.
(v) *Angina pectoris* may be caused by elevated right ventricular pressure or coronary arterial embolism as well as coexistent atheromatous coronary artery disease.
(vi) *Systemic embolism* from the left atrium occurs in 20% of patients not treated with anticoagulants and is recurrent in 25% of victims; 50% of clinical emboli are cerebral. Predisposing factors are atrial fibrillation and a large left atrium but the stenosis need only be mild.
(vii) *Ortner's syndrome* occurs in severe mitral stenosis. Marked dilatation of the pulmonary artery or left atrium may compress the left recurrent laryngeal nerve causing hoarseness.

Signs

The four cardinal auscultatory signs of mitral stenosis are heard when the valve cusps are still mobile (Table 8.4). As the cusps become rigid and calcified the loud first heart sound and opening snap disappear. As pulmonary artery pressure rises additional signs (Table 8.5) appear, and when severe the middiastolic murmur may be inaudible ('silent' mitral stenosis).

Differential diagnosis

Conditions which may mimic the auscultatory signs of mitral stenosis are listed in Table 8.3. They are readily differentiated by associated physical signs and echocardiography.

Investigations

(i) *Echocardiography* is the most useful investigation. It is diagnostic, estimates the severity of stenosis and gives information about the anatomy of the valve cusps. On M-mode echocardiography the diastolic closure rate of the anterior mitral cups (E–F slope) is reduced in rough proportion to the severity of stenosis. Fusion of the

Table 8.4

PHYSICAL SIGNS IN MITRAL STENOSIS

	Sign	*Explanation of sign*
Facies	Malar flush	Peripheral cyanosis and vasoconstriction due to low cardiac output
Arterial pulse	Normal or low volume	Normal or reduced stroke volume
Venous pressure	Normal	Normal right heart pressures
Apex beat	'Tapping'	Palpable first heart sound
Auscultation	Loud S1	Wide closing excursion
	Opening snap	Sudden tensing of stenotic valve leaflets at maximum opening excursion
	Rumbling apical diastolic murmur	Turbulent blood flow. Louder in left lateral position, after exercise, in expiration. *Length* of murmur correlates with severity of stenosis
	Presystolic murmur	In sinus rhythm transvalvular blood flow is accelerated by atrial contraction

anterior and posterior cusps, fibrosis and calcification may be detected. Two-dimensional echocardiography demonstrates the reduced mitral valve orifice area. Doppler echocardiography quantitates the transvalvular gradient.

(ii) *Chest X-ray*: left atrial dilatation is seen as a double outline on the right border of the heart shadow with elevation of the left main bronchus and enlargement of the left atrial appendage below the pulmonary artery on the left border. A lateral film is essential to show valve calcification. In the lung fields upper lobe blood diver-

Table 8.5

PHYSICAL SIGNS OF PULMONARY ARTERIAL HYPERTENSION

Sign	*Explanation of sign*
Left parasternal lift	Right ventricular hypertrophy Tricuspid regurgitation
Loud pulmonary component of second heart sound	Abrupt pulmonary valve closure due to high pulmonary artery diastolic pressure
Tricuspid regurgitation	Right ventricular dilatation
Graham–Steell murmur	Functional pulmonary regurgitation in severe pulmonary hypertension. Mimics aortic regurgitation

sion indicates pulmonary venous hypertension; when left atrial pressure exceeds 25 mmHg pulmonary oedema produces hazy shadowing, lymphatic (Kerley B) lines and effusions.

(iii) *The ECG* is of limited value. In sinus rhythm, left atrial enlargement is indicated by a bifid and prolonged (> 100 ms) P-wave in lead II and a dominant negative component in V1. Atrial fibrillation is more usually present, and right ventricular hypertrophy is seen if pulmonary arterial hypertension has developed.

(iv) *Cardiac catheterisation* is necessary if the severity of stenosis is in doubt and to assess multiple valve lesions or coexistent coronary artery disease. Left atrial (or pulmonary capillary wedge) pressure is increased and there is a diastolic pressure gradient across the mitral valve. Cardiac output is usually reduced. Pulmonary artery pressures may be increased.

Treatment

Medical

(i) *Digoxin* controls the ventricular rate after the onset of atrial fibrillation.

(ii) *Diuretics* alleviate breathlessness and venous congestion associated with fluid retention.

(iii) *Anticoagulants* are essential to reduce the risk of systemic embolism. Left atrial thrombosis develops because of stagnation of blood due to mitral obstruction and atrial fibrillation in a chamber diseased by rheumatic carditis. Embolism is common at the onset of atrial fibrillation and anticoagulation should be commenced urgently with intravenous heparin until oral therapy is established.

(iv) *Antibiotics* have a prophylactic and therapeutic role. Penicillin prophylaxis (benzathine penicillin 0·6–1·2 megaunits intramuscularly every 3 weeks) against recurrent acute rheumatic fever is given to patients under 21 years of age. Amoxycillin 3 g orally is given 1 h before dental extraction to prevent infective endocarditis. Chest infections, often precipitated by pulmonary congestion must be treated promptly with appropriate antibiotics.

Surgical

Mitral valve surgery is indicated for patients significantly disabled by symptoms despite medical treatment whose mitral valve area, calculated by two-dimensional echocardiography Doppler measurements, or cardiac catheterization is less than 1·0 cm^2 (normal 4–5 cm^2). Mitral valvotomy or percutaneous balloon valvuloplasty is suitable when the valve is still mobile, competent and not calcified. Mitral valve replacement is necessary if the cusps are calcified and immobile, and if there is significant mitral regurgitation. Lifelong anticoagulation is necessary after insertion of a mechanical prosthetic valve.

MITRAL REGURGITATION

Background

Mitral regurgitation is commonly associated with mitral stenosis in rheumatic heart disease. However, in the western world pure mitral regurgitation is due mainly to non-rheumatic causes.

Floppy mitral valve (page 232) is the commonest of these, but ischaemic heart disease and infective endocarditis are important. The mitral valve apparatus is a complex mechanism consisting of the mitral annulus, valve leaflets, the chordae tendinae and papillary muscles. Mitral regurgitation may be caused by anatomical faults in any of these structures (Table 8.6).

Disease processes resulting in mitral regurgitation may involve one or several of the anatomical faults in Table 8.6. Conditions causing mitral regurgitation are summarised in Table 8.7.

The circulatory changes and therefore the clinical presentation depends on the speed of onset and severity of mitral regurgitation. *Chronic* mitral regurgitation may be progressive, particularly when due to degenerative disease, but is often well tolerated for many years even when moderately severe. *Acute* mitral regurgitation is often severe and poorly tolerated. The commonest causes are ruptured chordae tendinae, necrosis or rupture of a papillary muscle and prosthetic valve dysfunction (Table 8.7).

Pathophysiology

Pure mitral regurgitation is associated with left ventricular

Table 8.6

ANATOMICAL FAULTS CAUSING MITRAL REGURGITATION

Structure	*Anatomical fault*
Mitral annulus	Dilatation Calcification
Valve cusps	Distortion, scarring Excessive leaflet area Perforation Congenital cleft
Chordae tendineae	Redundancy Contraction Rupture Myxomatous degeneration
Papillary muscles	Dysfunction Necrosis Rupture

Table 8.7

CONDITIONS CAUSING MITRAL REGURGITATION

Mitral valve prolapse	Floppy valve syndrome Dilated valve ring Ruptured chordae tendineae
Ischaemic heart disease	Papillary muscle dysfunction Papillary muscle necrosis and (rarely) rupture
Infective endocarditis	Ruptured chordae tendineae Leaflet perforation Cusp distortion by vegetations
Rheumatic heart disease	Scarring and deformity of cusps, chordae tendineae, and papillary muscles
Cardiomyopathies	Papillary muscle dysfunction in dilated and hypertrophic cardiomyopathy. Fibrosis and distortion of chordae and papillary muscles in endomyocardial fibrosis
Miscellaneous (ageing, hypertension, diabetes, Marfan's syndrome)	Annular calcification
Prosthetic valve dysfunction	Dehiscence of suture ring
Connective tissue defects (Marfan's, Ehlers–Danlos syndrome, pseudoxanthoma elasticum, osteogenesis imperfecta)	Degeneration of valve cusp tissue

volume overload (page 219) and a consequent increase in left ventricular output. *Chronic* mitral regurgitation allows time for compensatory dilatation of the left ventricle and atrium and produces a minimal increase in filling pressures. By contrast, *acute* mitral regurgitation presents a sudden volume overload to the left atrium and ventricle, the steep rise in pulmonary venous pressure often resulting in pulmonary oedema.

Systemic hypertension (increased afterload) markedly increases mitral regurgitation.

Symptoms

Acute mitral regurgitation presents with severe breathlessness or frank pulmonary oedema, often of abrupt onset. Progressive fatigue and breathlessness are typical of *chronic* mitral regurgitation, decompensation sometimes resulting from systemic hypertension.

Physical signs

Typical physical signs of chronic mitral regurgitation are shown in Table 8.8. In acute regurgitation the murmur may stop before the second heart sound. Mitral valve prolapse (page x) typically displays a midsystolic click and late systolic murmur.

Investigations

(i) *Chest X-ray*: the pulmonary vasculature reflects the elevation of left atrial pressure. In acute severe mitral regurgitation the heart size may be normal and pulmonary oedema is present. Chronic regurgitation produces dilatation of the left ventricle and left atrium, the latter sometimes aneurysmal. Pulmonary venous congestion may be present.

(ii) *The ECG* is of little value. It may show left atrial enlargement in sinus rhythm. Atrial fibrillation is common in rheumatic mitral regurgitation and when the left atrium is dilated.

(iii) *Echocardiography*, by contrast, is invaluable. It distinguishes between many of the causes of mitral regurgitation (see Table 8.6). Dilatation of the left atrium and left ventricle reflects the severity of regurgitation. Serial estimations of left heart chamber dimensions and left ventricular function assist in followup. In mitral regurgitation a normal ejection fraction may reflect impaired myocardial function, and a moderately reduced ejection fraction (40–50%) indicates severe left ventricular dysfunction which predicts a poor outcome to mitral valve replacement. Doppler echocardiographic techniques, particularly Doppler colour flow mapping, may offer a semiquantitative assessment of mitral regurgitation.

(iv) *Cardiac catheterisation* is used principally to detect coexis-

Table 8.8

PHYSICAL SIGNS IN CHRONIC MITRAL REGURGITATION

	Sign	*Explanation of sign*
Arterial pulse	Jerky	Normal volume, rapid upstroke pulse
Venous pressure	Normal	Normal right heart pressures unless pulmonary hypertension develops
Apex beat	Sustained, sometimes double. Systolic thrill	Left ventricular enlargement, sometimes with a palpable filling wave (S3)
Left parasternal palpation	Heave	Expansile left atrium in severe regurgitation
Auscultation	Soft or obscured S1	Pansystolic murmur present
	Apical pansystolic murmur radiating to the axilla; less often to aortic area, back, spine, cranium	Regurgitation starts with onset of LV systole and continues throughout systole
	Loud S3	Rapid diastolic inflow to LV from LA

LA = left atrium
LV = left ventricle
S1 = first heart sound
S3 = third heart sound

tent coronary artery disease. Large 'v' waves are present in the left atrial and pulmonary wedge pressure tracings, and sometimes in the main pulmonary artery tracing. Left ventriculography confirms the regurgitation of contrast medium into the left atrium.

Differential diagnosis

(i) *Tricuspid regurgitation* produces a pansystolic murmur in the lower sternal area. It is usually a manifestation of right heart failure in patients with pulmonary hypertension secondary to left heart lesions.

(ii) *Ventricular septal defect*: a *congenital* ventricular septal defect produces a pansystolic murmur maximal at the lower left sternal edge. In adults it is usually small (maladie de Roger) and of no haemodynamic consequence. An *acquired* ventricular septal defect due to ischaemic rupture of the muscular septum is a lifethreatening lesion presenting as a new pansystolic murmur early in the course of acute myocardial infarction. It is distinguished from acute mitral regurgitation using bedside right heart catheterisation, by demonstrating a left-to-right shunt at ventricular level. An accurate anatomical diagnosis is confirmed by left ventricular contrast angiography prior to surgical closure of the defect.

(iii) *Aortic valve disease*: the systolic murmur of aortic valve disease may be louder at the apex than at the upper right sternal edge. It is not pansystolic but ejection or midsystolic in timing.

Treatment

Acute mitral regurgitation

Urgent cardiac catheterisation and mitral valve replacement are mandatory since the mortality of this lesion without surgery is very high. Emergency treatment with diuretics and afterload reduction (nitroprusside, hydralazine) are essential preoperative measures.

Chronic mitral regurgitation

Medical treatment Mild mitral regurgitation is well tolerated. Antibiotic prophylaxis against infective endocarditis is required for dental and invasive procedures. Moderate mitral regurgitation with symptoms is treated with digoxin, diuretics and vasodilators to reduce afterload. Anticoagulation is given if atrial fibrillation is present.

Surgical treatment Surgery is indicated for severe mitral regurgitation producing symptoms refractory to medical treatment, progressive cardiomegaly or declining left ventricular function. Mitral valve replacement is usual but mitral valve repair is gaining popularity in suitable cases.

MITRAL VALVE PROLAPSE

Definition

Prolapse of one or both mitral valve cusps into the left atrium during ventricular systole.

Background

In 1961 Barlow and associates in South Africa demonstrated that apical midsystolic clicks and late systolic murmurs were associated with mitral valve prolapse. Many synonymous terms have been used—floppy valve syndrome, Barlow's syndrome, systolic click-murmur syndrome and mitral valve prolapse syndrome. Mitral valve prolapse is a non-specific finding which may be associated with many disorders of the mitral valve (Table 8.9).

Floppy mitral valve is due to myxomatous proliferation of the zona spongiosa of the valve leaflets. The leaflets become redundant—too big for the left ventricle—and the chordae tendinae elongate and weaken. Prolapse is most marked in late systole when left ventricular volume is smallest. The condition is common affecting 5–10% of the population with a female : male ratio of 3:1. There is a high incidence in tall, thin patients and those with a variety of minor congenital deformities of the thoracic cage.

Symptoms

The great majority of patients are asymptomatic. Anxiety, palpi-

Table 8.9

CONDITIONS ASSOCIATED WITH MITRAL VALVE PROLAPSE

Floppy valve syndrome
Ischaemic heart disease
Dilated cardiomyopathy
Hypertrophic cardiomyopathy
Atrial septal defects
Marfan's syndrome
Pseudoxanthoma elasticum

tations, non-specific chest pain and fatigue are common. Severe prolapse with symptomatic mitral regurgitation is rare.

Diagnosis

(i) *Auscultation*: single or multiple midsystolic clicks and a late systolic murmur are typical in patients with late systolic prolapse. Pansystolic prolapse results in a pansystolic mitral regurgitant murmur.

(ii) *Echocardiography*: in late systolic prolapse the M-mode echocardiogram shows an abrupt posterior movement of the mitral leaflets in midsystole coincident with the onset of the murmur. In pansystolic prolapse the systolic segment of the echogram shows a 'hammock-shaped' configuration.

(iii) *Left ventricular contrast angiography* is rarely required but can demonstrate prolapse of one or both mitral valve cusps.

Complications

(i) *Infective endocarditis* has a significant incidence. Antibiotic prophylaxis for dental and septic procedures is advised for all patients with both click and murmur.

(ii) *Systemic embolism* from non-infective platelet emboli occurs but there is no indication for routine anticoagulation.

(iii) *Ventricular ectopic beats*, and rarely *ventricular tachycardia*, fibrillation and sudden death rarely occur. Such patients are generally symptomatic young females with a documented systolic murmur and electrocardiographic T wave abnormalities in inferior leads.

Treatment

Asymptomatic patients should be reassured, but followed up to detect progressive mitral regurgitation if a murmur is present. Propranolol is effective for chest discomfort, and antiarrhythmic therapy must be considered for those with symptomatic ectopic beats or paroxysmal atrial or ventricular tachyarrhythmias detected by ambulatory electrocardiographic monitoring.

AORTIC STENOSIS

Background

Left ventricular outflow tract obstruction is most common at the aortic valve, but may occur as supravalvular stenosis (page 136), discrete subvalvular stenosis (page 136) and in hypertrophic cardiomyopathy (page 105).

The causes of aortic valvular stenosis are shown in Table 8.10. Most adults with isolated valvular stenosis have a congenitally bicuspid aortic valve. Rheumatic aortic stenosis is almost invariably accompanied by mitral valve disease.

Turbulence caused by congenitally abnormal aortic valve cusps causes leaflet damage, fibrosis, calcification and stenosis.

Pathophysiology

Aortic stenosis subjects the left ventricle to pure pressure overload (page 219). Left ventricular output is maintained by left ventricular hypertrophy. The normal aortic valve orifice area is about 3·0 cm^2 and stenosis is critical when it is reduced to 0·70 mm^2. Cardiac output is usually normal at rest and in severe stenosis the pressure gradient across the valve may be 100–150 mmHg. As the left ventricle fails cardiac output falls and the measured gradient may then suggest only mild stenosis (less than 50 mmHg).

When the severity of aortic stenosis is in doubt it is therefore necessary to measure both pressure gradient and cardiac output so that the valve area may be calculated.

Table 8.10

CAUSES OF VALVULAR AORTIC STENOSIS

Congenital
Unicuspid
Bicuspid
Tricuspid
Acquired
Rheumatic
Senile degenerative
Atherosclerotic (homozygous type II hyperlipidaemia)
Rheumatoid arthritis
Ochronosis

The 'booster pump' function of atrial contraction is particularly important in aortic stenosis providing the extra-diastolic stretch necessary for effective left ventricular contraction. The onset of atrial fibrillation may result in rapid and sometimes fatal decompensation.

Symptoms

Patients with mild aortic stenosis are asymptomatic. Even severe aortic stenosis may be asymptomatic for many years before the three cardinal symptoms—angina pectoris, effort syncope and congestive heart failure—appear, usually in the sixth decade.

Signs

The physical signs are summarised in Table 8.11.

Table 8.11

PHYSICAL SIGNS IN AORTIC STENOSIS

	Sign	*Explanation of sign*
Carotid pulse	Anacrotic; small volume, slow upstroke, late peak	Aortic valvular obstruction
Apex beat	Thrusting, palpable 'a' wave, displaced laterally in heart failure	Left ventricular hypertrophy, forceful atrial contraction. LV dilatation in CCF
Systolic murmur	Midsystolic, ejection type, sometimes with palpable thrill	Starts with LV ejection; ends before A2
Ejection click	Present in mild stenosis, absent in severe	Sudden halting of movement when valve is still pliable
Added sounds	S4 present	Atrial contraction
	S3 sometimes	Heart failure present

CCF = congestive cardiac failure
LV = left ventricle
S3, S4 = third and fourth heart sounds
A2 = aortic second sound

Investigations

(i) *ECG*: left ventricular hypertrophy is a sensitive indicator of the severity of aortic stenosis. 'Strain pattern' (T wave inversion in anterolateral leads) indicates severe left ventricular hypertrophy.

(ii) *Chest X-ray*: the heart size is often normal, despite the presence of severe aortic stenosis. Left ventricular enlargement denotes additional aortic regurgitation or left ventricular failure. Aortic valve calcification is seen in lateral films.

(iii) *Echocardiography*: M-mode echocardiography shows a reduced aortic valve opening measurement (normal 1·6–2·6 cm) but in severe stenosis the aortic valve echogram usually appears totally disorganised. Left ventricular hypertrophy and dilatation can be quantified. Two-dimensional echocardiography most accurately detects the presence of a bicuspid aortic valve. Doppler echocardiography may quantify the transvalvular pressure gradient.

(iv) *Cardiac catheterisation*: the definitive assessment of severity in aortic stenosis is by measurement of the systolic pressure gradient between the left ventricle and aorta: there is no fully reliable non-invasive method. The procedure should include measurement of cardiac output, calculation of aortic valve area, left ventriculography and selective coronary angiography.

Prognosis

Severe aortic stenosis is well tolerated for many years. The prognosis of untreated aortic stenosis is poor once symptoms appear. The approximate interval from the onset of symptoms to the time of death is 2 years for congestive cardiac failure, 3 years for syncope and 5 years for angina pectoris.

Treatment

Medical Antibiotic prophylaxis against infective endocarditis is mandatory. Patients with asymptomatic severe aortic stenosis should not undertake sudden, vigorous or athletic activity. Atrial fibrillation may occur in severe aortic stenosis or because of coexistent mitral valve disease, and is treated with digoxin. Symptomatic aortic stenosis is treated surgically.

Surgical

The indications for surgery are:

(i) *Children* with severe aortic stenosis, symptomatic or not. Aortic valvotomy with commissural incision relieves obstruction with low operative risk (less than 2%).
(ii) *Adults*: severe aortic stenosis (aortic valve area $<0{\cdot}75^2$) producing symptoms indicates aortic valve replacement. Aortic valvotomy is inappropriate in fibrotic and calcified valves. Opinions differ but aortic valve replacement is not generally advised in the absence of symptoms, even for severe stenosis.

AORTIC REGURGITATION

Background

The development of aortic valvular regurgitation may be acute or chronic with corresponding differences in the clinical features and management. Acute aortic regurgitation frequently requires urgent cardiac catheterisation and aortic valve replacement while chronic regurgitation may be well-tolerated for many years. However, surgical results are poor if aortic valve replacement is delayed until chronic volume overload has caused irreversible left ventricular damage and the challenge of management is to decide the proper timing of aortic valve replacement.

Pathology

The aortic valve is a less complicated structure than the mitral valve. Competent aortic valve closure depends upon the normal anatomy of the aortic root, the valve leaflets, and the subvalvular structures. Aortic regurgitation may be caused by pathological faults in any or all of these structures (Table 8.12).

Rheumatic valvular disease causes fibrotic distortion of the

Table 8.12

CAUSES OF AORTIC VALVULAR REGURGITATION

Cusps	Rheumatic Infective endocarditis Biscuspid Rheumatoid Trauma
Root	
inflammatory	Syphilis Ankylosing spondylitis Non-specific urethritis Rheumatoid
non-inflammatory	Dissecting aneurysm Marfan's syndrome Idiopathic Ehlers–Danlos syndrome Pseudoxanthoma elasticum
Subvalvar	Subaortic ventricular septal defect (Fallot type)

cusps. Infective endocarditis may destroy or perforate a leaflet and large vegetations can prevent proper cusp closure. Congenital biscuspid valves usually develop stenosis and regurgitation in adult life but the larger cusp may prolapse in childhood. Aortic regurgitation may be caused by a wide variety of inflammatory diseases causing aortic root distortion and non-inflammatory conditions resulting in aortic root dilatation. In Fallot's tetralogy a large subaortic ventricular septal defect borders the aortic valve cusps causing aortic regurgitation by loss of structural support.

Pathophysiology

Chronic aortic regurgitation results in left ventricular volume overload and increased left ventricular stroke volume. The ventricle adapts by dilatation and hypertrophy, sometimes to a massive degree, but end diastolic pressure is often near normal. Chronic volume overload is well-tolerated for many years, but as dilatation progressively increases the ventricle becomes stiffer, end diastolic pressure rises, stroke volume falls and heart failure eventually develops.

In *acute* aortic regurgitation the regurgitant blood enters a normal-sized left ventricle which has not had the opportunity to adapt by dilatation. Left ventricular end diastolic pressure rises steeply and acute pulmonary oedema may develop. Left ventricular diastolic pressure exceeds left atrial pressure early in diastole causing premature closure of the mitral valve, a useful sign of acute, severe aortic regurgitation which may be readily detected by M-mode echocardiography.

Symptoms

Patients with chronic severe aortic regurgitation may be asymptomatic for many years. Exertional breathlessness, orthopnoea, paroxysmal nocturnal dyspnoea are frequent presenting symptoms. Angina pectoris and uncomfortably forceful cardiac action are not uncommon. Patients with acute aortic regurgitation present with severe breathlessness, pulmonary oedema and cardiovascular collapse.

Physical signs

The characteristic signs of *chronic* severe aortic regurgitation are shown in Table 8.13 and reflect a large pulse volume with peripheral vasodilatation. Durosiez's sign is elicted by compressing the femoral artery with the stethoscope bell to cause partial obstruction. A systolic murmur is always produced, but an additional diastolic murmur due to reverse flow indicates moderate to severe aortic regurgitation. Hill's sign is present when the systolic blood pressure in the leg, measured using a wide thigh cuff, is greater than 40 mmHg higher than that in the arm. In normal subjects the difference is less than 20 mmHg. In assessing the severity of aortic regurgitation the loudness of the left parasternal diastolic murmur is of no value but its duration is very helpful, a long murmur indicating severe regurgitation. As left ventricular function deteriorates progressive shortening of the murmur occurs because pressures in the aorta and left ventricle equalise earlier as ventricular diastolic pressure rises. Subtle variations in the site and quality of the diastolic murmur provide useful aetiological clues. A right, rather than left, parasternal diastolic murmur suggests an aortic root abnormality such as aortic dissection or syphilitic disease. A harsh or musical murmur, sometimes with a diastolic thrill, suggests perforation of an aortic

Table 8.13

PHYSICAL SIGNS IN AORTIC REGURGITATION

	Physical sign	*Explanation of sign*
Corrigan's sign	'Collapsing' or 'waterhammer' pulse of rapid upstroke, high volume and quick collapse	Large stroke volume; collapse due to regurgitation and peripheral vasodilatation
De Musset's sign	Head nodding	Same
Quincke's sign	Nailbed capillary pulsation	Same
Hill's sign	Popliteal–brachial pressure difference > 40 mmHg (see text)	Same
Durosiez's sign	Femoral diastolic murmur (see text)	Retrograde flow in femoral artery
Bisferiens pulse	Bifid, high volume carotid pulse	Wide pulse pressure in dominant aortic regurgitation
Apex beat	Thrusting, diffuse, laterally displaced	Left ventricular hypertrophy and dilatation
Auscultation	Soft or absent A2	Regurgitant valve
	Parasternal diastolic murmur	Same
	Aortic systolic murmur	Increased flow
	S3 gallop	Developing left ventricular failure
Austin–Flint murmur	Apical rumbling diastolic murmur	Early partial closure of mitral valve in moderate/severe regurgitation

A_2 = aortic second heart sound S_3 = third heart sound

valve cusp in infective endocarditis (the 'seagull murmur') or an everted cusp in syphilitic disease. In *acute* aortic regurgitation many of the classical signs are diminished or absent. Systemic arterial pulse pressure widens little, the diastolic murmur is short and there is a prominent third heart sound. Sinus tachycardia with a low cardiac output state are usual.

Investigations

Table 8.14 contrasts the auscultatory, echocardiographic and haemodynamic findings in the chronic severe and acute severe aortic regurgitation.

Table 8.14

SEVERE AORTIC REGURGITATION: COMMON DIFFERENCES BETWEEN CHRONIC AND ACUTE

Feature	*Chronic*	*Acute*
Physical signs	As Table 8.13	Tachycardia Low cardiac output failure *Normal* pulse pressure
Echocardiogram		
Left ventricle		
internal diameter	Increased	Normal
wall motion	Increased	Normal
hypertrophy	Present	Absent
Mitral valve		
closure point	Normal	Premature
leaflet flutter	Often present	Often present
Cardiac catheter		
Left ventricular end diastolic pressure	Normal or increased	Marked increase
Aortic systolic pressure	Increased	Normal
Aortic diastolic pressure	Decreased	Normal
Angiographic regurgitation	Severe	Severe

(i) *Electrocardiogram*: left ventricular hypertrophy and left atrial enlargement are usual in chronic aortic regurgitation; in acute aortic regurgitation the ECG may be normal. P–R interval prolongation may suggest that regurgitation is caused by an inflammatory condition of the aortic root.

(ii) *Chest X-ray*: heart size reflects the severity and duration of regurgitation. Moderate to severe chronic regurgitation always causes cardiac enlargement, sometimes to a massive degree. In acute aortic regurgitation heart size may be normal. Left atrial enlargement suggests coexistent mitral valve disease or cardiac failure. Aortic valve calcification is often indicative of mixed stenosis and regurgitation. Dilatation of the ascending aorta is present, especially with coexistent aortic stenosis; aneurysmal dilatation suggests aortic root disease. Lung fields are normal until advanced left ventricular failure develops.

(iii) *Echocardiography* provides information on the diagnosis, severity and aetiology of aortic regurgitation:

(a) *left ventricle*: left ventricular diastolic diameter and systolic shortening are increased in chronic regurgitation and normal in acute regurgitation. Systolic shortening decreases as left ventricular function declines;

(b) *aortic valve*: the valve echogram may be relatively normal in pure aortic regurgitation. If stenosis coexists disorganisation and calcification of the valve are often seen. Vegetations are readily demonstrated in infective endocarditis;

(c) *mitral valve*: high frequency diastolic fluttering of the anterior mitral valve leaflet is a sensitive sign of aortic regurgitation of any severity, acute or chronic. It is caused by impact of the regurgitant jet of blood from the aorta onto the mitral leaflet. In acute aortic regurgitation premature closure of the mitral valve occurs. Severe regurgitation into the normal-sized left ventricle causes a steep rise in pressure and closure of the mitral valve in mid-diastole;

(d) *aortic root*: aneurysmal dilatation suggests that aortic root disease may be the cause of regurgitation.

(iv) Angiography: rapid injection (20–30 ml/s) of radiographic contrast medium into the aortic root confirms the presence and severity of regurgitation. Left ventricular size and function, and aortic root anatomy are also assessed.

Differential diagnosis

Table 8.15 shows the conditions from which aortic valvular regurgitation should be distinguished. The Graham–Steel murmur is a soft early diastolic murmur of functional pulmonary regurgitation due to severe pulmonary arterial hypertension.

Prognosis

Severe acute aortic regurgitation leads to early death in left ventricular failure. In chronic aortic regurgitation 75% of patients survive for 5 years and 50% survive for 10 years after diagnosis. Average survival after the onset of symptoms is 3 years, unless aortic valve replacement is performed.

Treatment

Acute aortic regurgitation

This requires prompt aortic valve replacement if it is severe. Parenteral antibiotic therapy should be given for 2 weeks for untreated infective endocarditis before surgery, if the patient

Table 8.15

DIFFERENTIAL DIAGNOSIS OF AORTIC REGURGITATION

Graham–Steell murmur
Aortic 'runoff' conditions ruptured sinus of valsalva persistent ductus arteriosus coronary arteriovenous fistula aortic-left ventricular tunnel
Ventricular septal defect with associated aortic regurgitation

remains haemodynamically stable. Premature mitral valve closure on the M-mode echocardiogram is a valuable indicator of the need for emergency aortic valve replacement.

Chronic aortic regurgitation

This may be well-tolerated for many years. If it is mild or moderate in severity only antibiotic prophylaxis against infective endocarditis is required. If the patient is symptomatic or has severe aortic regurgitation but is asymptomatic the problem is to decide the correct timing of surgery. Postoperative results are poor if surgery is delayed until irreversible left ventricular dysfunction has developed. No strict criteria are established but aortic valve replacement should be performed for mild or moderate effort breathlessness which persists despite treatment with digoxin and a mild diuretic, a progressive increase in radiological heart size, and evidence of deteriorating left ventricular systolic function on serial echocardiography.

If left ventricular function remains well-preserved aortic valve replacement results in marked symptomatic improvement and a reduction in heart size. The operative mortality rate is between 5 and 10%.

TRICUSPID VALVE DISEASE

Tricuspid Stenosis

Background

Acquired tricuspid stenosis is almost always rheumatic in origin and accompanies mitral and often aortic valve disease. Clinically important tricuspid stenosis occurs in 5% of patients with rheumatic heart disease, although it is more common in developing countries. The pathological changes in the valve cusps are similar to those in mitral stenosis. A pressure gradient across the tricuspid valve as low as 3–5 mmHg may be clinically significant and the diagnosis must be established by simultaneous pressure measurement in the right atrium and right ventricle. A poor outcome following mitral valve surgery may result from failure to detect important coexistent tricuspid stenosis.

Symptoms

The symptoms cannot be distinguished from those of the mitral stenosis which is invariably present. Fatigue and symptoms secondary to an elevated venous pressure may be present. Tricuspid stenosis may diminish the symptoms of pulmonary congestion in mitral stenosis.

Physical signs

The auscultatory signs closely mimic those of mitral stenosis but there are two important clues to the presence of tricuspid stenosis.

(i) In sinus rhythm the jugular venous pulse shows a prominent 'a' wave and a slow 'y' descent, both due to obstructed filling of the right ventricle.

(ii) The diastolic and presystolic murmurs of tricuspid stenosis are increased in intensity on inspiration because negative intrathoracic pressure increases systemic venous return.

Investigations

(i) *The ECG* in sinus rhythm shows right atrial enlargement with peaked P waves in leads II and V1 exceeding 2·5 mV in amplitude. Since mitral valve disease will also be present the electrocardiographic signs of biatrial enlargement are often seen, with P waves exceeding 100 ms duration in lead II and a tall P wave with a prominent negative terminal deflection in V1.

(ii) The *chest X-ray* shows cardiomegaly with marked prominence of the right heart border due to right atrial enlargement.

(iii) The *echocardiogram* of tricuspid stenosis closely resembles that of mitral stenosis.

(iv) *Cardiac catheterisation* confirms an elevated right atrial pressure with a large 'a' wave and slow 'y' descent. Simultaneous pressure measurement in the right atrium and ventricle confirms a diastolic gradient ranging from 2 to 10 mmHg depending on severity. Right atrial contrast angiography shows thickening and decreased mobility of the valve leaflets and a jet of contrast through the obstructed tricuspid orifice.

Treatment

Diuretics are effective if fluid retention is present but surgery is required for significant stenosis. Tricuspid valvotomy is performed if there is no significant tricuspid regurgitation but valve replacement may be necessary. A tissue valve is preferred to a prosthesis in the tricuspid position.

Tricuspid Regurgitation

Background

Tricuspid regurgitation is usually functional, resulting from right ventricular dilatation complicating right ventricular failure in a variety of pulmonary or cardiac diseases (Table 8.16). Direct organic involvement of the tricuspid leaflets usually follows rheumatic fever and leads to mixed stenosis and regurgitation. Staphylococcal infective endocarditis of the tricuspid valve is particularly noted in intravenous drug addicts. Metastatic carcinoid syndrome may affect the right heart with deposits of fibrous tissue on the ventricular endocardium and valve cusps leading to regurgitation.

Table 8.16

CAUSES OF TRICUSPID REGURGITATION

Functional
Mitral valve disease
Cor pulmonale
Right ventricular infarction
Eisenmenger's syndrome
Primary pulmonary hypertension
Organic
Rheumatic
Ischaemic
Infective endocarditis
Prolapsing cusp
Atrioventricular canal defect
Carcinoid syndrome
Ebstein's anomaly

Tricuspid regurgitation is well tolerated if pulmonary artery pressure is normal—indeed, the valve may be removed and not replaced in resistant infective endocarditis without serious consequence. Conversely, functional tricuspid regurgitation may often cause disabling symptoms of low cardiac output and systemic venous congestion.

Clinical features

Cardiac cachexia and jaundice are common. The cardinal physical sign of tricuspid regurgitation is a prominent expansile systolic 'cv' wave with a steep 'y' descent in the jugular venous pulse. Systolic pulsation of a tender liver and even of varicose veins may be seen. Oedema and ascites frequently develop. Auscultation reveals a third heart sound and a pansystolic murmur in the lower left parasternal or subxiphoid region. Both are accentuated by inspiration. In functional tricuspid regurgitation due to pulmonary arterial hypertension the pulmonary second heart sound is prominent.

Investigations

(i) *Electrocardiography* usually confirms atrial fibrillation.
(ii) *The chest X-ray* shows cardiomegaly due to right atrial and ventricular enlargement. The lung fields often reflect pulmonary venous and arterial hypertension in functional tricuspid regurgitation.
(iii) *The echocardiogram* demonstrates the features of right ventricular volume overload similar to that in atrial septal defect—increased right ventricular diameter and reversed interventricular septal motion. Two-dimensional contrast echocardiography involving the rapid injection of a saline bolus into an arm vein will usually demonstrate tricuspid regurgitation. Microbubbles are formed which are readily visible on echocardiography and are seen washing to and fro across the tricuspid valve and into the inferior vena cava and hepatic veins during systole. Doppler colour flow mapping is now the non-invasive method of choice for the demonstration of tricuspid regurgitation.
(iv) *On cardiac catheterisation* right atrial and right ventricular

diastolic pressures are raised. Right ventricular and pulmonary artery systolic pressures exceeding 60 mmHg favour functional tricuspid regurgitation. Contrast injection into the right ventricle demonstrates reflux into the right atrium.

Treatment

Bedrest and intensive antifailure therapy reduce right ventricular size and thereby diminish tricuspid regurgitation. Surgical correction of left-sided rheumatic valvular disease usually allows resolution of functional tricuspid regurgitation, but if severe organic tricuspid disease is present surgical repair or replacement of the valve may be necessary. Tricuspid valve replacement increases the morbidity and mortality of concomitant valve surgery, and any prosthesis will impose moderate stenosis in the tricuspid position.

PULMONARY VALVE DISEASE

The causes of pulmonary valve disease are listed in Table 8.17. Pulmonary stenosis is almost always congenital. Rheumatic fever is a rare cause, although a high incidence of pulmonary valve involvement is reported in populations living at high altitude such as Mexico City. Pulmonary regurgitation is usually due to dilatation of the valve ring secondary to pulmonary arterial

Table 8.17

CAUSES OF PULMONARY VALVE DISEASE

Pulmonary stenosis
Congenital (p. 134)
Rheumatic
Carcinoid syndrome
Pulmonary regurgitation
Funtional (Graham–Steell murmur)
Marfan's syndrome
Congenital
Surgically induced

hypertension of any cause—the resulting Graham–Steel murmur is a blowing parasternal early diastolic murmur resembling that of aortic regurgitation. Congenital causes include absent or malformed leaflets. Pulmonary regurgitation not infrequently follows surgical correction of pulmonary valvular or subvalvular stenosis, for example, total correction of tetralogy of Fallot.

Pulmonary valvular stenosis may be relieved by surgical valvotomy and by percutaneous transluminal valvuloplasty using a balloon catheter. Pulmonary regurgitation seldom requires specific treatment.

THE USE OF ARTIFICIAL CARDIAC VALVES

These may be of mechanical or tissue construction. Their relative merits are summarised in Table 8.18.

Prosthetic valve replacement commenced in 1960 with the caged ball valve followed by the low profile tilting disc designs. They are of proven durability but require lifelong anticoagulation to avoid thromboembolism. Tissue valves were developed to overcome this problem and the porcine heterograft was introduced clinically in 1965. They have a very low incidence of thromboembolism and long-term anticoagulation is not required. Their durability is less certain and there is a high failure rate due

Table 8.18

FEATURES OF ARTIFICIAL CARDIAC VALVES

Type—example	*Advantages*	*Disadvantages*
Mechanical Caged ball Tilting disc single leaflet bileaflet	Long experience Durable Predictable performance	Lifelong anticoagulants Thromboembolism Audible clicks Haemolysis
Tissue Porcine heterograft Bovine pericardium	No anticoagulation Little thromboembolism Inaudible No haemolysis	Uncertain durability High failure rate in children

to degeneration and calcification of the leaflets in children and adolescents. Tissue valves are particularly suitable for women of childbearing age since the risks of fetal haemorrhage and malformation due to warfarin are avoided. Surgical risks have diminished considerably but remain important. The operative mortality of single valve replacement in the aortic or mitral position is about 10%, for combined aortic and mitral valve replacement nearly 20% and for additional tricuspid valve replacement mortality is between 29% and 40%.

FURTHER READING

Braunwald E. (Ed) *Heart disease: A textbook of Cardiovascular Medicine (1988)* pp. 1023–1092. Saunders, Philadelphia.

Fowler N.O., Van der Bel-Kahn. (1979). Indications for surgical replacement of the mitral valve. *Am. J. Cardiol.*, **44,** 148.

Frank S., Johnson A., Ross J. (1973). Natural history of valvular aortic stenosis. *Br Heart J.*, **35,** 41.

Hansing C.E., Rowe G.G. (1972). Tricuspid insufficiency. A study of haemodynamics and pathogenesis. *Circulation*, **45,** 793.

Honey M., (1961). Clinical and haemodynamic observations on combined mitral and aortic stenosis. *Br Heart J.*, **23,** 545.

Hoshino P.K., Gaasch W.H. (1986). When to intervene in chronic aortic regurgitation. *Arch. Intern. Med.*, **146,** 349.

Odemuyiwa O., Hall R.J.C. (1986). Editorial: assessing the severity of valve stenosis. *Br. Heart J.*, **55,** 117.

Perloff J.K., Harvey W.P. (1960). The clinical recognition of tricupsid stenosis. *Circulation*, **22,** 346.

Roberts W.C., Perloff J.K. (1972). Mitral valvular disease. A clinicopathological survey of the conditions causing the mnitral valve to function abnormally. *Ann. Intern. Med.*, **77,** 939.

Selzer A., Cohn K.E. (1972). Natural history of mitral stenosis: a review. *Circulation*, **45,** 878.

Vela J.E., Conteras R., Sosa F.R. (1969). Rheumatic pulmonary valve disease. *Am J Cardiol.*, **23,** 12.

Wynne J. (1986). Mitral valve prolapse. *N. Engl. J. Med.*, **314,** 577.

Chapter 9

Diseases of the Pulmonary Circulation

NORMAL PUMONARY CIRCULATION

The mean pulmonary artery pressure at rest is between 12 and 17 mmHg. There is a small rise with exercise. In health the low vascular resistance is maintained by three factors.

(i) The pulmonary arteries are thin walled vessels and can easily distend to accommodate increased flow.

(ii) They have little vasomotor tone and changes in vascular resistance are mainly passive.

(iii) The volume of the pulmonary vascular bed is not constant but expands with an increased cardiac output. In the upright position, at rest, blood flow is mainly through the lower zones of the lungs but when cardiac output increases the capillary systems in the mid and upper zones open up and blood flow becomes uniform. The distribution of flow is explained by the effect of gravity on both arterial and venous pressure which are therefore greatest in the lower zones. Most of the vascular bed is within the parenchyma of the lungs and flow depends on the transmural pressure exerted by the alveoli as well as the arterial–venous pressure difference. The intravascular pressures exceed alveolar pressure in the lower zones at rest. When the cardiac output increases during exercise the arterial and venous pressures become greater than transmural alveolar pressure in the mid and upper zones.

PULMONARY HYPERTENSION

Definition

Pulmonary hypertension is present when the mean pulmonary artery pressure at rest is more than 20 mmHg (systolic 30 mmHg, diastolic 15 mmHg). Mild pulmonary hypertension is a mean pulmonary artery pressure of 20–30 mmHg, moderate 30–40 mmHg and severe above 40 mmHg.

Background

Massive pulmonary embolism or pneumothorax cause an acute rise in pulmonary artery pressure. This rarely exceeds 50 mmHg before the thin-walled right ventricle fails and death occurs.

Most disorders causing pulmonary hypertension (Table 9.1) are chronic and the pressure rises to systemic levels. The right ventricle adapts by hypertrophy and for a number of years maintains cardiac output until eventually it fails. Death is due to right ventricular failure. Some patients die suddenly with syncope, due to sudden reduction of cerebral blood flow, or with a cardiac arrhythmia.

Pregnancy worsens severe pulmonary hypertension and is contraindicated. If a woman with Eisenmenger's syndrome becomes pregnant the physiological rise in cardiac output cannot be accommodated in the diseased pulmonary circulation and the right-to-left shunt is increased with worsening cyanosis. The fetus fails to grow and usually aborts. Therapeutic abortion should be offered early in pregnancy.

Pathophysiology

The mechanisms that initiate a rise in pulmonary artery pressure are listed in Table 9.2. Whatever the underlying mechanism the prolonged elevation of pressure creates a vicious circle in the pulmonary arteries. High pressure causes structural changes in the walls of the arteries which perpetuate and accentuate pulmonary hypertension.

The larger pulmonary arteries are muscular, have an internal and external elastic lamina and a continuous muscle coat. Smaller arteries are partially muscular. The smallest are non-muscular with a single elastic lamina.

Table 9.1

CAUSES OF PULMONARY HYPERTENSION

(1)	Disorders associated with chronic hypoxia	(a)	Chronic bronchitis and emphysema
		(b)	Hypoventilation syndromes kyphoscoliosis neuromuscular disease obstruction of extrathoracic airways disturbance of the respiratory centre
		(c)	High altitude
(2)	Disorders of the lung parenchyma	(a)	Pulmonary fibrosis
		(b)	Cystic fibrosis
		(c)	Sarcoidosis
		(d)	Massive pneumothorax
(3)	Disorders of the pulmonary arteries	(a)	Primary pulmonary hypertension
		(b)	Scleroderma (CREST syndrome)
		(c)	Pulmonary vasculitis
		(d)	Peripheral pulmonary artery stenosis
		(e)	Pulmonary embolism
		(f)	Schistosomiasis
(4)	Disorders of the pulmonary veins		Pulmonary veno-occlusive disease
(5)	Disorders of the left heart	(a)	Left ventricular failure
		(b)	Mitral valve disease
		(c)	Cor triatriatum
		(d)	Left atrial myxoma
		(e)	Constrictive pericarditis
(6)	Congenital heart disease		Left-to-right shunts

The earliest pathological changes are reversible. These are medial hypertrophy of the muscular arteries. Further changes are usually irreversible. Intimal thickening is found in all but mild degrees of pulmonary hypertension. There is cellular proliferation producing an 'onion-skin' appearance. The collagen internal

Table 9.2

MECHANISMS WHICH ELEVATE PULMONARY ARTERY PRESSURE

Vasoconstriction—hypoxia
Raised pulmonary venous pressure—passive transmission
Increased blood flow
Loss of lung parenchyma
Obstruction of the pulmonary arteries
Disease primarily affecting the pulmonary vasculature

to the internal elastic lamina increases. These pathological changes occur in pulmonary hypertension of any aetiology.

More complex vascular lesions develop in primary pulmonary hypertension and Eisenmenger's syndrome. There is fibrinoid necrosis and dilatation or plexiform change, in which the small arteries dilate, have prominent endothelial proliferation and vein like side branches.

Alveolar hypoxia

The pulmonary arteries constrict when $Pa\text{O}_2$ falls beneath 7·3 kPa. This may be a direct effect of hypoxia on the vascular smooth muscle or hypoxia may mediate vasoconstriction by increasing levels of circulating vasoconstrictors such as prostaglandins, thromboxane A_2, serotonin or histamine. There is an individual variation in the hypoxic response.

The effect of alveolar hypoxia confined to one area of a lung is to divert blood to ventilated areas and hence to improve oxygenation. However, generalised hypoxia produces generalised vasoconstriction. It also causes secondary erythrocytosis and this adds to pulmonary vascular resistance when the haemocrit exceeds 55%.

Hypoxia is the mechanism for pulmonary hypertension with chronic bronchitis and emphysema and the hypoventilation syndromes. Low oxygen concentration in air at high altitude causes pulmonary hypertension. The mean pulmonary artery pressure at rest in residents in the Peruvian Andes (3650 m; 12 000 feet) is 28 mmHg. This gradually falls after descent to sea level.

Raised pulmonary venous pressure

Passive transmission of high left atrial pressure is the mechanism for pulmonary hypertension in disorders of the left heart. When this is chronically elevated above 20 mmHg—usually in patients with mitral stenosis, secondary structural changes develop in the pulmonary arteries and there is a disproportionate rise in pressure.

Increased flow

Pulmonary artery pressure is not very flow-dependent and physiological increases in cardiac output are usually balanced by an increase in vascular bed volume and a reduction in resistance. The capacity of the vascular bed is exceeded when there is a large left-to-right shunt and flow is more than four times normal. Pulmonary artery pressure rises and structural changes establish pulmonary hypertension.

Loss of lung parenchyma

The pulmonary artery pressure does not rise if one lung is removed if the other lung is healthy. It is probable that about two-thirds of the lung parenchyma must be lost to cause pulmonary hypertension. This can occur with severe pulmonary fibrosis, cystic fibrosis and sarcoidosis.

Obstruction of pulmonary arteries

Recurrent thromboemboli or the ova of schistosomiasis, which pass through the pulmonary arteries during their life cycle, may cause extensive obstruction of the pulmonary vasculature and pulmonary hypertension.

Disease primarily affecting the pulmonary vasculature

Pulmonary hypertension can be caused by vasculitis due to systemic lupus erythematosus, polyarteritis nodosa, Takayasu's disease and the unexplained changes described in the next section.

Unexplained Pulmonary Hypertension

Three pathological entities are recognised but can be difficult to differentiate in life.

(i) Primary pulmonary hypertension (plexogenic pulmonary angiopathy).
(ii) Recurrent peripheral thromboemboli.
(iii) Pulmonary veno-occlusive disease.

Primary pulmonary hypertension

This often affects young people; 75% are dead in 10 years. The diagnosis is not usually made until the irreversible plexiform changes have occurred. There are a number of recognised associations which may be clues to the aetiology (Table 9.3). The condition should be suspected in any patient who presents with shortness of breath, syncope during or immediately after excercise and angina without evidence of underlying heart disease.

Table 9.3

ASSOCIATIONS WITH PRIMARY PULMONARY HYPERTENSION

Association	*Mechanism*
Oral contraceptive use Pregnancy Postpartum period	Female hormones
Ingestion of aminorex fumarate fenfluramine *Crotalaria spectabilis* seeds (rats)	Drugs? like catecholamines or dietary toxic substance
Cirrhosis and portocaval shunts	Failure to degrade a metabolic product
Familial history	Genetic predisposition to pulmonary vasoconstriction
Autoimmune disease Raynaud's phenomenon	Abnormal vascular responses

Although it can occur in either sex or any age group it is commonest in young women. It often presents around the time of childbirth when cardiac work is increased. The symptoms and signs are those of pulmonary hypertension of whatever cause and are described in the next section.

Recurrent peripheral thromboemboli

These obstruct the lungs in a more patchy distribution. There are pathological differences with obstruction of the muscular and non-muscular arteries but only slight medial hypertrophy and no plexogenic lesions.

Pulmonary veno-occlusive disease

The radiological appearances are the most important in distinguishing pulmonary veno-occlusive disease. This is a syndrome of pulmonary venous hypertension and thus pulmonary oedema. The chest X-ray shows pulmonary oedema and septal lines without the pulmonary venous dilatation associated with left atrial hypertension.

Death usually occurs within two years of symptoms. Treatment for all unexplained pulmonary hypertension may be approached in the same way (see p. 371).

Diagnosis

The history, examination or investigations may reveal an underlying cause, for example, chronic bronchitis and emphysema, mitral stenosis or congenital heart disease. The diagnosis of unexplained pulmonary hypertension is made by exclusion of other causes.

Mild or moderate pulmonary hypertension is associated with few symptoms and signs. The symptoms of severe pulmonary hypertension are mainly due to the reduction of cardiac output. The earliest are breathlessness and fatigue. Syncope occurs because the rise in cardiac output with exercise is limited by the high resistance to outflow from the right ventricle. Loss of consciousness occurs typically during exercise but it can happen immediately after exercise due to pulmonary vasoconstriction. Angina of effort is the result of right ventricular hypertrophy and reduced coronary blood flow. The abnormal arteries may rupture

Table 9.4

SIGNS OF PULMONARY HYPERTENSION, RIGHT VENTRICULAR HYPERTROPHY AND FAILURE

	Sign	*Explanation*
Signs of an underlying condition, e.g. lung disease, congenital heart disease	–	–
Signs of pulmonary hypertension	Loud and palpable pulmonary second sound	High diastolic pressure in the pulmonary artery increases the force of closure
	Narrowed splitting of second sound	High pressure (*unless* bundle block is present)
	Pulmonary systolic murmur	Dilatation of the main pulmonary trunk
	Pulmonary diastolic murmur	Pulmonary regurgitation due to higher diastolic pressure in the pulmonary artery and dilatation of the pulmonary valve ring

Signs of right ventricular hypertrophy	Forceful parasternal heave	Increased force of contraction of right ventricle
	Prominent ‘a’ wave in jugular venous pressure	Increased force of contraction of right atrium
Signs of right ventricular failure	Jugular venous pressure elevated *both* in inspiration and expiration	High right atrial pressure
	Prominent ‘v’ wave	Tricuspid regurgitation
	Tricuspid systolic murmur	Tricuspid regurgitation due to dilatation of the tricuspid valve
	Right ventricular third sound	Rigid and failing right ventricle
	Peripheral oedema	Increasing venous pressure, renal and metabolic changes
	Hepatic tenderness and enlargement	Venous congestion
	Pulsatile liver	Tricuspid regurgitation

Table 9.5

INVESTIGATION OF PULMONARY HYPERTENSION

Investigations	*Abormalities*
Chest X-ray	Enlarged main pulmonary trunk Large central pulmonary arteries Small peripheral pulmonary arteries with an abrupt transition in arterial size Normal heart size until right ventricular failure
Electrocardiogram	Frontal plane QRS axis greater than 120° Dominant R wave in praecordial leads Inverted T wave in V_1–V_4 Right bundle branch block Tall, peaked 'p' waves
Echocardiogram	Pulmonary valve motion absent 'a' wave flat or reversed e–f diastolic closure accelerated opening Right ventricle hypertrophy reversed septal motion
Right heart catheter	Raised right atrial, right ventricular and pulmonary artery pressures. (These may be at systolic levels) Pulmonary capillary wedge pressure is often difficult to obtain but is low or normal Cardiac output is reduced

and cause haemoptysis. The enlarged pulmonary artery can press on the left recurrent laryngeal nerve causing vocal chord paralysis with hoarseness.

The signs of pulmonary hypertension depend on the severity and the response of the right ventricle. They are listed in Table 9.4.

Investigation will depend on the underlying aetiology but Table 9.5 shows the findings due to pulmonary hypertension itself as found in patients with primary pulmonary hypertension.

Treatment

If no underlying cause is found the aims of treatment are:

(i) To raise the cardiac output.
(ii) To reduce the pulmonary artery pressure so that progression of the damage in the arteries is limited.

Vasodilators are sometimes helpful. Each patient should be tested acutely during catheterisation. Either intravenous prostacyclin or nifedipine are used. Prostacyclin is safer because its effects can be immediately reversed if there is a catastrophic fall in systemic blood pressure. A good response is an increase in cardiac output and a fall in pulmonary artery pressure without a marked decrease in systemic pressure. Such patients should be treated with oral nifedipine. The long-term response is unpredictable but usually disappointing.

Anticoagulation may prevent secondary thromboembolism. Heart lung transplantation can now be considered for otherwise hopeless cases.

PULMONARY HEART DISEASE (COR PULMONALE)

Definition

Pulmonary heart disease is hypertrophy of the right ventricle resulting from diseases affecting the function and/or structure of the lung and its vessels except when these alterations are the result of diseases primarily affecting the left side of the heart or of congenital heart disease (World Health Organisation, 1963).

Background

This definition stresses the development of right ventricular hypertrophy but pulmonary heart disease is often first recognised clinically when there is right heart failure. The initial response to an increased afterload is for the right ventricle to dilate. If the rise in pulmonary artery pressure is acute the right ventricle soon fails. In chronic pulmonary hypertension the adaptive response is right ventricular hypertrophy and for a time this maintains a normal cardiac output. Eventually the right ventricular end diastolic pressure and volume become raised. Oedema formation is due to the elevation of venous pressure and renal and metabolic changes. Hypoxia exacerbates right ventricular failure and impairs left ventricular function.

The clinical causes of pulmonary heart disease are listed in Table 9.1, sections 1–4. By far the commonest is chronic airflow limitation due to chronic bronchitis and emphysema.

Chronic Airflow Limitation

Background

Three diseases are associated with chronic airflow limitation—asthma, chronic bronchitis and emphysema. Pulmonary heart disease is not associated with atopic asthma because the key to the development of pulmonary hypertension is hypoxia.

Chronic bronchitis and emphysema are common and in industrial areas account for a quarter of all cases of heart failure. The two diseases often coexist because the causative factors are the same—smoking and industrial air pollution.

Pathophysiology

Chronic bronchitis is a functional disorder characterised by excess mucus secretion from the tracheobronchial mucous glands, chronic cough and sputum production. Inflammatory changes in the bronchioles occur as a result of inhalation of smoke and cause airflow limitation. Emphysema is a pathological condition with dilatation and destruction of the air spaces distal to the terminal bronchiole. The distortion of the airways which follows destruction of the alveoli leads to limitation of airflow.

Although the underlying pathology is not distinct there are two clinical presentations. One group of patients hyperventilate and maintain a normal $Pa\text{CO}_2$ and a near normal $Pa\text{O}_2$. Emphysema predominates, they are pink and puffing ('pink puffers') and, because they do not have marked alveolar hypoxia, pulmonary hypertension and pulmonary heart disease are not common. In the second group there is widespread airflow limitation associated with chronic bronchitis. The widespread underventilation of perfused areas (ventilation/perfusion mismatch) results in a low Pao_2 and raised $Paco_2$. Hypoxia causes pulmonary hypertension and right heart failure occurs. These patients are blue and bloated ('blue bloaters').

Blue bloaters may have an inadequate response of the respiratory centre to hypoxia and so do not hyperventilate. However this is difficult to distinguish from the pure mechanics of severe airways limitation and a fixed thoracic cavity. These can make the blue bloater incapable of responding to a rise in $Paco_2$ even if respiratory drive is normal.

There are differences in respiration during sleep between the two groups. Respiration becomes irregular and responses to hypoxia and bronchopulmonary irritation are diminished during periods of rapid eye movement (REM) sleep. In blue bloaters the $Paco_2$ fails to as low as 3–4 kPa during REM sleep. Hypoxia is the trigger for development of pulmonary hypertension. These episodes are far less frequent in pink puffers and the difference may be due to respiratory drive or the reduction in the cough impulse producing further secretion-induced airway limitation in chronic bronchitis.

Clinical features

The signs of pulmonary hypertension are listed in Table 9.4. They are often masked by the hyperinflated lungs. The heart sounds may be heard best in the epigastrium. External jugular veins are engorged by movement of the accessory muscles of respiration and a high intrathoracic pressure often elevates the jugular venous pressure in expiration. When the right ventricle falls the jugular venous pressure remains high in inspiration.

Table 9.6 shows the major clinical differences between blue bloaters and pink puffers.

Treatment

The principles are as follows.

Treatment of the underlying lung disease

A respiratory infection often precipitates acute heart failure. Culture of the sputum and blood may isolate the organism but the commonest are *Streptococcus pneumoniae* and *Haemophilus influen-*

Table 9.6

CLINICAL FEATURES AND INVESTIGATION OF CHRONIC BRONCHITIS AND EMPHYSEMA

Clinical feature	*Blue bloaters*	*Pink puffers*
Breathlessness	Not short of breath	Very breathless
Cyanosis	Central cyanosis	Not cyanosed
Weight	Fat	Thin
Mental state	Relaxed	Anxious
Right heart failure	Common	Unusual
Investigation		
Haematocrit	Elevated	Normal
Pao_2	<6·6 kPa (normal 12–14·6)	>8·3 kPa
$Paco_2$	>6·6 kPa (normal 4·5–6·0)	<6·0 kPa
Sleep hypoxaemia	Falls in Pao_2 to 3–4 kPa may occur	Falls in Pao_2 are unusual
Chest X-ray	Cardiomegaly and normal sized lungs	Marked hyperinflation of lungs with a small vertical heart shadow
Respiratory function tests	Irreversible airways obstruction	Irreversible airways obstruction
	$\frac{\text{Forced expiratory volume, FEV}_1}{\text{Forced vital capacity, FVC}} < 75\%$	$\frac{FEV_1}{FVC} < 75\%$
	Total lung capacity normal	Total lung capacity increased
		Residual volume increased
	Elastic recoil normal or slightly impaired	Elastic recoil very reduced
	Diffusing capacity (transfer factor for carbon monoxide) normal or slightly impaired	Diffusing capacity reduced

The clinical presentation depends on the severity of disease. Table 9.6 lists the features and findings of investigations found in the two ends of the spectrum of presentation of chronic airways obstruction. It should be remembered [illegible]

zae. Both are sensitive to ampicillin. Chest physiotherapy should be routine. Bronchodilators are beneficial if the airflow limitation is partly reversible. Salbutamol can be given orally, by intravenous infusion or by a nebuliser. Central respiratory stimulants have little place but sedatives should be avoided. Smoking must be banned.

Treatment of hypoxia

Oxygen to reduce pulmonary hypotension is the most important therapy. Low doses (1–2 litres/min) of 100% oxygen are given through nasal catheters. The dose is titrated with arterial blood gases so that Pao_2 rises without a marked increase in $Paco_2$.

Intermittent positive pressure ventilation should only be used if it is judged that the patient has a reasonable chance of longer term survival—the preexacerbation clinical state must not have been too severe. It is delivered by an endotracheal tube and adjusted according to arterial blood gases.

Selected patients with chronic airways limitation will benefit from long-term oxygen therapy. They must have chronic respiratory failure (FEV persistently $<1{\cdot}5$ litres and Pao_2 persistently $<7{\cdot}3$ kPa) with or without peripheral oedema. They must have agreed *never* to smoke. Oxygen is made at home by an oxygen concentrator which converts air into a stream of 90% oxygen. It is delivered at a rate of 1–2 litres/min by nasal catheters. The patient must breathe oxygen for at least 15 h a day. Long-term treatment reduces pulmonary artery pressure.

Treatment of the right heart failure

Diuretics reduce oedema. Hypokalaemia must be avoided because alkalosis further reduces the sensitivity of the respiratory centre. Potassium-sparing diuretics, such as spironolactone can be combined with the loop diuretic.

Digoxin is contraindicated if there is sinus rhythm because these patients are particularly sensitive and develop digoxin-induced arrhythmias.

HYPOVENTILATION SYNDROMES

Chest Wall and Neuromuscular Disorders

Severe chest wall deformity (kyphoscoliosis, thoracoplasty) and neuromuscular disorders (poliomyelitis, Guillain–Barré syndrome, myasthenia gravis) are associated with hypoventilation and alveolar hypoxia. The changes are most severe during rapid eye movement (REM) sleep when the diaphragm is the main muscle of respiration. Patients with respiratory failure may be helped by the stimulant–antidepressant protryptiline 5–20 mg at night which reduces rapid eye movement sleep. Nocturnal respiratory support can be given by negative pressure ventilation using a Tunnicliffe jacket or pneumosuit.

Disturbances of the Respiratory Centre

Obesity—hypoventilation syndrome (Pickwickian syndrome)

This is extreme obesity with hypoventilation, daytime sleepiness, polycythaemia and pulmonary heart disease. There is a reduced ventilatory response to the inhalation of carbon dioxide. The treatment is weight reduction and respiratory stimulants.

Central sleep apnoea syndrome

Periodic apnoea occurs during sleep causing waking and sleep deprivation. Associated features are loud snoring, bed-wetting, morning headaches, daytime sleepiness and personality change. Nocturnal diaphragmatic pacing may be helpful.

Obstructive sleep apnoea

Intermittent apnoea during sleep occurs in some patients with enlarged tonsils and adenoids or acromegaly and hypothyroidism. The clinical features are similar to the central sleep apnoea syndrome. $Pa\text{o}_2$ is reduced and hypoxia induces pulmonary hypertension.

PULMONARY EMBOLISM

Background

In the United Kingdom there are 21 000 deaths due to pulmonary embolism a year. This is a condition in which death occurs early after the event, indeed 80% of all those who die do so within 4 h. Many have no warning symptoms or signs. Nearly all pulmonary emboli are the result of thrombi formed in the deep leg veins or pelvic veins. These fragment and after passing through the inferior vena cava and right heart, impact the pulmonary arteries. Fat, amniotic fluid or air are other rare causes.

Venous thrombi form because of three possible factors (Virchow's triad):

(i) Stasis of blood in the vein—the commonest cause.
(ii) Damage to the vessel wall.
(iii) Alteration in coagulability of the blood.

Locally the thrombus can disrupt the venous valves and cause varicose veins and the postphlebitic syndrome. There is a danger to life if it fragments. A massive pulmonary embolism occludes four-fifths of the pulmonary arterial tree. The pulmonary artery pressure rises up to 50 mmHg due to arterial obstruction and further reflex arterial constriction. Right ventricular dilatation and failure follows with acute reduction in cardiac output. In a small or moderate pulmonary embolism the clot quickly breaks up on impact and is mechanically remodelled. It is lysed over hours and days by endogenous fibrinolytic mechanisms. Blood exudes into the surrounding alveoli but actual tissue necrosis (pulmonary infarction) probably does not occur in more than 15% of cases.

Risk factors for venous thromboembolism

There are geographical differences in the prevalence. Venous thromboembolism is commoner in Europe and the United States compared with Asia and Africa. This may be due to variations in diet, pattern of disease and physical activity as well as race. Women are affected more often than men and it becomes commoner with increasing age—usually associated with heart

Table 9.7

RISK FACTORS FOR VENOUS THROMBOEMBOLISM

Immobility
Previous history of venous thromboembolism
Surgery (especially orthopaedic and gynaecological)
General anaesthesia
Trauma to the legs, pelvis or spine
Obesity
Varicose veins
Heart disease: congestive heart failure and venous stasis
Cancer: pancreas, lung, stomach, colon, uterus, breast, prostate
Pregnancy and puerperium
Oral contraceptives and oestrogen therapy
Blood group A
Antithrombin III deficiency
Plasminogen disorders
Vitamin K-dependent clotting factor infusions

disease or cancer. Smoking appears to protect against the development of venous thrombosis. Pulmonary embolism is uncommon in patients who are healthy and fully mobile. Any patient confined to bed for a few days may develop the disease. The risk factors are listed in Table 9.7.

Clinical features of deep vein thrombosis

Two-thirds of patients with deep vein thrombosis have no physical signs. Even extensive deep vein thrombosis may be 'silent' and the first evidence is a pulmonary embolism. The usual clinical features are listed in Table 9.8. The differential diagnosis is muscle strain, muscle cramps, pressure from bed rest, a haematoma, an intact synovial cyst in the calf (Baker's cyst) or synovial rupture of the knee joint. The diagnosis of an intact synovial cyst is made by palpation of the popliteal fossa but when it ruptures synovial fluid extravasates into the tissues of the calf and it is more difficult to differentiate from deep venous thrombosis. A history of sudden calf pain and swelling occurring during exercise is the typical history of synovial rupture. An arthrogram confirms the diagnosis.

Table 9.8

CLINICAL FEATURES OF DEEP VEIN THROMBOSIS

Due to venous obstruction	*Due to inflammation around thrombus*
Swelling of the leg over several hours	Pain
Dilatation of superficial veins	Tenderness over deep vein
Increase in skin temperature	Positive Homan's sign
Bluish discoloration of the skin	

Investigation of deep vein thrombosis

(i) *Doppler flow detector*: this demonstrates changes in the rate of venous flow. A transducer is placed over the femoral vein and the calf is squeezed. If the veins are patent there is a swishing sound. The technique is simple and 80% correct but can fail to detect a dangerous fresh clot which has not yet obstructed flow. It is the most commonly used screening test.

(ii) *Impedance plethysmography*: the volume of the calf during and after venous compression is measured by a strain gauge around the calf. A cuff is placed above the knee. It is a simple test and detects 80% of major thrombi but does not detect all calf vein thrombi.

(iii) *I^{125} Fibrinogen scanning*: potassium iodide is given so that the thyroid gland is saturated and will not take up radioactive iodine. Fibrinogen I^{125} is injected and is taken up by a forming or recently formed thrombosis. This can be detected by a scintillation counter. It is not accurate for clots above the middle of the thigh.

(iv) *Venography*: this is the only way to be sure of the diagnosis of a deep vein thrombosis and new low ionic contrast media have made it a safer investigation. A tourniquet around the ankle ensures that contrast enters the deep rather than superficial veins after injection into a vein on the foot. Calf vein opacification is increased by a tourniquet above the knee. The radiologist follows the contrast using an image intensifier and when the calf veins have been filled the knee tourniquet is released and the contrast floods the thigh and pelvic veins. A deep vein thrombosis is diagnosed if there is a filling defect in the contrast medium on more than one film or if a vein is completely occluded.

Prevention of venous thromboembolism

Prophylactic measures should be taken in high risk patients. The principles are:

(i) Reduce venous stasis (Table 9.9).
(ii) Reduce blood coagulability.

Full-dose heparin or oral anticoagulation is the most effective method but cannot be used in surgical patients because of the risk of massive haemorrhage. Low-dose heparin, 10 000 units every 12 h is the most widely used prophylaxis. The heparin must be injected carefully into a fold of skin on the anterior abdominal wall. It is effective in general surgery but not proven in the high-risk femoral fractures and hip replacements.

Dextran, a partly hydrolysed glucose polymer decreases platelet adhesiveness. Infusion of dextran reduces the frequency of fatal pulmonary embolism but may not be as effective as low-dose heparin in reducing deep vein thrombosis. Either a 10% solution of 40 000 molecular weight or a 6% solution of 70 000 molecular weight dextran can be used. It may cause an anaphylactic reaction and because it is a plasma expander it puts some patients at risk of pulmonary oedema.

Aspirin and dipyridamole alter platelet function but have not been shown to be effective in reducing venous thrombosis.

Table 9.9

METHODS FOR REDUCING VENOUS STASIS

Leg elevation: 15 cm above horizontal increases venous flow by 30%
Elastic stockings
Physiotherapy: exercises for the calf muscles
Intermittent pneumatic leggings
Passive leg exercise during surgery
Early mobilisation

Clinical features of pulmonary embolism

Reliance on clinical observations alone for diagnosis is often inaccurate. The presentation depends on the size of the embolism (Table 9.10). Pleuritic chest pain is due to pleural involvement. When a distal pulmonary artery is obstructed blood exudes into the alveoli and produces haemoptysis.

A large embolus impacts in the central pulmonary arteries and pleuritic pain is not necessarily a feature of this syndrome. The symptoms and signs are those of the haemodynamic disturbance and are due to:

(i) Acute right heart failure.
(ii) Acute reduction in cardiac output.
(iii) The ventilation/perfusion mismatch which leads to arterial desaturation and hyperventilation (blood gases—low Pao_2 and low $Paco_2$).

Massive pulmonary embolism may be followed by circulatory collapse, loss of consciousness and death within minutes.

Chronic Pulmonary Thromboembolism and Pulmonary Hypertension

Pulmonary hypertension and pulmonary heart disease due to recurrent or unresolved pulmonary thromboembolism is rare. Patients present with the symptoms and signs of pulmonary hypertension. They may have no history of a pulmonary embolism or evidence of deep vein thrombosis. Lung perfusion scans show major areas of underperfused lung and a pulmonary arteriogram confirms occlusions in proximal pulmonary arteries. Severe pulmonary hypertension is not reduced by anticoagulation and prognosis is poor. Late embolectomy or endartectomy procedures have been undertaken with some success.

Investigations

(i) *Plain chest X-ray*: this is abnormal in 75% of patients. Changes suggesting a pulmonary embolism are usually present within 12 h (Table 9.11). A normal chest X-ray

Table 9.10

CLINICAL FEATURES OF ACUTE PULMONARY EMBOLISM

Embolism	*Symptoms*	*Signs*	*Explanation of sign*
Small embolus	None	None	Too little lung damage
Embolus obstructing a distal pulmonary artery	Pleurisy	Pleural rub	Pleural involvement
	Haemoptysis	Crackles	Infarcted lung
	Shortness of breath	Fever	Restriction due to pleuritic loss of lung volume with elevation of the diaphragm or pleural effusion due to pulmonary infarction
		Shallow breathing	
		Dullness to percussion at base	

Embolus obstructing central pulmonary arteries	Angina	Jugular venous pressure elevated Normal pulmonary closure sound Tachycardia Gallop rhythm (summation of third and fourth sounds with tachycardia)	Acute right heart failure with dilatation *but* a pulmonary artery pressure 50 mmHg and no right ventricular hypertrophy High end diastolic pressure (III) Forceful atrial contraction (IV)
	Apprehension Mental confusion Syncope Sudden death	Low blood pressure Small volume pulse with sharp upstroke	Acute fall in cardiac output
	Breathlessness	Tachypnoea Hyperventilation Cyanosis	Ventilation/perfusion mismatch

Table 9.11

CHEST X-RAY IN PULMONARY EMBOLISM

X-ray abnormality	*Percentage of patients*	*Explanation*
Pulmonary opacities (wedge shape uncommon) These may evolve to atelactic streaks.	40	Loss of lung volume, alveolar haemorrhage and pulmonary infarction
Pleural effusion	30	Infarcted lung with pleural involvement
Pulmonary vessel changes Distended proximal pulmonary artery Abrupt tapering to an occluded vessel Oligaemia	40	Obstruction of a major pulmonary artery
Cardiac enlargement	9	Dilatation of right ventricle due to increased afterload
Pulmonary oedema	Occasional	Increased blood flow through remaining perfused vessels

does not exclude the diagnosis and changes are frequently missed.

(ii) *Electrocardiogram*: this remains normal after a small pulmonary embolism. With a large embolism 85% of patients have an abnormality. The diagnostic patterns are:

(a) S wave lead 1, Q wave in lead 2 and T wave inversion in lead 3 (S1 Q3 T3 pattern) plus right ventricular T wave inversion (T inverted in V1–V4).

(b) S1 Q3 T3 plus right bundle branch block.

Other patients show non-specific changes of tachycardia, T wave inversion and ST segment depression. About 5% of patients develop atrial fibrillation.

(iii) *Arterial blood gases*: the changes are non-specific but reflect the underperfused but ventilated lung (an increase in physiological dead space). There is a reduction of Pao_2 and $Paco_2$.

(iv) *Ventilation–perfusion lung scans*: regional perfusion of blood in the lungs can be shown by trapping radioactive particles in the arterial-capillary bed. The agent of choice is technetium 99^m albumin microspheres with a particle size of 20–40 μ. They are injected intravenously into a supine patient and in a normal lung are uniformly distributed. The lungs are scanned with a gamma camera. The fragments are removed by macrophages in the circulation and only 0·1% of the pulmonary capillaries are occluded by the technique. It is very unlikely that lung function will be made worse. A normal perfusion scan virtually excludes a pulmonary embolism but the test is not specific. Perfusion defects may result from other lung pathology, such as emphysema, tumour. However large defects, especially lobar defects are most likely to be due to pulmonary embolism.

Specificity is improved by demonstrating a ventilation–perfusion mismatch. In pulmonary embolism the defect in perfusion clearly exceeds that of ventilation but in chronic lung disease the defects are matched. Ventilation is assessed by scanning after inhalation of an inert gas, either xenon 133, xenon 127 or krypton 81.

Gamma camera images should be taken in six projections—anterior, posterior, both laterals and two obliques.

(v) *Pulmonary angiogram*: this is the most specific test. It has a low mortality but a significant morbidity so it is reserved for selected patients. A sharp cutoff in a vessel of 2·5 mm or more in diameter is diagnostic. Areas of oligaemia and asymmetry of blood flow occur.

Medical treatment

The aims of treatment are to prevent pulmonary embolism in patients with deep vein thrombosis and to prevent a recurrence in patients with a small or moderate pulmonary embolism. In massive pulmonary embolism efforts must be made to maintain cardiac output and in selected patients to lyse or remove the

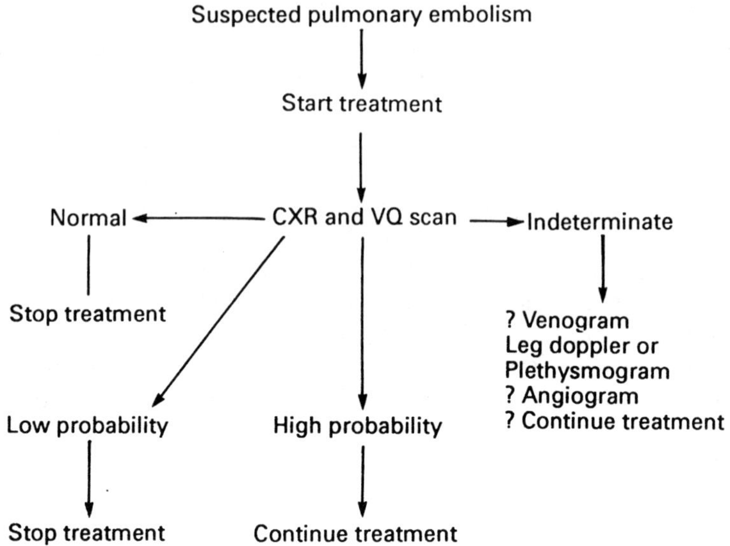

Massive pulmonary embolism: cardiovascular support and oxygen

Fig. 9.1. Management of suspected pulmonary embolism

vascular obstruction. Medical treatment should be tried first, and the management is outlined in Figure 9.1.

Anticoagulant therapy

Intravenous heparin should be started on suspicion of a pulmonary embolism; 40 000 units daily by intravenous continuous infusion is the usual initial dose except in elderly patients or those weighing less than 50 kg when the dose is reduced to 30 000 units. After the first day the dose is adjusted to maintain the partial thromboplastin time to two to three times the control.

Warfarin treatment can be started at the same time and should overlap intravenous heparin for 3 days or longer until the international normalised ratio is between two and three times normal. Warfarin 10 mg is given as the first dose and further doses decided by measurement of the international normalised ratio from 16 hours after the first, second and third daily dose. A flexible regime avoids overanticoagulation. Oral anticoagulants should be given for 3–6 months. Lifelong warfarin treatment is recommended for patients who have a second pulmonary embolism.

Lytic therapy

Treatment with streptokinase or urokinase should be reserved for carefully selected patients (Table 9.12).

Streptokinase is a purified streptococcal exotoxin. It combines with plasminogen in a 1:1 ratio and this complex activates the production of plasmin from the plasminogen left over in the plasma. This lyses fresh fibrin clots. Therapy should be monitored to achieve the most effective levels. Thrombin time should be maintained between two and three times normal. The usual dose is 600 000 units given intravenously over 30 min and followed by a constant infusion of 100 000 units/h for 48 h. Thereafter heparin is given in the usual way.

There is a high risk of haemorrhage. Sensitivity reactions may occur and hydrocortisone is often added to the initial infusion to suppress these.

Urokinase is a protein synthesised by kidney cells. It can be extracted from urine for commercial use but the process is

Table 9.12

INDICATIONS FOR LYTIC THERAPY

Immediately for critically ill patients with a combination of these clinical findings: Extreme shortness of breath Cold peripheries Hypotension Poor urine output Hypoxia with central nervous symptoms
Later in a small group initially treated with heparin who have survived 24 h but who do not make a usual haemodynamic recovery
Patients with pre-existing cardiac or pulmonary disease in whom spontaneous resolution will be delayed

complex and the drug is expensive. It is a direct activator o plasminogen and it is not antigenic. There is no good evidenc that it is more effective in the treatment of pulmonary embolism.

Other measures

Oxygen should be given to relieve hypoxaemia. Intravenous diamorphine will reduce pain and anxiety.

Surgical treatment

Embolectomy

Most patients with massive pulmonary embolism who survive the immediate crisis can be satisfactorily treated medically. Embolectomy requires cardiopulmonary bypass and for the majority of patients this means transfer to a cardiothoracic centre. Travelling is bad for patients suffering massive pulmonary embolism. They should only be moved in exceptional circumstances, which are:

(i) Failure to respond to streptokinase therapy.
(ii) A major contraindication to thrombolytic therapy.

Venous interruption

Of patients who have suffered a pulmonary embolism 80% have more clot in their leg or pelvic veins. There is no evidence that interrupting procedures reduce the risk of recurrence. This risk is about 3–5%. Operations themselves have a mortality of between 5–10%. Various procedures are available from insertion of an umbrella filter in the inferior vena cava to plication with sutures or ligation. These should be reserved for patients with:

(i) A major contraindication to anticoagulant therapy.
(ii) With major recurrences of emboli despite adequate anticoagulation.

Thromboembolism in Pregnancy

Pulmonary embolism is the second commonest cause of maternal death (after hypertensive disease). About three in every 1000 pregnant women are affected. Anticoagulant treatment presents additional risk to both mother and fetus.

Heparin does not cross the placenta. The main problems are bleeding and bone demineralisation in the mother. Demineralisation is thought to be due to a reduction in vitamin D levels and crush fractures may occur in women treated for over 3 months.

Warfarin is teratogenic and increases the risk of abortion. The embryopathy occurs in 5% of women given warfarin in the first trimester of pregnancy. It comprises abnormalities of the cartilage and bones, chondrodysplasia punctata, nasal hypoplasia and abnormalities of the central nervous system. Serious bleeding in the mother is common after 36 weeks.

Patients who develop pulmonary embolism or deep vein thrombosis should be anticoagulated for the remainder of the pregnancy and for 6 weeks after delivery. A suggested regime is intravenous heparin infusion up to 13 weeks and after 36 weeks of pregnancy, the dose of heparin being carefully monitored by a haematologist. The concentration is measured by the protamine sulphate neutralisation test. Oral heparin may be substituted in the intervening weeks and controlled by frequent prothrombin estimations. Neither heparin nor warfarin are secreted into breast milk and breastfeeding is safe.

Women with previous thromboembolism have a relatively low risk of recurrence (about 5–10%) in a further pregnancy. This must be balanced against the risk of anticoagulation. Bone demineralisation has occurred in patients taking only 10 000 units of heparin daily. Routine prophylaxis is not recommended for the patient who has had one previous thromboembolism.

FURTHER READING

Benatar S.R., Immelman E.J., Jeffery P. (1986). Pulmonary embolism (review). *British Journal of Diseases of the Chest*, **80**, 313–34.

Benotti J.R., Dalen J.E. (1984). The natural history of pulmonary embolism. *Clinics in Chest Medicine*, **5**, 403–10.

Coon, W.W. (1984). Venous thromboembolism. Prevalence, risk factors and prevention. *Clinics in Chest Medicine*, **5**, 391–402.

Fennerty A.G., Renowden S., Scolding N., Bentley D.P., Campbell I.A., Routledge P.A. (1986). Guidelines to control heparin treatment. *British Medical Journal*, **292**, 579–580.

Fennerty A., Dolben J., Thomas P., Backhouse G., Bentley D.P., Campbell I.A.,

Routledge P.A. (1984). Flexible induction dose regimen for warfarin and prediction of maintenance dose. *British Medical Journal*, **288**, 1268–1270.

Oakley C.M. (1985). Editorial: management of primary pulmonary hypertension. *British Heart Journal*, **53**, 1–4.

Thadani U., Burrow C., Whitaker W., Heath D. (1975). Pulmonary veno-occlusive disease. *Quarterly Journal of Medicine*, **173**, 133–159.

Chapter Ten

Heart Failure

Definition

Heart failure is a clinical syndrome consisting of the symptoms and signs which develop when the heart is unable to generate an output sufficient to meet the metabolic needs of the body.

Circulatory failure is a wider term and encompasses abnormalities of the heart, the volume or distribution of blood resulting in inadequate blood supply to the vital organs (Table 10.1).

Acute circulatory collapse is called shock. If it results from cardiac dysfunction it is termed cardiogenic shock.

Causes of heart failure

These can be divided into myocardial failure and non-myocardial disease (Table 10.2). The commonest causes are myocardial failure due to ischaemia or hypertension. The failure may be precipitated or aggravated by a secondary cause (Table 10.3). Heart failure is not by itself an adequate clinical diagnosis. The cause and any precipitating factor should always be stated.

Incidence and prognosis

Advanced heart failure affects about a quarter of a million people in the United Kingdom. It is a major cause of death. The prognosis is not good. The Framingham study in the United States showed that 50% of patients with chronic heart failure were dead within 5 years and 90% within 10 years. Recent advances in both the medical and surgical management may improve the outlook. New developments are the use of vasodilators, angiotensin-converting enzyme inhibitors and cardiac transplantation.

Table 10.1

CAUSES OF CIRCULATORY FAILURE

- Heart failure
- Low plasma volume
  - bleeding (rapid loss of 30% blood volume)
  - fluid loss, vomiting, diarrhoea
- Inappropriate distribution of blood
  - septicaemia
  - metabolic or toxic
    - overdose
    - liver failure
    - renal failure
    - repiratory failure
    - beriberi
  - endocrine
    - diabetic ketoacidosis
    - Addisonian crisis
    - phaeochromocytoma
    - thyrotoxic crisis
  - anaphylaxis
  - neurological
    - spinal cord injury
    - stroke with autonomic dysfunction
  - malignant hyperthermia

Table 10.2

CAUSES OF HEART FAILURE

Myocardial failure	*Non-myocardial causes*
Ischaemic heart disease	Valvular heart disease
Systemic hypertension	Congenital heart disease
Cardiomyopathy	Pericardial disease
Myocarditis	Cardiac tumours

Table 10.3

PRECIPITATING CAUSES OF HEART FAILURE

Arrhythmias: tachyarrhythmia, bradyarrhythmia, atrioventricular dissociation

Systemic infection: pneumonia

Infective endocarditis

Pulmonary embolism

Inappropriate drugs:
beta-blockers and other antiarrhythmic agents with negative inotropic effects
indomethacin, phenylbutazone and non-steroidal anti-inflammatory agents (NSAIDs) that cause sodium retention

Sodium and water overload, intravenous infusion

Withdrawal of adequate diuretic treatment

Thyrotoxicosis

Pathophysiology

There are four determinants of performance of the normal heart:

(i) Preload.
(ii) Afterload.
(iii) Contractility.
(iv) Heart rate.

Preload

This is the length or the passive stretch of myocardial fibres at the end of diastole. It equates to the ventricular end diastolic volume. Frank and Starling showed that the capacity of the ventricle to vary its force of contraction is dependent on its initial size. The force of the contraction depends on the initial muscle length. The higher the preload the more forceful is the contraction of the heart muscle fibres. Understretching (hypovolaemia) leads to a depression of myocardial performance. In these circumstances increasing preload will improve performance. This can be achieved by increasing circulatory volume. Atrial contraction, if properly timed, increases ventricular filling and preload. Normal atrial systole improves cardiac performance. An assessment of left ventricular preload can be indirectly obtained by measuring the pulmonary capillary wedge pressure.

Afterload

This is the force per unit area or tension developed in the wall of the ventricle during the ejection of blood that must be generated to maintain stroke volume. It is dependent upon (i) the peripheral vascular resistance which is the impedence to ventricular ejection and (ii) the size of the ventricular cavity derived from the law of Laplace which states that tension is the product of pressure in a sphere and its radius. Thus, the more dilated the ventricle, the larger the radius and the greater the tension which must be developed to achieve a given intra-cavity pressure.

Contractility

This is the force with which the myocardial fibres can contract independently of either the preload or afterload or heart rate. It is accepted that an increase in contractility occurs physiologically under increased sympathetic drive and can be achieved pharmacologically by giving drugs such as digoxin (inotropic agents). If preload and afterload are constant then cardiac performance will improve if contractility increases (a positive inotropic effect).

Heart rate

This is an important mechanism for increasing cardiac output and is under the control of the sympathetic and vagus nerves. It is affected by circulating catecholamines. When left ventricular and diastolic volume is maintained by increased venous return, as in exercise, cardiac output increases with an increase in heart rate. If heart rate is fixed, for instance in patients with heart block, then a maximal cardiac output during exercise cannot be achieved.

COMPENSATORY MECHANISMS FOR AN ABNORMALITY OF CARDIAC FUNCTION

The important compensatory mechanisms are:

(i) Neurohumoral changes.
(ii) The Frank–Starling mechanism.
(iii) Local factors affecting the arterioles.
(iv) Myocardial hypertrophy.

These compensatory mechanisms are interrelated and all have a limited potential. They eventually become detrimental to the patient with the failing heart.

The sympathetic tone is increased and the levels of circulating catecholamines are elevated in heart failure. In acute heart failure the effect is a positive inotropic and chronotropic response, but the changes are less obvious in chronic heart failure when there is apparent downgrading of the cardiac receptor sites. The peripheral effects of increased sympathetic activity are systemic arteriolar constriction and activation of the renin–angiotensin system. Angiotensin II is a potent vasoconstrictor and stimulates aldosterone secretion from the adrenal zona glomerulosa. Aldosterone increases the reabsorption of sodium in the proximal renal tubule and expands plasma volume.

Local factors such as hypoxia and histamine cause vasoconstriction of the arterioles.

The net effect of these compensatory mechanisms is to increase both pre and afterload on the heart.

The stretched cardiac muscle contracts with a greater force according to the Frank–Starling mechanism. However, this compensatory mechanism breaks down when the increases in pressure have no further effect on cardiac output. The pressure rise will lead to either pulmonary or systemic venous congestion and pulmonary or peripheral oedema is produced. When the myocardial fibres are maximally stretched the atroventricular valves are also stretched. Functional incompetence develops and this results in a further fall in forward stroke volume.

Chronic pressure or volume overload causes the myocardium to hypertrophy in an attempt to maintain systolic wall tension. When the stimulus is predominantly a pressure overload, for example, hypertension or aortic stenosis, the muscle mass increases without cavity dilatation. In chronic volume overload, for example, aortic or mitral regurgitation the myocardial fibres stretch and increase in mass. The cavity dilates and wall thickness is little changed.

For a time the hypertrophy allows the ventricle to compensate for the increased work.

Ultimately pathological hypertrophy leads to decreased contractility. This is due to left ventricular diastolic dysfunction as a result of impaired diastolic filling.

PULMONARY OEDEMA

Left heart failure produces pulmonary oedema. When the pulmonary capillary pressure exceeds plasma oncontic pressure

Table 10.4

CAUSES OF PULMONARY OEDEMA OTHER THAN LEFT VENTRICULAR FAILURE

Increased pulmonary capillary pressure
- Mitral stenosis

Decreased plasma oncotic pressure due to hypoalbuminaemia
- Renal disease
- Hepatic disease
- Other causes of protein loss such as enteropathies or skin diseases

Increased negative interstitial pressure due to rapid removal of a pneumothorax

Altered alveolar capillary membrane permeability due to:
- Inhaled toxins
- Aspiration of gastric contents
- Radiation
- Drugs, such as nitrofurantoin
- Shock lung with trauma

Lymphatic insufficiency

Unknown causes
- High altitude
- Neurogenic, such as head injury
- Narcotic overdose
- Eclampsia

(about 23 mmHg) water is forced out of the capillaries into the interstitial spaces of the lung, eventually filling the alveoli with disruption of the alveolar capillary membrane. Pulmonary oedema is a complication of disorders other than left heart failure and these are listed in Table 10.4.

CLINICAL PRESENTATION OF HEART FAILURE

Acute Heart Failure

The patient is breathless, has pulmonary oedema, is cyanosed and peripherally constricted. An acute cause will usually be found, such as myocardial infarction or acute valvular dysfunction. Patients with chronic heart failure may have episodes of acute exacerbation.

Chronic Heart Failure

Breathlessness is the major symptom. The other symptoms and signs result from the reduced cardiac output and from venous congestion with oedema.

Circulatory Collapse Due to an Abnormality of Cardiac Function (Cardiogenic Shock)

This is characterised by a low blood pressure, reduced or no urine output and very marked peripheral constriction.

Symptoms of heart failure

Shortness of breath

The most important symptom of left heart failure is breathlessness. The degree of respiratory distress depends upon the severity of heart failure. The progression is:

(i) Dyspnoea on exertion.
(ii) Orthopnoea.
(iii) Paroxysmal nocturnal dyspnoea.

Table 10.5

NEW YORK HEART ASSOCIATION FUNCTIONAL CLASSIFICATION

Class 1	No limitations. Patients are able to undertake ordinary physical activity without symptoms
Class 2	Slight limitation of physical activity. These patients are all right at rest but become short of breath, fatigued or develop angina with ordinary physical activity
Class 3	Marked limitation of physical activity. There are no symptoms at rest but ordinary physical activity quickly produces symptoms
Class 4	Symptoms are present even at rest

(iv) Dyspnoea at rest.
(v) Acute pulmonary oedema.

The New York Heart Association Classification is often used to grade functional impairment (Table 10.5).

Cough

Patients in heart failure often have a non-productive cough. It occurs under the same circumstances as dyspnoea and is caused by pulmonary congestion.

Orthopnoea

This is shortness of breath that develops while lying down and which is relieved by sitting or standing.

Paroxysmal nocturnal dyspnoea

These attacks are acute exaggerations of orthopnoea. They usually awaken the patient with extreme gasping for breath and a feeling of suffocation. The patient may wheeze and this is called cardiac asthma. It is caused by congestion of the bronchial mucosa.

Other symptoms of heart failure are listed in Table 10.6.

Table 10.6

GENERAL SYMPTOMS OF HEART FAILURE

Symptom	*Explanation*
Lethargy and weakness	Low cardiac output
Tiredness of the legs when walking	Reduced blood flow in muscles due to increased resistance in arterioles
Confusion	Hypoxia and hypotension
Extreme anxiety and restlessness with acute heart failure	Hypoxia and hypotension
Insomnia	Hypoxia and hypotension
Nocturia	Change in diurnal rhythm of urine production which is suppressed during the day when the patient is upright and increased at night while supine
Oliguria	Marked fall in renal perfusion in severe heart failure
Upper abdominal pain	Liver congestion
Anorexia, sickness, constipation	Congestion of the bowel
Loss of weight (cardiac cachexia)	Severe anorexia

Physical signs of heart failure

The patient with acute heart failure gasps for breath. There may be pink frothy sputum, cyanosis, tachycardia and obvious peripheral vasoconstriction. Profuse sweating is common.

Lung signs

In acute heart failure crepitations are heard over both lung fields. They result from transudation of fluid into the alveoli. There may be wheeze and this can lead to diagnostic confusion with bronchial asthma. In very severe heart failure Cheyne–Stokes respiration may be present.

In chronic heart failure the crepitations are most frequently heard at the bases of the lungs and they may be associated with pleural effusions. These are usually bilateral but if unilateral the effusion is on the right side. Crepitations are frequently heard in cigarette smokers and patients with respiratory disease. By themselves they do not establish the diagnosis of left ventricular failure.

Additional heart sounds

These are the most reliable signs in the diagnosis of heart failure.

The *third heart sound* occurs during the period of rapid filling of the ventricles. It may be physiological in people up to the age of 40. It is rarely heard after this age unless there is pathology which causes early rapid filling of the ventricles, that is, heart failure in which the elevated venous pressure causes the rapid flow.

The *fourth heart sound* is produced by contraction of the atria and is heard at the end of diastole in conditions which hinder the filling of the ventricles such as left ventricular failure.

When there is tachycardia the third and fourth heart sounds cannot be identified separately and are heard as one—a *summation gallop*.

Pulsus alternans

Pulsus alternans is a regular rhythm with alternate strong and weak beats. It may be detected either by palpation or sphygmomanometry in very severe left ventricular failure. It is due to an alteration in stroke volume due to the incomplete recovery of failing myocardial fibres.

Systemic venous hypertension

This is detected by examination of the jugular venous pulse. Two observations should be made:

(i) The height of the pulse in the neck.
(ii) The type of wave form.

In sinus rhythm an 'a' and a 'v' wave will be seen. The 'a' wave is caused by venous distension due to right atrial systole. It is not present in atrial fibrillation. The 'v' wave results from the rise in right atrial pressure when blood flows into the right atrium at the time when the tricuspid valve is shut. The liver often enlarges before oedema develops. Compression of a congested liver produces expansion of the jugular vein. This is because the right heart cannot easily accept this increased venous return in heart failure. The sign is known as hepatojugular reflux.

Oedema

Oedema occurs in the dependent parts of the body. It accumulates over the sacrum in bedridden patients and in ambulant patients at the feet and ankles. In very chronic severe congestive heart failure oedema becomes generalised (anasarca). It may then be associated with the development of ascites and large pleural effusions.

INVESTIGATION OF HEART FAILURE

The cause of heart failure often cannot be made without some investigation (Table 10.7). Investigations are also useful to monitor the effects of treatment.

Chest X-ray

This is the best investigation to confirm the presence of left heart failure. It is also a useful guide to the severity of failure—although there may be a timelag between development and

Table 10.7

INVESTIGATION OF HEART FAILURE

Chest X-ray
Electrocardiogram
Blood tests
Echocardiogram
Radionuclide studies
Right heart catheterisation
Left heart catheterisation

resolution of changes as judged radiologically compared to the clinical condition. The heart size and shape is best evaluated with a frontal (posterior–anterior) film, a penetrated film and a left lateral film.

Redistribution of blood flow (upper lobe blood diversion)

When the pulmonary capillary pressure is elevated to 12–18 mmHg flow to the lower lung fields is reduced due to vasoconstriction. This is caused by perivascular oedema and the effect is most at the bases because hydrostatic pressure is greater there. Flow to the upper lung fields is increased and the diameter of the upper lobe blood vessels eventually becomes greater than those in the lower lobes.

Kerley B-lines (septal lines)

These lines are found in the lower lung fields. They occur in the periphery and extend to the surface of the lung. They are caused by fluid accumulating in the interstitial spaces. The pulmonary vessels become enlarged and their radiographic shadows become blurred.

Kerley A-lines are also produced by interstitial fluid. They are not limited to the basal areas and often originate from the hilum but do not extend to the pleural surface.

Alveolar oedema

When the pulmonary capillary pressure rises acutely above 23 mmHg filling of the alveolar spaces can occur. Confluent patchy densities radiate outwards from the mediastinum—the 'batswing' appearance.

Electrocardiogram

This is usually abnormal in the presence of heart failure and is useful in establishing the presence of rhythm disturbance, myocardial damage and ventricular hypertrophy. T-wave inversion is caused by an abnormality of repolarisation but should not necessarily be equated to ischaemia.

Blood Tests

It is essential to monitor the urea and electrolytes in the management of heart failure. Estimation of haemoglobin and serum thyroxine may be indicated if anaemia or thyrotoxicosis is suspected. Blood cultures to exclude infective endocarditis should alway be taken in patients with heart failure and a murmur.

Echocardiogram

Echocardiography is non-invasive and extremely useful. The size of the cardiac chambers, ventricular wall thickness, contractility, valve function and disease can be assessed. Left ventricular ejection fraction can be calculated. Two-dimensional echocardiography provides additional information about regional wall motion and can be used to demonstrate a ventricular aneurysm. Pericardial effusion can be identified.

Radionuclide Studies

Two types of study are commonly performed.

Gated pool imaging

Gated blood pool imaging uses red cells labelled with technetium 99 (multigated nuclear angiogram—MUGA scan). The first pass through the heart may be studied to exclude a significant left-to-right shunt. The blood pool study or nuclear angiogram builds up cycles of cardiac action by gating the pictures to the electrocardiogram. The ejection fraction and parameters of systolic and diastolic function may be calculated, the ventricular size and segmental wall motion may be studied and ventricular aneurysms detected. The investigation may be combined with exercise which will reveal wall motion abnormalities in patients with ischaemic heart disease.

Thallium myocardial perfusion scan

This may demonstrate that ischaemia is the cause of heart failure.

Right Heart Catheterisation via a Subclavian Vein

A Swan–Ganz balloon catheter can be advanced into the pulmonary artery and inflation of the balloon will float and wedge the catheter tip in a small pulmonary artery branch. The 'pulmonary capillary wedge pressure' is an indirect measurement of left atrial pressure which in turn usually reflects left ventricular end diastolic pressure. This technique can be used to confirm the presence of heart failure and is often useful in monitoring the acute effects of treatment. If the mean pulmonary capillary wedge pressure equates to the end diastolic pulmonary artery pressure, the catheter can be left in the pulmonary artery for pressure measurements.

Left Heart Catheterisation and Coronary Arteriography

This invasive investigation is reserved for patients in whom other investigations have failed to elucidate the cause of heart failure. It is usually a prerequisite when cardiac surgery is contemplated. For instance, clinical examination, electrocardiography and echocardiography may have established that aortic stenosis is the cause of heart failure. Many cardiac surgeons would still demand a coronary arteriogram to exclude significant coexistent coronary artery disease.

MANAGEMENT OF ACUTE HEART FAILURE

The following steps are taken:

(i) The patient should be sat upright and given 100% oxygen by nasal catheters.

(ii) Intravenous diuretic: a loop diuretic, such as either frusemide or bumetanide, should be injected intravenously. Symptoms are often relieved before any diuretic effect. This is due to vasodilatation and a reduction in ventricular preload. Huge doses do not need to be used in patients who have not been exposed to diuretic therapy and 40 mg of frusemide will often suffice. Larger doses may compromise ventricular filling by too great a reduction in preload.

(iii) Intravenous morphine 5–10 mg or diamorphine 5 mg can be given cautiously to anxious patients but should be avoided in the elderly or exhausted. Opiates act centrally, relieving anxiety, and reducing sympathetic activity. This results in vasodilatation and a further reduction in ventricular preload.

(iv) Vasodilators: nitrates are effective in the reduction of pulmonary oedema and should be used in patients with an elevated jugular venous pressure. Their main action is to dilate the venous capacitance bed but they also dilate the pulmonary and coronary circulations.

(v) Aminophylline can be a useful drug when there is marked bronchospasm complicating pulmonary oedema. However, it should be given with great caution (250 mg over 10 min) as it may induce life-threatening arrhythmia.

(vi) Reduction in blood volume: removal of a pint ($1\frac{3}{4}$ litres) of blood or temporary tourniquets around the thighs (not more than 30 min) produces an acute reduction of ventricular preload which is occasionally beneficial in emergency treatment.

(vii) Positive pressure ventilation can clear pulmonary oedema which is resistant to other measures, but will often cause a fall in systemic blood pressure.

(viii) Intra-aortic balloon counter pulsation: mechanical circulatory assistance should only be used when there is a surgically correctable cause of acute heart failure—for instance in the preparation for surgery of a patient with an acute ventricular septal defect.

(ix) Correction of precipitating factors (see Table 10.3): effective measures to control rhythm disturbance in particular are of extreme importance.

MANAGEMENT OF CIRCULATORY COLLAPSE

This will depend upon the clinical diagnosis. Blood pressure and tissue perfusion can be easily assessed. Treatment, however, often requires knowledge of the filling pressure of the left ventricle. These questions must be answered:

(i) Has the circulation collapsed because the pump is failing as a result of myocardial dysfunction (cardiogenic shock)?

or

(ii) Is the pump failing because of inadequate ventricular filling?

The jugular venous pressure relates only to right ventricular filling and can be misleading in reflecting left ventricular function. To be confident about adjustments in treatment the pulmonary capillary wedge pressure or pulmonary artery end diastolic pressure must be monitored using a Swan–Ganz catheter.

Circulatory collapse due to haemorrhage, septic or anaphylactic shock requires volume expansion with intravenous fluids.

Cardiogenic shock is most often caused by massive myocardial infarction involving 40% or more of the left ventricular mass. In these circumstances the ventricle contracts poorly and left ventricular filling pressure is generally increased. This is a critical medical emergency and should be managed in an intensive or coronary care unit. The clinician must always be clear about what can be achieved and many patients will inevitably die.

Left ventricular performance must be helped by making sure that the preload and afterload are optimal.

The ideal left ventricular filling pressure is at the upper limit of the normal range, that is about 18 mmHg. If it is greater than this but blood pressure is being maintained then a vasodilator should be given. If both blood pressure and tissue perfusion are reduced then an inotropic agent (dopamine and/or dobutamine) should be infused to increase ventricular contractility. If possible a vasodilator should be added to reduce peripheral vasoconstriction. The primary aim is to increase cardiac output, usually with an increase in myocardial contractility. Pulmonary function should also be improved by reducing the pulmonary capillary pressure to relieve pulmonary oedema. Increases in renal and cerebral blood flow will lead to an improved urine output and mental state.

MANAGEMENT OF CHRONIC HEART FAILURE

The possibility of a surgically correctable lesion should be considered. This would make early investigation mandatory. Examples are: aortic stenosis, postinfarction ventricular septal defect, valve destruction due to infective endocarditis.

Systemic hypertension is an important cause of heart failure and high blood pressure should be treated.

Treatment principles

General measures

Appropriate restriction of activity should be advised. Patients should stop smoking and reduce their salt intake.

Diuretics

A thiazide diuretic or a combination with a potassium-sparing diuretic, such as amiloride or triamterene, should be given to patients in mild heart failure. In more severe cases a loop diuretic will be necessary. The serum potassium should be monitored to avoid hypokalaemia which can induce arrhythmias. It is essential to clear pulmonary oedema but overzealous attempts to remove all peripheral oedema at the expense of increasing uraemia should be resisted.

Vasodilator therapy

This represents a major change in the conventional approach to chronic heart failure. Diuretics remove fluid but are potentially detrimental because they stimulate the renin–angiotensin system which leads to more vasoconstriction. Plasma volume is reduced, glomerular filtration is reduced and blood urea rises. Vasodilator therapy is aimed at improving the haemodynamics of the failing heart and can often allow a reduction in the total dosage of diuretic. They should probably be introduced into the treatment regime sooner rather than later. Venous dilators reduce preload and arteriolar dilators the afterload. Angiotensin-converting enzyme inhibitors increase serum potassium levels and should not be given concurrently with potassium-sparing diuretics. The dose-limiting factor is hypotension. Renal and coronary blood flow will be compromised if the arterial pressure is reduced to beneath 90/60 mmHg.

Digoxin

Everyone agrees that digoxin should be given to patients in rapid atrial fibrillation. Control of the rate of atrial fibrillation and improved ventricular filling increases cardiac output. There is still controversy about the use of digoxin in the presence of sinus rhythm. Many patients do not benefit and will of course be exposed to the toxic effects of the drug. It would seem sensible not to give digoxin at first to patients in sinus rhythm. If diuretics and vasodilator therapy fail then a cautious trial of digoxin is worthwhile.

Other inotropic agents

The beneficial effect of dopamine and dobutamine appears to be largely restricted to acute administration. Long-term infusions are usually ineffective although intermittent 24 h infusions may be tried. Inotropic drugs with vasodilating properties like amrinone or milrinone are more effective but have troublesome side-effects. Xamoterol is a $beta_1$ receptor partial agonist which increases cardiac output in chronic, moderate or mild cardiac failure.

Antiarrhythmic agents

Sudden death is common in patients with chronic ischaemic heart failure, often due to ventricular arrhythmias. Conventional antiarrhythmic drugs have a negative inotropic effect and may worsen heart failure. Amiodarone is less likely to depress left ventricular function and should be considered for some patients. Ambulatory electrocardiographic recordings are useful in patient selection.

Surgery for cardiac failure secondary to coronary artery disease

Patients with heart failure and a left ventricular aneurysm caused by myocardial infarction may benefit from aneurysm resection and revascularisation. Other patients with overt heart failure are not usually considered for surgery. However, the prognosis of patients with diminished left ventricular function associated with atheromatous disease in all three main coronary artery branches is improved by coronary artery bypass surgery.

CARDIAC TRANSPLANTATION

The first human-to-human heart transplant was performed in 1967 by Professor Christiaan Barnard in Cape Town. The procedure is now offered to an increasing number of patients with a wide variety of heart disease (Table 10.8). Younger patients do better and the operation is mainly confined to patients under the age of 55. The timing of surgery is difficult. The patient must be judged to have terminal heart failure but the operation should not be delayed until irreversible renal, liver and lung damage has occurred. Survival has improved, due mainly to the introduction of percutaneous transvenous endomyocardial biopsy to diagnose acute rejection and to improved immunosuppressive agents, particularly cyclosporin A. The 1 and 2 year survival rate is now 80%.

Table 10.8

INDICATIONS FOR CARDIAC TRANSPLANTATION

Dilated cardiomyopathy
Ischaemic heart disease with resistant heart failure and a dilated hypodynamic left ventricle
Hypertrophic cardiomyopathy with resistant heart failure
Congenital heart disease which is otherwise inoperable but not with increased pulmonary resistance. Cardiopulmonary transplantation is being developed for patients with pulmonary hypertension

PREVENTION OF HEART FAILURE

The commonest cause of chronic heart failure is coronary artery disease with myocardial infarction. Intervention within the first 6 hours of a heart attack (Table 10.9) may reduce the size of the

Table 10.9

PRESERVATION OF THE MYOCARDIUM IN AN ACUTE HEART ATTACK

Early and effective pain relief
Early admission to a coronary care unit: correction of cardiac arrhythmias
Early thrombolysis, peripheral venous administration of streptokinase
Percutaneous transluminal coronary angioplasty

infarct and the incidence of heart failure. The most important developing treatment is the advent of thrombolysis followed by coronary angioplasty.

FURTHER READING

Dollery C.T., Corr L. (1985). Drug treatment of heart failure. *British Heart Journal*, **54**, 234–242.

Francis G.S. (1985). Neurohumoral mechanisms involved in congestive heart failure. *American Journal of Cardiology*, **55**, 15A–21A.

Lipkin D.P., Poole-Wilson P.A. (1985). Treatment of chronic heart failure: a review of recent drug trials. *British Medical Journal*, **291**, 993–996.

McKee P.A., Castelli W.P., McNamara P.M., Kannel W.B. (1971). The natural history of congestive heart failure: the Framingham Study. *New England Journal of Medicine*, **285**, 1441–1446.

Chapter Eleven

Drugs and the Heart

INOTROPIC AGENTS

These are drugs which increase the force of contraction of the heart. Calcium ions are the final link in the excitation–contraction process of muscle and the tension developed in the myocardial fibres is dependent on the amount of calcium present. Inotropic agents increase calcium delivery. They are classified in Table 11.1.

Table 11.1

CLASSIFICATION OF INOTROPIC DRUGS

Digitalis glycosides	
Sympathomimetic amines	
alpha and beta-agonists	Noradrenaline Adrenaline Dopamine
$beta_1$ agonists	Dobutamine Prenalterol Xamoterol
$beta_1$ and $beta_2$ agonists	Isoprenaline
$beta_2$ agonists	Salbutamol Pirbuterol
Phosphodiesterase inhibitors	Aminophylline Amrinone Milrinone
Glucagon	
Calcium	

Digitalis Glycosides

Glycosides are compounds of plant origin, made up of a sugar combined to a steroid nucleus and a lactone ring (Table 11.2). William Withering first described the effects and hazards of digitalis in 1785.

Digoxin is the most commonly used glycoside and is extracted from the dried leaves of *Digitalis lanata* plants grown commercially in the Netherlands.

Mechanism of action

The cardiac glycosides inhibit sodium–potassium (Na–K) adenosine triphosphatase (ATPase) in the sarcolemma (the sodium pump). Sodium accumulates in the cells and displaces bound calcium ions which produce a positive inotropic effect.

The antiarrhythmic action is due to the effects on the heart and indirectly on the autonomic nervous system.

The cardiac effects are:

(i) The refractory period in the conducting tissues is increased. This causes slowing of the ventricular response to atrial fibrillation and flutter. The P–R interval is prolonged in sinus rhythm.
(ii) The refractory period in the atria and ventricles is decreased (Q–T interval shortens).

Toxicity is also related to the inhibition of ATPase activity. Sodium replaces intracellular potassium which results in a loss of

Table 11.2

PLANT ORIGIN OF DIGITALIS GLYCOSIDES

Drug	*Plant*
Digoxin	*Digitalis lanata*
Lanatoside C	*Digitalis lanata*
Digitoxin	*Digitalis purpura*
Ouabain	*Strophanthus gratus* seeds

membrane potential and increased excitability and automaticity in the atrial and ventricular myocardial cells. Digitalis and potassium compete for the digitalis binding sites on the cell membranes. With hypokalaemia digoxin fills more of the binding sites and toxicity occurs.

Pharmacokinetics

The digitalis glycosides have very different pharmacokinetics.

Digoxin

In the past there has been wide and dangerous variation in bioavailability due to differences in manufacture. A new standard for bioavailability was set in 1975 and now all brands conform.

Bioavailability of digoxin is 90%. Absorption through the duodenum is rapid and it is therefore no better to give digoxin parenterally than by mouth. It is excreted largely unchanged by the kidney. The micro-organism *Eubacterium lentum* can inactivate digoxin in the gut and changes in bowel flora, for instance by concurrent use of antibiotics, can alter blood levels. The plasma half-life is 36 h.

Digitoxin

This is completely absorbed and is either metabolised or excreted in the gut. This means that blood levels are not altered by poor renal function. Digitoxin has an enterohepatic circulation and 25% is recycled. Cholestyramine binds with the glycoside in the gut and prevents reabsorption.

The plasma half-life is 5 days. If a patient forgets a dose there is little change in the plasma levels.

Lanatoside C

This glycoside is less well absorbed than digoxin and is converted to digoxin in the gut. There is greater variation in bioavailability.

Ouabain

It is not absorbed and must be given intravenously. The peak effect is obtained within 2 h. Elimination is mostly through the kidneys and the plasma half-life is 18 h.

Clinical uses and management of digoxin therapy

Digoxin is the treatment of first choice in:

(i) Patients with atrial fibrillation or flutter and a rapid ventricular response.
(ii) Patients with heart failure and atrial fibrillation.

Other indications have lessened with the development of new antiarrhythmic drugs and different approaches to the management of heart failure. Acute heart failure should be treated first with diuretics and vasodilators. The role of digitalis in patients with chronic heart failure and sinus rhythm remains debated. The practical approach is to reserve digitalis therapy for those who fail to respond satisfactorily.

Table 11.3

FACTORS WHICH ALTER THE EFFECT OF DIGOXIN

Cause	Mechanism
Increased effect	
Renal failure	Reduced clearance
Old age	Reduced clearance
Myxoedema	Reduced clearance
Spironolactone and triamterene	Inhibits renal tubular secretion
Hypokalaemia (diuretics, beta$_2$ stimulators)	Increased sensitivity
Hypoxia	Increased sensitivity
Quinidine, flecainide, amiodarone, verapamil	Drug interactions ?displacement from myocardium
Decreased effect	
Gastrointestinal upset	Reduced absorption
Malabsorption	Reduced absorption
Metoclopramide	Speeds gut transit time
Antacids	Adsorb digoxin and retain it in the gut
Thyrotoxicosis	Increased clearance
Phenylbutazone, phenytoin, rifampicin	Drug interactions

Treatment with digoxin is normally started with a loading dose of 0·5 mg orally. This is followed by 0·25 mg at 8 h and 0·25 mg at 16 h. The usual maintenance dose is 0·25 mg daily but this must be reduced in elderly patients or when renal function is impaired. The factors altering the effect of digoxin are listed in Table 11.3.

There are certain clinical situations where digoxin is contraindicated or when it must be given with special care. These are listed in Table 11.4.

Table 11.4

CONTRAINDICATIONS TO TREATMENT WITH DIGITALIS

Condition	*Reason*
Digitalis toxicity	Absolute contraindication. Digitalis treatment must be stopped until toxicity resolves
Heart block	First and second degree atrioventricular block may be converted to complete heart block
Direct current cardioversion	Ventricular fibrillation can be precipitated if the patient is digitalis toxic. (Ideally stop digoxin treatment 48 h before cardioversion)
Acute myocardial infarction	Digitalis glycosides should be reserved for patients with atrial fibrillation/and heart failure. Given to patients in sinus rhythm there is at least a theoretical risk that digoxin may do harm by increasing the infarct size
Hypertrophic obstructive cardiomyopathy	The inotropic effect worsens outflow obstruction
Pulmonary heart disease with hypoxia	Hypoxia increases sensitivity
Wolff–Parkinson–White (W–P–W) syndrome	The anterograde conducting pathway may be accelerated

Toxicity

Digitalis has a low therapeutic index—in other words, the difference between the plasma and tissue level which produces an optimal beneficial effect or causes toxicity is small. Great care must be taken to adjust the dose according to clinical observations and when indicated by measurement of the steady state plasma digoxin concentration. Evidence for toxicity is listed in Table 11.5.

Treatment of digitalis toxicity The patient should not be given more digitalis glycoside until toxicity has resolved. The plasma electrolytes must be measured and hypokalaemia corrected. Supraventricular arrhythmias often respond to beta-blockade. Temporary cardiac pacing may be required for heart block.

A massive digitalis overdose is life-threatening. Fab-fragments of digoxin specific antibodies are now available from poison centres. These are intact antibodies isolated from sheep antisera which are cleaved into fab-fragments. Digoxin binds with these and the plasma level falls sharply.

In digitoxin toxicity cholestyramine should be given to prevent enterohepatic circulation.

Table 11.5

TOXICITY OF DIGITALIS GLYCOSIDES

Extracardiac manifestations
Fatigue and profound muscle weakness
Nausea, vomiting, diarrhoea and abdominal pain
Yellow-green vision
Headache
Cardiac manifestations
Ventricular bigeminy
Tachyarrhythmias
Bradycardia and atrioventricular conduction disturbances
Electrocardiographic changes
Arrhythmias
Decreased T-wave amplitude
S–T segment depression (inverted tick sign)
Increase in U-wave amplitude
Shortening of the Q–T interval

Measurement of plasma digoxin

Digoxin is measured by a radioimmunoassay. The therapeutic range of digoxin is 1–2 ng/ml. (Match the plasma digoxin level with the serum potassium.) Blood should be taken 4–6 h after the last dose was given. The measurement can be useful in:

(i) The diagnosis of an overdose of digoxin.
(ii) The diagnosis of toxicity.
(iii) To assess drug compliance.
(iv) Where there appears to be therapeutic failure.

Sympathomimetic Amines

The endogenous and synthetic sympathomimetic amines have different effects due to their relative specificity for the adrenoceptors. The cardiovascular responses are classified in Table 11.6.

Table 11.6

CLASSIFICATION OF ADRENOCEPTORS

Adrenoceptor	*Site*	*Effect of stimulation*
$Alpha_1$	Postsynaptic	
	Vascular smooth muscle	Vasoconstriction
	Myocardium	Weak positive inotropic
$Alpha_2$	Presynaptic	Decreased sympathetic outflow in the CNS
$Beta_1$	Myocardium	Positive inotropic and chronotropic response
$Beta_2$	Vascular smooth muscle	Vasodilatation
Dopaminergic	Renal and mesenteric vascular beds	Vasodilatation

Dopamine

Dopamine is the naturally occurring immediate precursor of noradrenaline and has the following actions:

(i) Directly stimulates $beta_1$ receptors.
(ii) Releases noradrenaline from sympathetic nerve terminals which stimulates $beta_1$ receptors.
(iii) At low doses it activates specific dopaminergic receptors causing vasodilatation in the renal and mesenteric vascular beds.
(iv) At high doses it stimulates $alpha_1$ receptors causing vasoconstriction.

Dopamine is given by intravenous infusion starting at a dose of 0·5 μg/kg/min and increased in 2 μg/kg/min increments every 15 minutes. Stimulation of renal dopaminergic receptors and increase in renal blood flow is achieved with doses of between 2 μg/kg/min and 6 μg/kg/min. $Alpha_1$ mediated vasoconstriction occurs with >8 μg/kg/min. Tachycardia, arrhythmias, headache and anxiety occur with moderate to high doses (>6 μg/kg/min).

Dobutamine

This is a synthetic analogue of dopamine. It has a direct effect on the $beta_1$ receptors but it does not release noradrenaline nor does it have an action on the dopamine receptors. Therefore it does not alter renal blood flow. Its advantage is that it produces less tachycardia than dopamine and is safer in patients with myocardial infarction. The usual dose is 2·5 μg/kg/min increasing to 15 μg/kg/min.

These two inotropic agents may be used in combination.

Orally active $beta_1$ stimulants, Xamoterol

Xamoterol is a cardioselective $beta_1$ partial agonist and has a positive inotropic effect when sympathetic tone is low. This is the first $beta_1$ partial agonist that is orally active. It occupies the beta 1 receptors in the myocardium and in mild or moderate heart failure, its agonist activity may increase cardiac output by 10–25%. On exercise it attenuates the increase in heart rate which may make it particularly useful in patients with mild heart failure accompanied by angina pectoris. Xamoterol is contraindicated in severe heart failure when sympathetic tone is high.

Beta$_2$ agonists

Salbutamol and pirbuterol, which is seven times more specific for beta$_2$ receptors than salbutamol, have been shown to produce an acute rise in cardiac output largely due to a reduction in peripheral resistance. They are effective acutely but induce serious arrhythmias.

Phosphodiesterase Inhibitors

An alternative approach to myocardial stimulation is to increase cyclic adenosine monophosphate (cAMP) by inhibiting the degrading enzyme, phosphodiesterase. The methyl xanthines (such as aminophylline) produce a positive inotropic effect by this mechanism. Their use is limited by the high incidence of arrhythmias.

The dipyramides, amrinone and milrinone, are being investigated. They are thought to work by inhibiting phosphodiesterase. Amrinone has produced serious side-effects including thrombocytopenia.

Clinical uses of non-digitalis inotropic agents

The major use is in the management of cardiogenic shock. Careful haemodynamic monitoring is essential. There is some evidence that ischaemic damage may be accelerated.

Tachyphylaxis occurs during long-term treatment with sympathomimetic amines due to down-regulation of cardiac beta$_1$ receptors and limits their usefulness. Intermittent intravenous infusions of dobutamine, given for 48 h every week, may overcome this and produce some long-term benefits in chronic congestive heart failure.

VASODILATORS

This group of drugs have very different pharmacological properties and produce vasodilatation by a number of mechanisms (Table 11.7). Drugs which dilate veins increase the volume of the

Table 11.7

CLASSIFICATION OF VASODILATORS

Mechanism of action	*Vasodilator*	*Predominant site of action*
Direct vascular smooth muscle relaxation	Morphine	Veins
	Nitrites (amyl nitrite)	Veins and arteries
	Nitrates	Veins and arteries
	Sodium nitroprusside	Arteries and veins
	Hydralazine	Arteries
	Diazoxide, minoxidil	Arteries
$Alpha_1$ (postsynaptic) adrenoceptor blockade with accumulation of cyclic AMP in vascular smooth muscle	Prazosin	Arteries and veins
	Terazosin	Arteries and veins
	Lidoramin	Arteries and veins
	Phentolamine	Arteries and veins
	Phenoxybenzamine	Arteries and veins
	Labetalol	Arteries and veins (also a beta-blocker)
$Alpha_2$ (presynaptic) stimulation in the brain stem with inhibition of synaptic outflow	Methyldopa	
	Clonidine	
Calcium slow channel blocker	Nifedipine	Arteries (±veins)
	Verapamil	Arteries (+veins)
	Diltiazem	Arteries (±veins)
	Nicardipine	Arteries (±veins)
Angiotensin converting enzyme inhibitors	Captopril	Arteries (±veins)
	Enalapril	
$Beta_2$ receptor agonists	Salbutamol	Arteries and veins
	Pirbutol	
Stimulation of AMP accumulation in vascular smooth muscle	Prostacyclin	Arteries (±veins)
	Prostaglandin E	

Table 11.8

THERAPEUTIC USE OF VASODILATATION

Clinical disorder	*Commonly used drugs*
Stable angina pectoris	Nitrates Calcium slow channel blockers
Coronary artery spasm	Nitrates Calcium slow channel blockers
Chronic hypertension	Hydralazine Prazosin Indoramin Labetalol Clonidine Nifedipine Verapamil Angiotensin converting enzyme (ACE) inhibitors
Hypertensive crises	Sodium nitroprusside Diazoxide and minoxidil Phentolamine Labetalol Nifedipine
Heart failure	Nitrates Hydralazine Prazosin Nicardipine Angiotensin converting enzyme (ACE) inhibitors

capacitance vessels, reduce preload and ventricular filling pressure. Drugs which dilate arteries and arterioles decrease the systemic vascular resistance (afterload). Most affect both the arteriolar and venous beds to some extent.

Clinical uses

Vasodilators are used in a wide variety of cardiovascular conditions (Table 11.8). Some have additional therapeutic effects which are discussed separately (see specific drugs).

Direct dilators of vascular smooth muscle

Nitrates

Both short-acting and long-acting nitrates have an important role in the prophylaxis and treatment of angina pectoris. They produce peripheral venous dilatation and thus a reduction in venous return to the heart (preload). Arteriolar diltation also occurs with consequent reduction in afterload. Left ventricular work and myoc ardial oxygen demand are reduced.

Nitrates dilate large coronary arteries and can prevent spasm in coronary arteries with or without atheromatous plaques. Small intramural coronary arteries are also dilated and this may lead to a redistribution of blood flow to ischaemic areas.

Sublingual glyceryl trinitrate gives rapid relief of an acute attack of angina but its effect lasts for about 30 min. The 300 μg tablet is appropriate for initial treatment when there is no tolerance to side-effects; 500 μg tablets are usually prescribed for long-term prophylaxis and treatment. An aerosol spray has the advantages of not degrading like an opened bottle of tablets (these should be replaced after 8 weeks), and in old people who may have difficulty in salivating to dissolve the tablet.

Sustained release and transcutaneous release preparations of glyceryl trinitrate have a prolonged effect. Long-acting nitrates (isosorbide mononitrate, isosorbide dinitrate) have been shown to have haemodynamic benefits in heart failure and confer longer protection against angina.

Side-effects of the nitrates include tachycardia, severe headache, hypotension and syncope. Intermittent treatment results in a reproducible cardiovascular effects, but continuous high blood levels of nitrates leads to a decrease of the pharmacological effects (tolerance). To prevent nitrate tolerance it is esential that dosing schedules should be designed to provide a period of at least several hours each day when nitrate levels are low.

Sodium nitroprusside

Intravenous sodium nitroprusside is reserved for emergency situations—hypertensive crises, and the control of blood pressure in patients presenting with a dissecting aortic aneurysm. The infusion (0·5 μg/kg/min increasing to up to 8 μg/kg/min) should not continue for more than 48 h because nitroprusside is converted into cyanmethaemoglobin and free cyanide which can accumulate and become toxic.

Hydralazine

Intravenous hydralazine is used for hypertensive emergencies including pre-eclampsia. For the long-term oral treatment of hypertension it is best to combine it with a beta-blocking agent to reduce reflex tachycardia. Systemic lupus erythematosus is an important side-effect at doses above 100 mg/day. The drug is metabolised by acetylation in the liver and then excreted in the urine. Slow acetylators are more likely to develop the lupus syndrome.

Diazoxide and minoxidil

Diazoxide has been used for hypertensive emergencies but a lower dose than previously recommended should be given to avoid severe hypotension (30–100 mg intravenously). Chronic treatment produces diabetes. Both diazoxide and minoxidil cause hirsutism, sodium retention and often gross oedema. Patients may require large doses of diuretics to counter this side-effect. Long-term treatment should be reserved for the exceptional patient with resistant hypertension.

Alpha-adrenoceptor blockers

Prazosin

Prazosin is a quinazoline derivative which selectively blocks postsynaptic alpha$_1$-receptors in the walls of blood vessels. It affects both the arteries and veins. It is well absorbed by the gut and is metabolised in the liver. It does not cause a reflex tachycardia but first-dose hypotension and syncope may be a problem. An initial dose of 0·5 mg by mouth is recommended and this should be given in the evening so that the patient spends the next few hours in bed.

Prazosin is established as a long-term treatment for hypertension. It is used in refractory heart failure but tachyphylaxis can occur. (Tachyphylaxis is the requirement for increasing doses of a drug to produce the same clinical effect.)

Terazosin is similar in structure to prazosin but has a longer half-life.

Labetalol

The beta-blocking activity means that labetalol is contraindicated in heart failure. It is used to treat chronic hypertension and hypertensive emergencies.

Phentolamine

Both $alpha_1$ and $alpha_2$ (presynaptic)-adrenoceptors are blocked. The major use of phentolamine is the acute treatment of hypotensive cases in phaeochromocytoma, monoamine oxidase interaction and clonidine withdrawal; 5–10 mg is injected intravenously.

Phenoxybenzamine

This is a longer-action oral alpha-blocker. It is prescribed with a beta-blocking agent to control hypertension due to phaeochromocytoma.

Indoramin

This is an effective hypotensive agent but its use is limited by drug-induced lethargy.

CALCIUM SLOW CHANNEL BLOCKERS

Mode of action

These drugs act by inhibiting the inflow of calcium ions across the cell membrane of myocardial fibres and vascular smooth muscle fibres during excitation.

They are a heterogeneous group of drugs which differ from each other in chemical structure, the mechanism of action at cellular level and overall cardiocirculatory action. All induce vasodilatation as a result of smooth muscle relaxation. Vasodilatation occurs mainly in the arteries, both coronary and peripheral. The dilator effect in the coronary arteries is particularly useful in coronary artery spasm. Some calcium slow channel blockers (nifedipine, nicardipine and diltiazem) have been shown to improve cerebral perfusion due to cerebral vascular dilatation.

The principal haemodynamic difference between the calcium slow channel blockers is the presence or absence of concomitant cardiodepressive effects.

The cardiac action potential consists of five phases (see Figure 1 Chapter 2). When a cardiac cell is stimulated there is a rapid influx of sodium ions through the fast sodium channel—phase 0, rapid depolarisation. The fast channel is rapidly inactivated. Depolarisation activates a second inward current of positive ions, in particular calcium, through a slow channel. This channel is slowly inactivated and it maintains the action potential plateau. This calcium influx is selectively inhibited by the calcium slow channel blockers of the verapamil type. Contractility, impulse conduction and heart rate are reduced. These effects diminish myocardial oxygen consumption and are of benefit in patients with angina pectoris. Verapamil and diltiazem, but not the calcium slow channel blockers of the dihydropyridine series (nifedipine and nicardipine), have an antiarrhythmic activity. The atrioventricular node is slow channel dependent and these drugs decrease automaticity or prevent re-entry in this region.

Clinical uses

The major clinical applications are summarised in Table 11.9.

Nifedipine is safely combined with beta-blocking agents and the two can be used with benefit in the treatment of chronic stable angina and hypertension. Verapamil and diltiazem taken with a beta-blocker may produce adverse effects from combined depression of the atrioventricular node. Severe bradycardia and asystole can occur. Intravenous verapamil should be avoided in patients taking a beta-blocker.

Nifedipine is probably the drug of first choice for treatment of hypertensive emergencies because it does not reduce cerebral blood flow (reset at higher autoregulation limits in sustained hypertension) despite the fall in systemic pressure.

The antiarrhythmic effects of verapamil and diltiazem are discussed on page 322.

Side-effects

Nifedipine has the most potent vasodilating effect (ten times more

Table 11.9

CLINICAL USES OF CALCIUM SLOW CHANNEL BLOCKERS

Clinical use	*Calcium slow channel blocker*	*Mechanism*
Stable angina	Nifedipine, nicardipine, verapamil, diltiazem	Coronary and peripheral vasodilatation (reduced afterload)
Coronary artery spasm	Nifedipine, nicardipine, verapamil, diltiazem	Coronary vasodilatation
Hypertension	Nifedipine, verapamil	Peripheral vasodilatation
Hypertensive crises	Nifedipine	Peripheral vasodilatation
Heart failure	Nifedipine, nicardipine	Peripheral vasodilatation (reduced afterload and preload)
Paroxysmal supraventricular tachycardia (acute)	Verapamil, diltiazem	Block of slow channel conduction in A–V node (class IV action)

Prophylaxis of supraventricular tachycardia (chronic treatment)	Verapamil, diltiazem	Block of slow channel conduction in atrioventricular node (class IV action)
Atrial flutter and fibrillation (slowing of ventricular response)	Verapamil, diltiazem	Block of slow channel conduction in atrioventricular node (class IV action)
Hypertrophic cardiomyopathy	Verapamil	Improvement in systolic and diastolic ventricular function due to changes in contractility with calcium channel blockade
Cardiopulmonary bypass—? protection of the myocardium	Nifedipine	Prevention of calcium ion accumulation in myocardial cells preserves function
Raynaud's phenomenon	Nifedipine, verapamil	Peripheral arterial vasodilatation
Migraine	Nifedipine	Cerebral arterial vasodilatation
Pulmonary hypertension	Nifedipine	Pulmonary arterial vasodilatation

than verapamil and diltiazem) and therefore it causes more side-effects due to vasodilatation. Ankle oedema is produced by peripheral vasodilatation and should not be misinterpreted as heart failure. The negative inotropic effects are greatest with verapamil. They are usually offset by vasodilatation and reflex increased sympathetic activity but may further depress left ventricular function when this is already impaired.

Verapamil suppresses renal elimination of digoxin and increases serum digoxin levels. The dose of digoxin should be reduced when the drugs are used in combination.

Table 11.10 shows the side-effects of the four commonly used drugs.

Table 11.10

SIDE-EFFECTS OF CALCIUM SLOW CHANNEL BLOCKERS

Effect	*Nifedipine*	*Nicardipine*	*Verapamil*	*Diltiazem*
Headache	++	++	+	+
Skin flushing	++	++	+	−
Ankle oedema	++	+	+	−
Hypotension and dizziness	++	+	+	+
Constipation	−	−	++	−
Atrioventricular block (avoid with conduction defects)	−	−	+	+
Heart failure	−	−	+	−

ANGIOTENSIN CONVERTING ENZYME (ACE) INHIBITORS

The original ACE inhibitor, teprotide, was derived from the venom of a South American snake, *Bothrops jararaca.* Three synthetic orally active drugs are now available, captopril, enalapril and lisinopril.

Mode of action

The octapeptide, angiotensin II, is formed by the action of converting enzyme on the inactive precursor decapeptide, angiotensin I. Angiotensin II constricts arterioles, enhances sympathetic activity and causes sodium retention by a direct renal action and by release of aldosterone. Converting enzyme inhibition reduces the plasma renin and angiotensin I.

Angiotensin I converting enzyme is the same enzyme as kinase II. Inhibition prevents degradation of the vasodilator peptide, bradykinin. Increased levels of bradykinin cause direct vasodilation (Figure 11.1).

In contrast to other vasodilators which cause sodium retention, the fall in aldosterone levels following the reduction in angiotensin II promotes a mild diuresis.

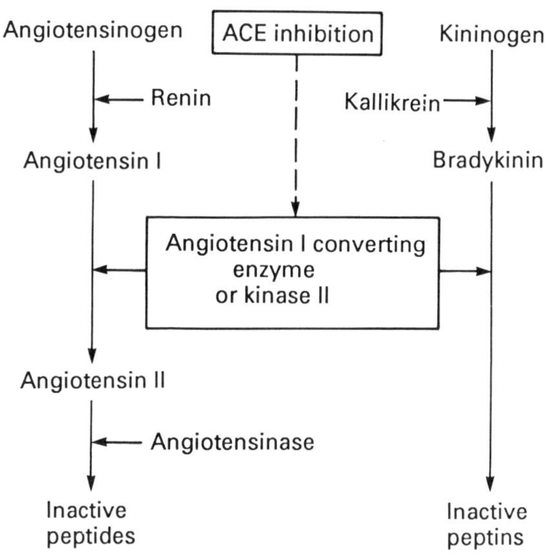

Fig. 11.1. The sites of action of ACE inhibition

Captopril

Captopril is well absorbed from the gut and maximum blood concentrations are achieved within 1–5 h. It is excreted by the kidneys and accumulates in patients with renal failure.

An initial dose of 6·25 mg three times daily is recommended.

Side-effects are relatively few if the total daily dose is nc increased above 150 mg/day.

Enalapril

Enalapril is a prodrug, and is converted to the active compounc enalaprilat in the liver. The peak plasma level is achieved abou 3 h after ingestion and it has a longer-lasting effect than captopri and therefore can be given once a day. It is also excreted in th urine and must be used with caution in patients with renal failure.

Lisinopril

This is a long acting, once daily derivative of enalapril but does not require hydrolysis in the liver so its effect does not depend on hepatic metabolism.

Clinical uses

In heart failure

The results with ACE inhibitors are more encouraging than those with any other vasodilator. They produce haemodynamic improvement which makes a substantial difference to a patient's life. Quality of life has been shown to be increased but of great interest is some evidence that they may improve prognosis.

In hypertension

ACE inhibitors reduce blood pressure. An additional fall may be obtained by adding a diuretic. Although it might be expected that the antihypertensive effect would be most clearly seen in hypertension due to renal artery stenosis with high plasma renin levels, the drugs are potent in patients with essential hypertension.

Side-effects

The first dose of an ACE inhibitor can produce a rapid fall in blood pressure. The risk is greater if the patient is also taking a diuretic and can be reduced if the first dose is small and diuretics are withheld on the first day of treatment.

Ace inhibitors suppress aldosterone and so may increase plasma potassium. Potassium-sparing diuretics and potassium supplements should not usually be given with them.

The molecule of captopril contains a sulphydryl grouping (like D-penicillamine) and some adverse effects (skin rashes, taste disturbance, proteinuria and neutropenia) may be related to this. Proteinuria occurs in 2% of patients treated with captopril although most have pre-existing renal disease. The nephrotic syndrome is reported but is rare. Proteinuria should be monitored during treatment. Neutropenia has usually been associated with underlying collagen disease.

Enalapril and lisinopril have no sulphydryl group and adverse reactions are even more uncommon. As with captopril, hypotension may be a problem. An interesting side effect of ACE inhibitors is a 'dry' or 'tickling' unproductive cough which persists with treatment.

ANTIARRHYTHMIC AGENTS

Classification

The classification based on electrophysiological effects was introduced by Vaughan Williams and depends on an understanding of cardiac muscle potential (Figure 11.2).

Class I agents

These drugs inhibit the fast inward current of sodium which causes the rapid phase of depolarisation. The maximum rate of depolarisation is therefore slowed. They are subdivided into three subgroups.

- (i) *Class Ia* (quinidine, procainamide, disopyramide) also widen the action potential.
- (ii) *Class Ib* (lignocaine, mexiletine, tocainide) shorten the action potential.
- (iii) *Class Ic* (flecainide, encainide, lorcainide, propafenone) do not affect duration of action potential.

Class II agents

These are beta-blockers that neutralise or block the effects of catecholamines. Phase 4 of the action potential is flattened.

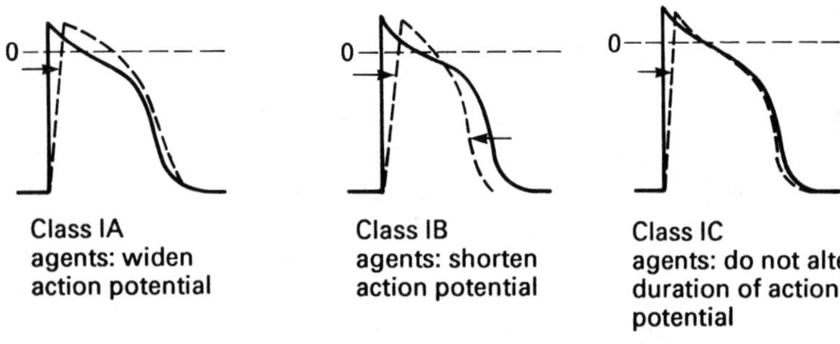

All class I agents inhibit fast sodium channel and reduce maximal rate of rise of phase 0

0
Class II
agents: flatten phase
4 of action potential
Class III
agents: widen duration of
action potential; rate of
depolarisation is unaltered
Class IV
agents: depress plateau
of action potential

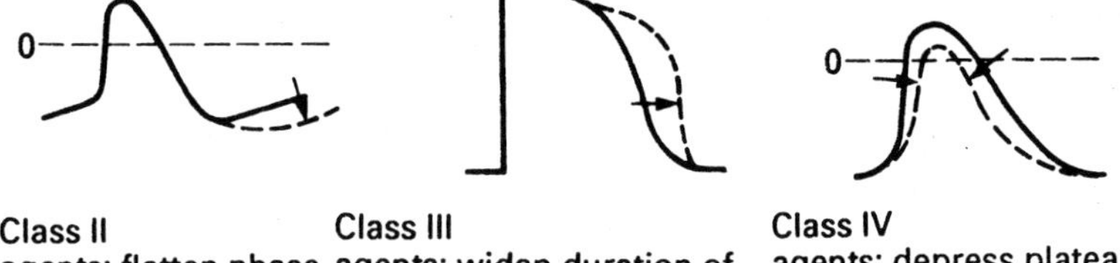

Fig. 11.2. Electrophysiological effects of antiarrhythmic agents

Class III agents

Amiodarone, sotolol—a beta-blocker—and bretylium have some class III effect; the action potential is prolonged but the rate of depolarisation is unaltered.

Class IV agents

These include verapamil and diltiazem; the transport of calcium into the cell is impaired and the plateau of the action potential is depressed.

This classification is useful in the basic understanding of the action of antiarrhythmic agents (Table 11.11).

Proarrhythmic effects of antiarrhythmic drugs

Antiarrhythmic drugs have the potential to aggravate an existing arrhythmia or precipitate a new arrhythmia. This side-effect is

Table 11.11

CLASSIFICATION OF ANTIARRHYTHMIC DRUGS ACCORDING TO SITES OF ACTION

Site	Drugs
Sinoatrial node	Digoxin, beta-blockers, Class IV drugs
Atrium	Classes Ia, Ic drugs, beta-blockers, class III drugs
Accessory pathways	Classes Ia, Ic, III drugs
Atrioventricular node	Digoxin, class Ic drugs, beta-blockers, class IV drugs
Ventricles	Class I, III drugs

common to all antiarrhythmic drugs including the beta-blockers. The incidence varies between 5 and 15%. It appears to be more likely in patients with serious ventricular arrhythmias but age, sex and left ventricular function do not predict a proarrhythmic effect. The arrhythmias range from increased ventricular ectopic beats to potentially lethal torsade de pointes ventricular tachycardia.

Specific Drugs

Class Ia

Quinidine

This is an alkaloid which was isolated from cinchona bark. Quinidine is used for the long-term prophylaxis of supraventricular and ventricular arrhythmias. It is well absorbed from the intestine and metabolised in the liver. The half-life is about 8 h but there is marked individual variation. Slow release quinidine formulations produce better therapeutic levels. Serum quinidine concentrations should be measured in long-term treatment (therapeutic levels—3–6 mg/l).

Side-effects The common initial side effects are usually gastrointestinal and in approximately one third of patients the drug will have to be stopped. The serious side effects are cardiac and occur during long term treatment. These are pro-arrhythmic effects and conduction delays. The major direct effect is depression of conduction with prolongation of QRS. Stop the drug if the QRS extends by 50% or 25% in the presence of an interventricular conduction defect or if it exceeds 0·14 seconds.

There is a risk of QT prolongation and consequent ventricular tachycardias. No patient with an initial QT interval of 0·4 seconds or hypokalaemic should be given quimidine. In long term treatment the drug should be stopped if there is significant prolongation of the QT interval (exceeds 0·6 seconds).

It is esential to monitor the electrocardiogram regularly during treatment.

Other side effects are:

(i) Tinnitus, dizziness, diarrhoea, blurring of vision (cinchonism).
(ii) Thrombocytopenic purpura.
(iii) Interaction with digoxin, it reduces renal excretion of digoxin.
(iv) Interreaction with warfarin, quinidine increases anticoagulation.

Procainamide

The indications are acute treatment and short-term prophylaxis of supraventricular and ventricular arrhythmias. Procainamide is well absorbed and metabolised to N-acetyl procainamide. Its half-life is 3 h and that of its metabolite is 8 h. Excretion is mainly to the kidneys.

Side-effects These are:

(i) Hypotension after intravenous injection.
(ii) Ventricular tachycardia.
(iii) Lupus erythematosus syndrome with fever and joint pains. This is most common in slow acetylators but the risk is high in all patients after 6 months' treatment and so limits the long-term use.

Disopyramide

This is useful for the long-term prophylaxis of supraventricular and ventricular arrhythmias.

The drug is absorbed through the intestine; 50% is bound to plasma protein and 50% is metabolised. Excretion is partly through the kidneys and the dose should be reduced in renal failure.

Side-effects These are:

(i) Like quinidine it may precipitate ventricular tachycardia and ventricular fibrillation.
(ii) Related to its anticholinergic action: dry mouth, blurred vision, retention of urine. Disopyramide is contraindicated in patients with prostatism or glaucoma.

Class Ib

Lignocaine

Lignocaine is the drug of first choice in the acute treatment of ventricular tachycardia, ventricular fibrillation and multiple ventricular ectopic beats associated with myocardial infarction. It is no longer routinely prescribed prophylactically for ectopic beats after a heart attack because the negative inotropic effect may extend infarct size.

It is metabolised in the liver and the half-life is 30 min.

Side-effects These are, most importantly, central nervous system effects, initially confusion, difficulty in speaking, progressing to generalised convulsions.

Mexiletine

Mexiletine is used for the long-term prophylaxis of ventricular arrhythmias. It is absorbed by the intestine and metabolised in the liver. The half-life is 8 h.

Side-effects These include: severe nausea and vomiting in 20% of patients, and arrhythmogenic effects.

Tocainide

Indications are the acute and long-term prophylaxis of ventricular arrhythmias.

The drug is well absorbed from the gut but can also be given intravenously in acute treatment. It is part metabolised and part excreted by the kidneys.

Side-effects These are gastrointestinal symptoms and central nervous system symptoms including paraesthesiae and tremor.

Class Ic

Flecainide

Flecainide is useful for treatment of supraventricular arrhythmias, in particular the re-entrant tachycardia of Wolff–Parkinson–White (W–P–W) syndrome and ventricular arrhythmias.

It is readily absorbed, some bound to plasma protein, and it is excreted by the kidneys. The half-life is 20 h.

Side-effects These are:

(i) Negative inotropic effect.
(ii) Conduction defects may be worsened.
(iii) Proarrhythmic effects.
(iv) Increases the rate of digoxin absorption.
(v) Markedly increases the pacing threshold in patients with implanted cardiac pacemakers resulting in loss of pacing.

Class III

Amiodarone

Amiodarone was first introduced as an antianginal agent but it has a powerful antiarrhythmic action against a wide spectrum of arrhythmias. Given intravenously it is useful in the acute treatment of supraventricular, nodal and ventricular tachycardias including tachyarrhythmias associated with the Wolff–Parkinson–White (W–P–W) syndrome and ventricular fibrillation. Orally it is used in prophylaxis against supraventricular and ventricular arrhythmias. It is particularly useful for treatment of paroxysmal atrial fibrillation. There is some evidence that amiodarone may prevent sudden death in patients with hypertrophic obstructive cardiomyopathy. It is often successful when other antiarrhythmic agents have failed. However, it has troublesome side-effects, should be reserved for difficult rhythm disturbances, and should not usually be a first-line treatment. It does have less negative inotropic effect than other powerful antiarrhythmic agents and can be given to patients with reduced left ventricular function.

The drug accumulates and has a very long half-life of 35–40 days. The full therapeutic effect is not achieved for several days. Paradoxically intravenous amiodarone is active within minutes (the injectable-like effect). Amiodarone contains iodine and has structural similarities to thyroxine.

Side-effects These are related to total dose and therefore become commoner with length of treatment. They are listed in Table 11.12.

Table 11.12

SIDE-EFFECTS OF AMIODARONE

Side-effect	*Comment*
Corneal microdeposits	Unimportant; occurs in 100% treated patients
Photosensitivity dermatitis	Sometimes unpleasant and severe
Blue discoloration of the skin	Cosmetic
Hyperthyroidism/ hypothyroidism	Monitor thyroid functions; ? stop treatment or treat thyroid disorder
Hepatic dysfunction	Uncommon but important. Monitor liver function tests and stop treatment if these become abnormal
Peripheral neuropathy	Stop treatment
Pulmonary alveolitis	Serious, stop treatment and treat with steroids
Proarrhythmic effect	Like other antiarrhythmic agents, stop treatment
Drug interactions	Potentiates warfarin and digoxin. Reduce dose of these drugs
Intravenous amiodarone	Irritates veins—give by a long line into central vein

Bretylium

This drug is recommended for ventricular fibrillation which has failed to respond to lignocaine. It is given by either intramuscular or intravenous injection. Bretylium is excreted in the urine and the half-life is 10 h.

Side-effect The main one is important postural hypotension.

Class IV

Verapamil and diltiazem

Intravenous verapamil is often the treatment of choice for acute supraventricular tachycardias. It should not be used to terminate atrial fibrillation in the Wolff–Parkinson–White (W–P–W) syndrome because of the risk of accelerated antegrade conduction through the bypass tract. Both drugs are used in prophylaxis of supraventricular arrhythmias and for slowing the ventricular response in atrial fibrillation.

DIURETICS

A diuretic drug increases urine volume. Those in common use act directly on the nephron (Table 11.13). Other drugs produce a diuresis indirectly—for example, digoxin and theophylline by

Table 11.13

MAIN SITES OF ACTION OF THE DIRECT ACTING DIURETICS

Diuretic	*Site of action*
Carbonic anhydrase inhibitors (acetazolamide)	Proximal tubule
Loop diuretics (frusemide, bumetanide, ethacrynic acid)	Loop of Henle
Thiazide diuretics	Distal tubule
Aldosterone antagonists (spironolactone) Potassium-sparing agents (triamterene, amiloride)	Distal tubule

increasing renal blood flow, dopamine by dilating the renal arteries and mannitol by increasing the osmotic pressure of the glomerular filtrate.

Thiazide and Related Drugs

This group includes two newer compounds, indapamide and xipamide which are related to chlorthalidone. Metolazone is a quinazoline sulphonamide diuretic which is chemically related to both thiazides and frusemide.

Thiazides act on the distal tubule by inhibiting sodium and chloride reabsorption. They increase sodium excretion by about 10% of the filtered load. The onset of action is within 1–2 h and the effect lasts up to 24 h. K^+, Cl^- and HCO_3^- are lost in the urine with Na^+. Thiazides have additional vasodilator effects possibly mediated through prostaglandins.

Loop Diuretics

Frusemide, bumetanide, ethacrynic acid and piretanide are highly effective and can increase sodium excretion by up to 30%. Their main site of action is in the ascending limb of the loop of Henle. Chloride transport is inhibited and therefore sodium reabsorption is reduced. Cyclo-oxygenase inibitors like indomethacin block the diuresis suggesting that this is mediated by prostaglandins. Given orally the onset of action is within 1 h and the effects last for 6 h. By intravenous injection a diuresis is produced within 5 min.

Loop diuretics dilate the venous capacitance vessels and, given intravenously, reduce preload acutely.

Aldosterone Antagonists

Aldosterone acts on the distal tubules causing an increase in sodium reabsorption in exchange for potassium. Aldosterone antagonists compete with aldosterone for its receptor with the result that sodium reabsorption is inhibited. They are particularly effective when secondary hyperaldosteronism has developed in heart failure or is due to treatment with loop or thiazide diuretics.

Other Potassium-sparing Diuretics

Triamterene and amiloride act on the distal tubules to inhibit sodium reabsorption. They are not specific aldosterone antagonists and are weak diuretics used in combination with thiazides or loop diuretics to help conserve potassium.

Clinical uses

Acute left venticular failure

Intravenous frusemide or bumetanide are primary treatment. The marked venodilator effects and reduction in ventricular preload produce a clinical improvement before the onset of a diuresis. There is also an acute reduction in plasma volume due to the diuresis.

Chronic heart failure

Diuretics reverse the sodium and water retention which occurs as a result of the changes in renal physiology due to renal hypoperfusion. Thiazides and loop diuretics reduce the peripheral vascular resistance and ventricular afterload which improves ventricular performance.

Spironolactone and the other potassium-sparing diuretics are not used alone in the treatment of heart failure but are of value in combination with loop or thiazide diuretics. A synergistic action between metolazone and frusemide is well-recognised in patients with gross oedema resistant to large doses of the loop diuretic.

Hypertension

Thiazide diuretics and spironolactone are potent hypotensive agents. The fall in blood pressure is due to a reduction in total peripheral resistance. The hypotensive action does not parallel diuretic potency and loop diuretics are probably less useful in the long term treatment of hypertension. Diuretics have a flat dose response curve and little is gained by increasing the dose of bendrofluazide above 5 mg/day or chlorthaladone above 25 mg/day. Side-effects are minimised with low dose treatment. The antihy-ertensive effect of a thiazide can be demonstrated within 24 h.

Side-effects

Hypokalaemia

Loop and thiazide diuretics predispose to hypokalaemia particularly in elderly patients and those on a strict weight-reducing diet when intake of potassium is inadequate. Hypokalaemia is not usually a problem in fit hypertensive patients. The effects of severe hypokalaemia are muscle weakness, depression, constipation and severe cardiac arrhythmias.

Diuretic/potassium combination tablets contain only a small dose of potassium (7–12 mmol) which it too little to prevent or correct hypokalaemia in patients at risk.

Hyperkalaemia

Potassium-sparing diuretics may cause hyperkalaemia especially if renal function is impaired. This induces serious arrhythmias. The risk is lessened if these diuretics are used in combination with loop diuretics.

Hyponatraemia

This is seen in two circumstances.

(i) It results from a natriuresis without an equivalent loss of water in waterlogged patients. Dilutional hyponatraemia is treated by fluid restriction and improvement of heart failure.
(ii) In non-oedematous patients, often elderly, given inappropriate diuretic therapy. This is often the combination of proximal and distal-acting diuretics. Symptoms are weakness, nausea, anorexia and confusion. Treatment is fluid restriction and if necessary hypertonic saline.

Metabolic alkalosis

This results from excessive loss of chloride in the urine and is enhanced by hypokalaemia. Tetany and confusion occur with severe alkalosis.

Hypocalcaemia

Loop diuretics (not thiazides) cause the loss of calcium ions. Hypocalcaemia leads to tetany.

Hypomagnesaemia

Excretion of magnesium ions is enhanced by thiazides and loop diuretics. Digoxin toxicity is more likely.

Impaired glucose tolerance

The deterioration in glucose tolerance is slow and develops after many years of treatment. Abnormal glucose tolerance curves have been demonstrated in 20% of patients on chronic treatment. Diuretics should be avoided as a first-line treatment in diabetic hypertensive patients.

Hyperuricaemia

Urinary uric acid excretion is decreased and acute gout may be precipitated.

Hyperlipidaemia

Diuretics increase serum triglyceride and low density lipoproteins, so may enhance the risk of coronary disease.

Impotence

The Medical Research Council trial of the treatment of mild hypertension has shown that diruetics can produce impotence; 22% of men said they had this complaint after 2 years' treatment.

BETA-ADRENOCEPTOR BLOCKING AGENTS

The concept of a receptor mechanism was first suggested by Langley in 1905 and in 1948 Alquist confirmed the presence of two distinct receptors in the tissues—alpha-receptor and beta-receptors. In 1967 Lands *et al.* showed that one group of beta-receptors (beta$_1$) caused cardiac stimulation and enhanced lipolysis while the other group ($beta_2$) mediated vasodepression and bronchodilatation. In 1964 propranolol became the first commercially available drug to block the beta-adrenoceptor site. Ten beta-blocking drugs are currently marketed in the United Kingdom and there is one further compound which possesses both alpha-adrenoceptor and beta-adrenoceptor blocking activity (labetalol). Some are produced as fixed-dose combinations with diuretics and as slow-release formulations.

Pharmacological and physiological activities

These drugs have different pharmacological activities:

(i) *Cardio-selectivity*: drugs which block $beta_1$ receptors preferentially are called cardioselective.
(ii) *Partial agonist activity* (intrinsic sympathomimetic activity): some agents cause some excitation as they block the adrenoceptor site.
(iii) *Membrane stabilising activity*: some drugs have local anaesthetic properties.
(iv) *Lipid solubility*: lipophilic beta-blockers gain access to the brain and are more likely to be extensively metabolised in the gut and liver (first-pass effect).

These differences between drugs are of marginal importance in clinical practice. Cardioselective agents are relatively safer, but not safe, in patients who have bronchospasm and have less effects on peripheral blood flow. Gluconeogenesis after hypoglycaemia is mediated through $beta_2$-adrenoceptors in the liver. Cardioselective agents have a less profound effect on this recovery mechanism and are preferred for diabetic patients.

Partial agonist activity is associated with less profound bradycardia at rest and less effect on peripheral blood flow.

The most lipid soluble beta-blockers (propranolol, oxprenolol, metoprolol and timolol) gain access to the brain and are more likely to be associated with central nervous system side-effects such as bad dreams and relief of anxiety.

Mechanisms of action

Angina

The antianginal effect is mediated by blockage of $beta_1$-receptors leading to a reduction in heart rate, myocardial contractility and systemic blood pressure which diminish myocardial oxygen requirement.

Hypertension

The precise mechanism remains unknown. The fall in cardiac ouput is poorly correlated to reduction in blood pressure. In the majority of patients total peripheral resistance is reduced. All beta-blockers inhibit the renin–angiotensin system but there is again no correlation with blood pressure response. Basal plasma catecholamine concentrations are not altered by beta-blockade.

Clinical uses

(i) *Angina pectoris*: the efficacy of beta-blockers in stable angina pectoris is well established and they remain the mainstay of medical treatment. They are not so helpful in unstable angina or in patients with coronary artery spasm (nitrates and calcium antagonists are preferred).

(ii) *After myocardial infarction*: in carefully selected patients there is now clear evidence that there is a reduction in mortality in the year after myocardial infarction if a beta-blocking agent is taken. Large trials suggest that death is reduced by about 25% during that time. The incidence of non-fatal reinfarction is also reduced.

(iii) *Hypertension*: beta-blockers are a first-line treatment. The dose–response curve is relatively flat making management easier and allowing for sensible combination with diuretic agents.

(iv) *Arrhythmias*: paroxysmal supraventricular tachycardias related to emotion or exercise and ventricular arrhythmias may respond.

(v) *Hypertrophic cardiomyopathy*: beta-blockers improve haemodynamics and symptoms but there is no evidence that they prevent sudden death.

(vi) *Other indications*:thyrotoxicosis, phaeochromocytoma (in combination with alpha-blockade), migraine, anxiety and glaucoma.

Table 11.14

SIDE-EFFECTS OF BETA-BLOCKING AGENTS

Cardiovascular	Heart failure Bradycardia Proarrhythmic effects Raynaud's phenomenon Tired legs on exercise Intermittent claudication Withdrawal syndrome
Respiratory	Bronchospasm
Central nervous system	Vivid dreams Hallucinations Increased sense of wellbeing
Gut	Dyspepsia Bowel disturbance
Metabolic	Prolongs hypoglycaemia and masks symptoms of hypoglycaemia in diabetics Elevation of serum lipoproteins

Table 11.15

CONTRAINDICATIONS TO TREATMENT WITH BETA-BLOCKADE

Any evidence of heart failure

Conducting tissue disease (sinoatrial disease, heart block)

Bronchospasm or a history of asthma

Severe peripheral vascular disease

Unstable diabetes

Side-effects

These are listed in Table 11.14 and the contraindications to treatment in Table 11.15.

Sudden withdrawal of beta-blocking agents from patients with ischaemic heart disease can provoke worsening angina, arrhythmias or infarction. It is wise to reduce the dose of short-acting beta-blockers over a period of days. The risk of withdrawal of the long-acting beta-blockers, such as atenolol, seems negligible.

PLATELET INHIBITING DRUGS

The composition of a thrombus is dependent on the rate of blood flow. Venous thrombi which form in slow flow have a fibrin base. They are treated or prevented by anticoagulants which interfere with the formation of fibrin. Thrombi in fast-flowing arteries result from an interaction between an abnormal vessel wall and platelets. This process is not affected by anticoagulants and is treated with platelet-inhibiting drugs.

Sequence of Events resulting in an Arterial Thrombus

Damaged endothelium

This is caused by:

(i) Blood turbulence particularly at branching points.
(ii) Arterial graft sites.
(iii) Balloon angioplasty.

Platelet adhesion and activation

Platelets adhere to the damaged surface. Exposed collagen in the vessel wall activates the platelet membrane. Two processes then occur:

Table 11.16

CLINICAL USES FOR ANTIPLATELET DRUGS

Arterial grafts
After angioplasty
Unstable angina
Transient ischaemic attacks
Prosthetic heart valves (in combination with anticoagulants)
Primary and secondary prevention of coronary heart disease (see Chapter x)
? Pregnancy-induced hypertension

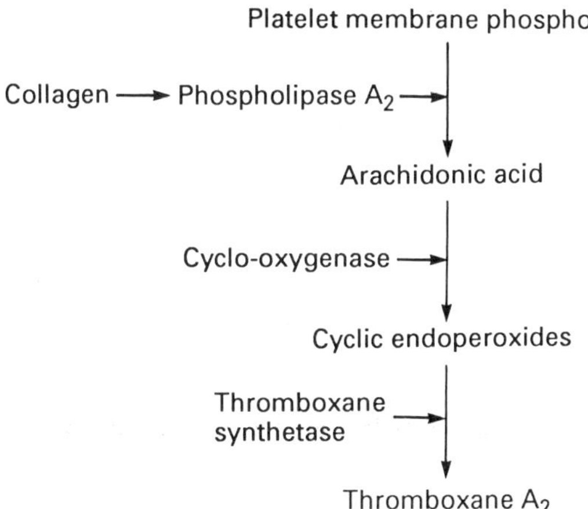

Fig. 11.3. Formation of thromboxane A_2

(i) Collagen induces platelet contraction which increases intraplatelet cytoplasmic calcium.

(ii) Collagen activates the membrane phospholipase A_2. Thromboxane A_2 is generated through this prostaglandin pathway (Fig. 11.2). Thromboxane A_2 increases the intraplatelet cytoplasmic calcium. Some thromboxane A_2 and adenosine diphosphate (ADP) are released from the platelet.

Platelet aggregation

The increase is cytoplasmic calcium and the release of thromboxane A_2 and adenosine diphosphate make platelets sticky and cause them to aggregate. Fibrin is incorporated into the platelet aggregation and an arterial thrombus is formed.

Prostacyclin

This is the main prostaglandin metabolite in vascular tissue. It is the most potent inhibitor of platelet aggregation and is present in undamaged endothelium of blood vessels (Fig. 11.4). Prostacyclin increases platelet cyclic adenosine monophosphate (cAMP). This decreases intraplatelet cycloplasmic calcium and the stickiness of the platelet. Thrombosis may occur when there is an imbalance

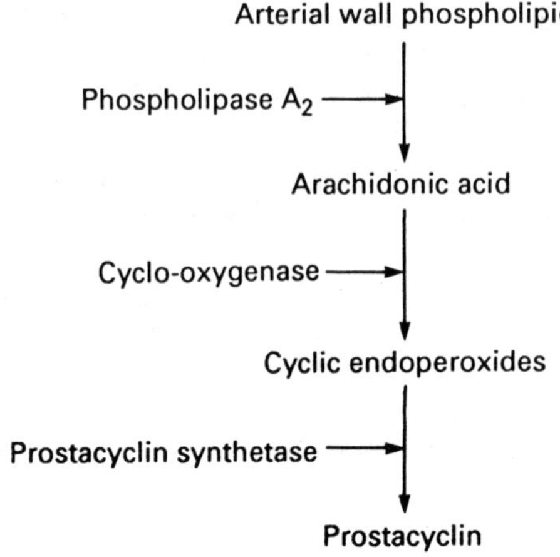

Fig. 11.4. The arterial wall prostaglandin pathway

between the production of thromboxane A_2 and prostacyclin by the vessel wall.

Cyclo-oxygenase

This enzyme is present in both platelets and in the arterial wall. It is acetylated and inhibited by aspirin. In the platelet the effect is permanent. In the arterial wall it is temporary because the cells can synthesise more enzyme.

Platelet Inhibiting Drugs (Used Clinically)

These are the main drugs used:

(i) Aspirin.
(ii) Sulphinpyrazone (Anturan).
(iii) Dipyridamole (Persantin).

Mechanism of action

Aspirin inhibits cyclo-oxygenase. The dose which blocks production of platelet thromboxane A_2 but has little effect on the production of arterial wall prostacyclin is disputed. Low doses (less than 75 mg/day) are currently favoured.

Sulphinpyrazone is a uricosuric agent. Like aspirin it inhibits cyclo-oxygenase but the inhibition is competitive.

Dipyridamole has a different site of action and blocks the phosphodiasterase enzyme which breaks down platelet adenosine monophosphate.

Aspirin and dipyridamole are frequently used in combination. The clinical uses are listed in Table 11.16.

FURTHER READING

Campbell R.W.F. (ed.) (1987). Clinical usefulness of antiarrhythmic drugs. *European Heart Journal*, **8**, Suppl. A.

Chamberlain D.A. (1985). Editorial: digitalis: where are we now? *British Heart Journal*, **54**, 227–233.

Dollery C.T., Corr L. (1985). Drug treatment of heart failure. *British Heart Journal*, **54**, 234–242.

Ellrodt A.G., Singh B.N. (1984). The role of slow-channel blockers in cardiovascular disease. *Recent Advances in Cardiology*, ed. Rowlands D.J., pp. 117–168. Edinburgh: Churchill Livingstone.

Lands A.M., Arnold A. and McAnliff J.P. (1967). Differentiation of receptor systems activated by sympathomimetic amines. *Nature*, **214**, 597–8.

Withering W. (1985). *An Account of the Foxglove and Some of its Medical Uses—Practical Remarks on Dropsy and Other Disease.* Birmingham. E.G.J. and J. Robinson.

Chapter Twelve

Systemic Arterial Hypertension

Background

Blood pressure is the product of the cardiac output and the resistance to flow within the small arteries and arterioles.

Hypertension is not easy to define because it is not a distinct disease. In any population the distribution of blood pressure is unimodal and so there is no cutoff between normal and high pressure. Hypertension is just the high end of this continuous range. The World Health Organisation has defined hypertension as a systolic blood pressure of more than 160 mmHg and/or a diastolic blood pressure of more than 95 mmHg. This is not synonymous with the need to treat and for any individual it is practical to define hypertension as the level of blood pressure at or above which treatment will be beneficial. Current advice is that patients with a diastolic blood pressure above 100 mmHg should be treated.

In most populations the level of blood pressure increases with age but there are individual trends. Those with the highest pressure in infancy tend to stay at the top throughout life. Those with the lowest pressure have a lesser rise and tend to stay at the bottom end of the distribution of pressure. This phenomenon is called 'tracking'. The track may be genetically determined.

Continuous ambulatory monitoring of blood pressure has demonstrated considerable physiological variations. There is a diurnal rhythm with the lowest pressures occurring during sleep and the highest in mid-morning. There are acute rises with both psychological and physical activity. The defence or alerting response is important in the interpretation of the level of blood pressure. Repeated measurements become less stressful and there is a regression of pressure towards the mean. Similar fluctuations

Table 12.1

IDEAL CONDITIONS FOR MEASUREMENT OF BLOOD PRESSURE

(1) The conditions should be reproducible
(2) The patient should be at rest for 3–5 min before measurement
(3) Either sitting or supine position is acceptable
(4) The cuff should be level with the heart
(5) The arm must be supported to prevent isometric exercise
(6) The midline of the bladder should be over the brachial artery (direct counterpressure is being applied)
(7) Avoid venous congestion from tight clothing or incomplete deflation from previous measurement
(8) Raise the pressure in the sphygmomanometer until the brachial pulse is obliterated (overinflation causes pain)
(9) Slow deflation (2 mm/s) is essential to avoid error
(10) The observer's eyes should be at the level of the mercury meniscus to overcome parallax error
(11) Standing and lying pressure must be measured if the patient is taking hypotensive agents which cause postural hypotension
(12) Do not hurry

of both systolic and diastolic pressure occur in both normal and hypertensive subjects.

Measurement of blood pressure

It is important that this measurement should be made by experienced observers, using adequate apparatus and under standardised conditions (Table 12.1).

Endpoint criteria

Figure 12.1 shows the five auscultatory phases (described by Korotkoff, a surgeon from St Petersburg in 1905). Most current trials use the disappearance of sounds, phase V, as the endpoint for diastolic pressure. This compares more accurately with intra-arterial diastolic pressure and is a more definite endpoint than phase IV. However, when there is a high cardiac output, such as in children, pregnant women, anxiety, aortic regurgitation and thyrotoxicosis, the sounds may not disappear and the level of pressure at which the sounds muffle (IV) must be recorded as diastole.

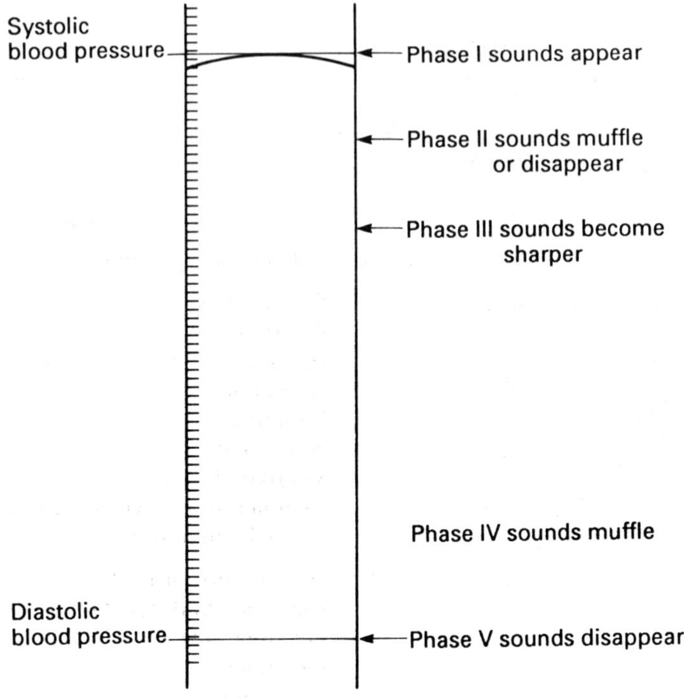

Fig. 12.1. Korotkoff sounds

Observer bias is an important source of error and the pressure should be recorded without prior knowledge of previous measurements. Sphygmomanometers which 'blind' the reading reduce observer bias (Hawksley random zero and London School of Hygiene and Tropical Medicine sphygmomanometers).

Equipment

Mercury sphygmomanometers are more accurate than aneroid sphygmomanometers. If aneroid instruments are used they should be calibrated regularly against a mercury sphygmomanometer. Most electronic sphygmomanometers are inaccurate.

All equipment should be carefully maintained. A common problem is dirt in the deflation valves which leads to an uncontrollable rate of fall of mercury.

The cuff should be long enough to encompass the arm. For

obese people a 36 mm bladder size should be used to avoid an artificially high reading.

ESSENTIAL HYPERTENSION

Of hypertensive patients 95% have essential hypertension. The cause is not agreed and the theories on pathogenesis remain unsatisfactory. Factors that may be important can be considered under three headings:

(i) Genetic background.
(ii) Environmental factors.
(iii) Physiological control mechanisms.

Genetic Background

This can be either familial or racial.

(i) *Familial trait:* hypertension often runs in families. There is a good correlation between blood pressures of relatives. In one study it was shown that for every 1 mm by which the diastolic pressure of a hypertensive patient exceeded the expected level the first degree relative's blood pressure was 0.4 mm higher than the expected level. This familial association could be the result of shared genes or shared environment or a combination of both. The importance of the genetic factor is shown in studies of twins, as identical twins have similar blood pressures. An infant's blood pressure at 3 months correlates with subsequent pressures at least up to the age of 8.

(ii) *Race:* there are important differences in blood pressure between racially distinct groups. The rise in blood pressure with age that is observed in western countries is absent among some primitive populations (Pacific atoll Polynesians, Aborigines, Kenyan nomads, Congo pygmies). However, when these people move to other areas they tend to lose their immunity to hypertension. This suggests that their environment is more important than their genetic makeup. In America the blood pressure of black people rises more rapidly than that of whites. This suggests the possibility of a genetic factor, although again there are environmental differences particularly in socioeconomic status.

Environmental Factors

These are as follows:

(i) *Salt intake:* the relationship of salt intake and hypertension remains hotly debated. There is experimental, epidemiological, and clinical evidence suggesting a causal connection.

(ii) *Stress:* mice placed in social conflict cages become hypertensive presumably due to overactivity of the sympathetic nervous system. After a time the hypertension will persist even though the stress is removed. Studies in man are conflicting and none have firmly established that stress is an important predisposing factor.

(iii) *Alcohol:* there is an association between high alcohol consumption (more than 35 g/day) and hypertension.

(iv) *Smoking and caffeine:* cigarette-smoking and caffeine ingestion increase the blood pressure acutely (important in outpatient clinic assessment) but they do not appear to have a chronic pressor effect.

(v) *Obesity:* population studies suggest a positive correlation between obesity and blood pressure.

(vi) *Temperature:* there appears to be an inverse relationship between ambient temperature and blood pressure. Blood pressures of servicemen stationed in hot climates is *lower* than the level of those living in colder areas.

Physiological Control Mechanisms

Blood pressure is maintained within normal limits by complex homeostatic mechanisms which control the cardiac output and peripheral resistance (Table 12.2).

Cardiac output is usually normal in established hypertension

Table 12.2

CONTROL MECHANISMS FOR BLOOD PRESSURE

Blood pressure	
Cardiac output	× *Total peripheral resistance*
Myocardial contractility and heart rate	Intrinsic autoregulation
Plasma volume	Autoimmune nervous system
	Circulatory humoral factors
	Renal–renin–angiotensin system
	? Prostaglandins
	? Kallikrein–bradykinin system
	Atrial natriuretic peptides
	Local factors
	Tissue metabolites, such as lactic acid, carbon dioxide
	? Prostaglandins, kallikrein–bradykinin system

although this does not rule out the possibility of an initial elevation which triggers reflex changes increasing total peripheral resistance. Abnormalities of intrinsic autoregulation, autonomic nervous system activity and circulatory humoral factors have been considered.

Abnormalities

Intrinsic autoregulation

Arteriolar smooth muscle dilates or contracts in direct response to the perfusion pressure. A reduction of pressure results in dilatation and an increased flow, while an increase leads to constriction and a reduced flow. Intrinsic autoregulation maintains a constant blood flow over a range of blood pressure. There is no evidence that a change in total body autoregulation is a primary abnormality in hypertension but high blood pressure leads to vascular adaption which alters the capacity for resistance vessels to dilate and restrict.

Autoregulation of the cerebral circulation is particularly important. In normotensives this control mechanism is active between mean arterial pressures of 60–140 mmHg. These levels are reset upwards in sustained hypertension and the brain may become underperfused if the blood pressure is reduced below the adapted lower limit.

Autonomic nervous system

Normal blood pressure control and its minute-to-minute variations are related to the activity of the autonomic nervous system. This is controlled by the vasomotor centre in the brain-stem which receives information from the higher cerebral centres and from circulatory baroreceptors.

Acute stimulation of the central nervous system causes an acute rise in blood pressure. However, it does not appear that overactivity of the sympathetic nervous system causes essential hypertension. No clearcut differences in circulatory catecholamine levels can be demonstrated between normotensives and hypertensives.

Baroreceptors are situated in the adventitia of the carotid sinuses and the aortic arch. They respond to stretching and therefore to the rate of change of blood pressure. The afferent pathway from the carotid sinus is through the IXth cranial nerve and from the aortic arch through the vagus nerves and sympathetics. An increase in baroreceptor activity inhibits the sympathetic outflow from the vasomotor centre and excites the vagal centre. If blood pressure rises, the arterial wall is stretched, baroreflex firing increases, diminished sympathetic activity causes vasodilatation, increased vagal activity causes cardiac slowing and the result is a decrease in arterial pressure. Conversely a lowering of pressure has the opposite effects leading to a reflex rise in pressure. This system acts as a 'buffer' to acute changes. Baroreflex activity diminishes and is reset at a higher pressure range with age and hypertension. These changes are thought to be the result of high blood pressure rather than the cause of essential hypertension.

Circulatory humoral factors

The important systems are described but there is no evidence for a consistent abnormality in patients with essential hypertension.

Renin–Angiotensin System

This is probably the most important renal control mechanism (Fig. 12.2).

Renin is an enzyme which hydrolyses renin substrate to form angiotensin I. The substrate is a glycoprotein synthesised by the liver. Most circulating renin comes from the juxtaglomerular apparatus of the kidney. Secretion is controlled by two receptors:

(i) A *baroreceptor* which is situated on the afferent arteriole of the glomerulus. This is sensitive to changes in perfusion pressure and responds to a decrease in pressure by increasing renin secretion. Stimulation of the renal beta-receptors increases renin release and stimulation of alpha-receptors inhibits renin release.

(ii) A *chemoreceptor* situated in the macula densa which responds to changes in the tubular sodium and chloride load. Extracellular fluid volume depletion leads to an increase in renin secretion.

Angiotensin I is an inactive decapeptide which is converted to the active octapeptide, angiotensin II, by a converting enzyme. This is a membrane-bound protein which is present in highest concentrations in the pulmonary vascular endothelium. The conversion takes

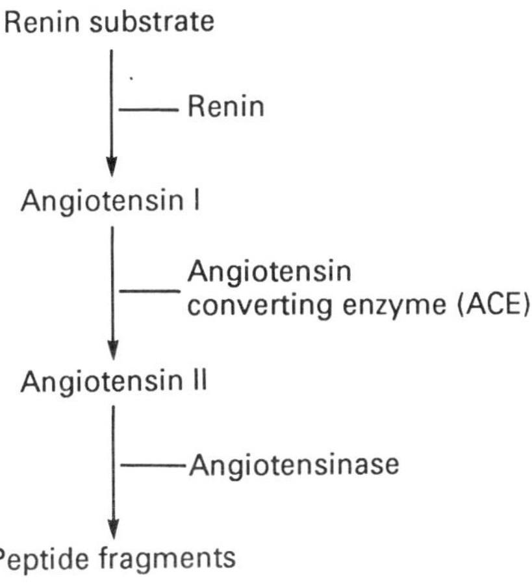

Fig. 12.2. The renin–angiotensin system

Table 12.3

ACTIONS OF ANGIOTENSIN II

Direct vasoconstrictor action on arteriolar smooth muscle
Stimulation of the adrenal zona glomerulosa causing increased secretion of aldosterone and sodium retention
Direct renal action causing sodium retention
Effect on the central nervous system increasing sympathetic efferent activity

place in the lungs. (Converting enzyme is the same as kinase II which converts bradykinin to inactive peptides.)

Angiotensin II is the main effector hormone (Table 12.3). It has a short half-life and is degraded into angiotensin III, a heptapeptide, and other inactive breakdown products. Angiotensin II directly stimulates the zona glomerulosa cells of the adrenal cortex to produce aldosterone. Other stimuli for aldosterone production are the potassium ion and adrenocorticotrophic hormone. Aldosterone acts at a specific segment of the distal renal tubule to increase the reabsorption of sodium.

Other Renal Hormones

Prostaglandins are produced in the renal medulla and may act locally on the renal arterioles. Most are removed in the pulmonary circulation but some prostacyclin may enter the systemic circulation and cause peripheral vasodilatation.

The enzyme kallikrein is formed in the distal renal tubule and acts on the alpha$_2$-globulin, kininogen, to form bradykinin. This peptide has local vasodilator and natriuretic properties. It remains unknown whether this system (Fig. 12.3) has systemic vasodilator effects.

Atrial Natriuretic Peptides

Three forms of peptides which are released from specific intracel-

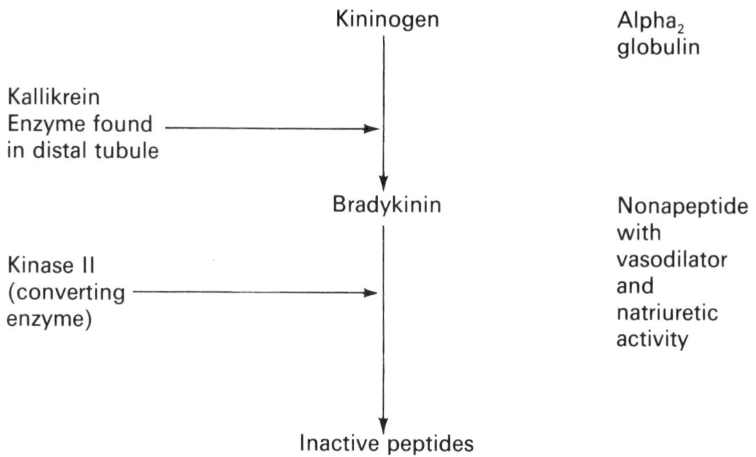

Fig. 12.3. Kallikrein–bradykinin system

lular granules in the atrial wall are now recognised. These are alpha, beta and gamma human (h) atrial natriuretic peptides and they have potent natriuretic and vasodilator properties. Atrial distension may be the stimulus for release of ANP and they may therefore participate in a negative feedback system controlling plasma volume and blood pressure.

SECONDARY HYPERTENSION

A cause for hypertension can be identified in about 5% of cases (Table 12.4). The commonest causes are pregnancy, oral contraceptive agents and renal disease. The underlying pathophysiological mechanism is understood in some cases (Table 12.5).

Renal Hypertension

Virtually all types of renal disease can be associated with hypertension. The classic form of hypertension which can be cured by surgery is renal artery stenosis which resembles the 'Goldblatt' model in which renal ischaemia and overproduction of renin was produced by a clip on the renal artery.

Table 12.4

CAUSES OF SECONDARY HYPERTENSION

Renal hypertension

Renovascular disease

Unilateral renal disease
- Pyelonephritis
- Obstruction
- Tuberculosis
- Tumour, including renin-secreting tumour
- Cyst

Bilateral renal disease
- Glomerulonephritis
- Pyelonephritis
- Analgesic nephropathy
- Obstruction
- Polycystic disease
- Collagen vascular disease
- Diabetes
- Gout
- Renal transplant

Endocrine hypertension

Primary aldosteronism
Cushing's syndrome
Congenital adrenal enzyme deficiencies
Phaeochromocytoma
Hyperparathyroidism
Acromegaly

Coarctation of the aorta

Drugs

Oral contraceptive pill
Liquorice and carbenoxalone
Non-steroidal anti-inflammatory agents (NSAIDS)
Monoamine oxidase inhibitors (MAOI) interaction with tyramine
Clonidine withdrawal

Pregnancy

Table 12.5

MECHANISMS INVOLVED IN SECONDARY HYPERTENSION

Mechanism	*Secondary hypertension*
Increased renin	Renovascular disease Renin-secreting tumour
Increased sodium and fluid retention	Chronic renal disease Sodium-retaining drugs
Increased catecholamines	Phaeochromocytoma MAOI interaction with tyramine Clonidine withdrawal
Increased mineralocorticoids	Primary aldosteronism Liquorice and carbenoxalone Congenital adrenal hyperplasia

Renovascular hypertension

This is the cause of hypertension in 0.5% of patients. The pathology is listed in Table 12.6. Renovascular hypertension is not easy to distinguish from essential hypertension, but Table 12.7 shows clinical clues which may help identify patients. Extensive investigation should be limited to these selected patients. The best predictor is a continuous abdominal bruit but this may occur with essential hypertension.

Screening and diagnostic tests are summarised in Table 12.8.

Table 12.6

CAUSES OF RENOVASCULAR HYPERTENSION

Cause	*Features*
Renal artery atheroma	Two-thirds of the cases Mainly middle-aged men Affects proximal renal artery
Renal artery dysplasia (commonest form is medial fibromuscular dysplasia)	Women under 35 Affects distal two-thirds of artery Abdominal bruit is common
Renal artery embolism and thrombosis	Associated with mitral stenosis Sudden onset of hypertension
Renal arteritis	Takayasu's disease Polyarteritis nodosa

Table 12.7

CLINICAL FEATURES OF RENOVASCULAR HYPERTENSION

Continuous abdominal bruit, especially upper quadrants
Female hypertensives under age 35 years
Sudden development or worsening of hypertension at any age
Hypertension refractory to usual medical treatment
Hypertension with unexplained renal impairment
Evidence of occlusive disease in other major vascular territories

An intravenous urogram or renal ultrasound is essential prior to renal angiography to exclude renal parenchymal disease. A combination of rapid sequence urography and nuclear imaging is the most accepted screening procedure.

Management

The management of renovascular hypertension depends on the aetiology, the age of the patient and the response to medical treatment. Percutaneous transluminal renal angiography (PTRA) or surgical revascularisation is appropriate for young patients, in particular those with fibromuscular hyperplasia; 60% of these patients will be cured and avoid long-term drug therapy. The complication rate of PTRA (puncture site haematoma, occlusion or dissection of the renal artery) is less than 5%. Surgical revascularisation has a similar success rate. Techniques include saphenous vein bypass, splenorenal bypass or hepatorenal bypass and endartectomy. Patients with atheromatous renovascular hypertension should be initially treated medically. Angiotensin-converting enzyme inhibitors should be used with caution and avoided if bilated renal artery disease is suspected. This is because ACE inhibition can open intrarenal shunts which bypass the glomeruli. An acute fall in glomerular filtration and renal failure may occur.

Unilateral renal disease

Nephrectomy improves or cures blood pressure in only about 30% of patients with unilateral hydronephrosis, chronic pyelonephritis or tuberculosis. There is no good correlation between split renal vein renin measurements and the result of surgery. A

Table 12.8

SCREENING AND DIAGNOSTIC TESTS FOR RENOVASCULAR HYPERTENSION (RVH)

Investigation	*Comment*
Rapid sequence intravenous urogram	*Limited sensitivity and specificity* Suggestive features: Decreased renal size (1.5 cm difference) Delay in early nephrogram and pyelogram of more than 1 min Increased density of pyelogram Ureteric notching due to collaterals
Nuclear imaging First-pass curve analysis after bolus intravenous injection of technetium 99^{m} (DTPA)	*Limited sensitivity and specificity*
? after captopril	Captopril increases renal blood flow in RVH and may increase sensitivity
I^{131} hippuran renogram	Difference in peak time of over 1 min is regarded as abnormal
Plasma renin activity	Casual measurement is of little value. Accuracy improved if sodium intake is controlled
Digital subtraction angiography	Less invasive than an arterial punctive but renal arterial branches are not visualised
Renal arteriography Flush aortogram followed by selective studies	*The definitive investigation* Atheroma typically produces a stenosis in the proximal 2 cm of the renal artery. Fibromuscular hyperplasia affects the more distal artery, often producing a 'string of sausages' appearance
Renal vein renin ratios	Overall data suggest that the ratio does not accurately predict the outcome of surgery

nephrectomy should only be recommended when there is a good urological reason for it.

Renin-secreting tumours

Hypertension due to an intrarenal haemangiopericytoma arising from the juxtaglomerular apparatus is rare but important. Surgical removal of the tumour is curative. Patients are usually young, have severe hypertension, hypokalaemia and high urinary potassium loss. The tumour is small and the diagnosis is made by demonstrating a high renin level in the renal vein of a kidney with no evidence of renal artery stenosis or parenchymal disease. Wilms' tumours may also secrete renin and cause hypertension.

Bilateral renal disease

Urinalysis is usually abnormal in patients with renal parenchymal disease.

In acute poststreptococcal glomerulonephritis, hypertension is common. Fluid overload can lead to hypertensive encephalopathy and death. Fluid intake must be restricted until the diuretic phase.

Chronic bilateral renal diseases are the commonest cause of hypertension apart from pregnancy and oral contraceptive use. It is particularly important in end-stage renal failure because it accelerates the destruction of remaining renal function. It is important to separate control of the blood pressure and impaired renal function. Sodium retention can be dangerous if the kidneys do not retain sodium normally. The best approach is to manage hypertension with hypotensive drugs. Any deterioration in renal function associated with a fall in blood pressure is usually temporary. Renal dialysis is rarely required for control of hypertension.

Prolonged ingestion of analgesics (aspirin, paracetamol, phenacetin) causes renal papillary necrosis. The condition should be suspected in any patient presenting with features of 'chronic pyelonephritis'.

Hypertension is common in patients who receive renal transplants, and many require hypotensive medication.

Endocrine Hypertension

Primary aldosteronism

There are two forms:

(i) Aldosterone-producing adenoma (Conn's syndrome). This is a benign tumour which produces aldosterone autonomously and is found in up to 80% of cases with primary aldosteronism.
(ii) Multinodular hyperplasia of the adrenal glands of unknown cause.

Excess aldosterone causes increased sodium reabsorption and potassium secretion in the distal renal tubule. The plasma volume expands and the hypertension is purely volume-dependent. The sodium and fluid retention does not proceed indefinitely. As the plasma volume expands the proximal reabsorption of sodium is reduced by an unknown 'escape' mechanism. This compensates for the excess distal reabsorption, and sodium output then equals input, but the equilibrium is reached at the expanded plasma volume. Potassium loss continues with an increased loss of hydrogen ions and the progressive development of hypokalaemic alkalosis.

Diagnosis

The diagnosis of primary aldosteronism should usually only be considered if the serum potassium is less than 3.2 mEq/l in a patient not taking diuretics. The hypertension used to be described as mild but it can be severe. Symptoms are due to the biochemical disturbance (hypokalaemic alkalosis) and are muscle weakness, rarely paralysis, paraesthesiae and tetany. Longstanding hypokalaemia induces changes in the renal tubules causing resistance to vasopression and polyuria and polydipsia (nephrogenic diabetes insipidus).

Differential diagnosis

Primary aldosteronism must be differentiated from secondary aldosteronism which is much more common and caused by severe hypertension with renal involvement or diuretic treatment. Pseudoaldosteronism occurs with ingestion of large amounts of liquorice or carbenoxolone. The active substance in both is glycerrhizinic acid which is structurally and physiologically similar to aldosterone. Table 12.9 shows a stepped plan for investigation. The distinction between adenoma and hypoplasia is difficult. Quadric analysis of the biochemical data, adrenal vein aldosterone levels and adrenal scanning (I^{131}-19-iodocholesterol) have been used. The latter is the simplest test and if a discrete adenoma is demonstrated then surgical removal is recommended. This results in a cure in 80% of cases. Otherwise the treatment is medical using spironolactone in doses of up to 400 mg/day to control the hypertension and biochemical disturbance.

Table 12.9

STEPS IN THE INVESTIGATION OF ALDOSTERONISM

Investigation	*Result*	*Conclusion*
Serum K^+	$<3{\cdot}2$ mEq/litre	Consider aldosteronism, cease diuretic, liquorice or carbenoxolone ingestion (Step 2)
24 h urine K^+ while patient is taking normal salt intake no potassium supplement no diuretic	<30 mEq/day	Likely to be due to previous diuretic therapy or loss of K^+ with diarrhoea
	>30 mEq/day	Step 3
Plasma renin activity after patient has taken potassium supplements for 3 weeks 'salt-free' diet for previous 5 days	Plasma renin activity not suppressed	Secondary aldosteronism
	Plasma renin activity suppressed	Primary aldosteronism (Step 4)
Plasma aldosterone	High	Differentiate adenoma from bilateral hyperplasia (Step 5)
Adrenal scan with I^{131}-19-iodocholesterol	Discrete tumour	Consider surgery
	Bilateral uptake	Spironolactone

Congenital adrenal hyperplasia

Two of the inherited adrenocortical enzyme deficiencies are associated with hypertension. These are:

(i) 11-beta-hydroxylase deficiency.
(ii) 17-alpha-hydroxylase deficiency.

In both normal cortisol synthesis is impaired, there is a compensatory rise in ACTH and the result is congenital adrenal hyperplasia. Mineralocorticoids are produced in excess and cause hypertension.

Presentation

11-beta-hydroxylase deficiency This is usually recognised in infancy with the child becoming virilised or pseudo-hermaphrodite in a female. Virilisation occurs because the enzyme defect does not interfere with the pathways of production of adrenal androgens, which like mineralocorticoids are produced in excess.

17-alpha-hydroxylase deficiency This enzyme is also present in the gonads so that a defect not only affects steroid synthesis but also gonadal synthesis of androgens and oestrogens.

Sexual development is abnormal but may not be obvious until puberty when secondary sex characteristics do not develop and females have primary amenorrhoea.

Treatment

Cortisol replacement is given in sufficient quantity to suppress ACTH excess. The dose has to be judged carefully because excess will produce Cushing's syndrome. Blood pressure will fall to normal. Patients with 17-alpha-hydroxylase deficiency also need androgen or oestrogen replacement therapy.

Cushing's syndrome

The mechanism of hypertension is unclear and levels of renin and aldosterone are usually normal. Cortisol increases vascular reactivity to catecholamines.

The majority of patients have bilateral adrenal hyperplasia as a result of hypersecretion of ACTH (Cushing's disease). In 20% of cases there is an adrenal adenoma or carcinoma and 10% of cases are caused by an ectopic ACTH-secreting tumour such as in oat cell carcinoma of the bronchus.

The characteristic findings are truncal obesity, a rounded face, skin bruising, purple striae, muscle weakness and wasting. Menstrual irregularities and hirsutism occur in females. The diagnosis is confirmed by finding elevated levels of plasma cortisol.

Phaeochromocytoma

This tumour arises from chromaffin tissue and secretes varying proportions of adrenaline, noradrenaline, dopamine and other catecholamine precursors. Some 90% are situated in the adrenal medulla, 10% of these are bilateral and 10% are malignant. Those arising from extra-adrenal chromaffin tissue are called paraganglionomas and are found in the neck, thorax, periaortic area, the hila of the kidneys and the bladder wall. Associated conditions are listed in Table 12.10.

Clinical features

The majority of patients have hypertension at all times but in 50% of cases there are intermittent abrupt superimposed rises in blood pressure. These are caused by a sudden surge of catecholamines from the tumour. Attacks of postural hypotension may

Table 12.10

ASSOCIATIONS WITH PHAEOCHROMOCYTOMA

Family history: autosomal dominant, 5% of cases
Neurofibromatosis: 5% of cases
Multiple endocrine syndrome (MEN) II (Sipple syndrome)
Medullary carcinoma of thyroid
Hyperparathyroidism
Multiple endocrine syndrome (MEN) III
Multiple mucosal neuromas
Medullary carcinoma of thyroid
Marfanoid appearance
Von Hippel–Lindau syndrome
Cerebellar haemangioblastoma
Angiomatous change in retinal vessels

occur if the tumour is secreting mainly adrenaline or dopamine rather than noradrenaline.

Typically the hypotensive paroxysms are associated with headache, sweating, skin pallor, palpitations and tremor. Glycosuria occurs after an attack. Occasionally they are complicated by acute left ventricular failure, angina or myocardial infarction. The attacks are usually spontaneous but can be precipitated by palpation of the abdomen, pregnancy, physical exercise and procedures like an intravenous urogram. The symptoms can easily be misinterpreted as acute anxiety or thyrotoxicosis.

Table 12.11

INVESTIGATION OF A PHAEOCHROMOCYTOMA

Investigation	*Comments*
24 h urine for estimation of metanephrines or vanillylmandelic acid (VMA) or catecholamines	High levels in phaeochromocytoma Urinary metanephrine estimation is the best screening test Metanephrines increased by MAOI and sympathomimetic agents Metanephrines decreased by X-ray contrast containing methylglucamine VMA increased by some foods including bananas, chocolate, coffee VMA increased by MAOI Free catecholamines—false positive with methyldopa and labetolol
Plasma catecholamines (radioenzymatic method)	Usually high
Ultrasound of adrenals	Detect tumours in the adrenal glands
CT scanning	
Selective arteriography	
Venous sampling for catecholamines at various levels of vena cava	Detection of tumours outside the adrenal glands
Scan with ^{131}metaiodobenzylguanidine	

The investigations for diagnosis and localisation of the tumour are outlined in Table 12.11.

Treatment

(i) *Acute episodes:* the patient should be given the alpha-blocker phentolamine 1–5 mg intravenously every 5 min until the pressure falls. An alternative is the alpha-blocker and beta-blocker, labetalol, given by intravenous infusion.

(ii) *Medical management and preparation for surgery:* the alpha-blocker, phenoxybenzamine, should be given by mouth at a dose starting at 10 mg twice daily and increased until the blood pressure is controlled. Propranolol 80–160 mg twice daily is then added to control tachycardia. Beta-blockers should never be given alone because the alpha-receptors are left unopposed and intense vasoconstriction results.

(iii) *Surgery:* this is the definitive treatment. The major problems are acute rises in blood pressure when the tumour is handled and precipitous falls in pressure which occur soon after its removal. It is essential to both alpha-block and beta-block the patient prior to surgery. During the operation the intra-arterial pressure should be monitored and acute rises can be treated with intravenous sodium nitroprusside. The patient should be transfused with blood or plasma to maintain central venous pressure at about 5 cm H_2O thus avoiding hypovolaemic shock.

(iv) *Malignant phaeochromocytoma:* patients with inoperable tumours can be treated with alpha-methyltyrosine. This inhibits the enzyme tyrosine hydroxylase in the synthesis of catecholamines and offers some palliation.

Hyperparathyroidism

About half of the patients with primary hyperparathyroidism have high blood pressure. The mechanism may be that vascular smooth muscle contractility is increased by high levels of serum calcium ions. Excess of calcium also impairs renal function. This may be irreversible and removal of the parathyroid adenoma does not always result in a fall in blood pressure.

Acromegaly

Hypertension occurs in some cases. It is suggested that growth hormone has a trophic action on vascular smooth muscle and thus increases vascular resistance.

Coarctation of the Aorta

This is a congenital narrowing of the aorta. The most common site is just distal to the origin of the left subclavian artery with a shelf-like obstruction where the ductus arteriosus connected the aorta and pulmonary artery *in utero*. There are associated abnormalities in 80% of cases, including a bicuspid aortic valve (in 50%), patent ductus arteriosus, ventricular septal defect and mitral disease. Berry aneurysms of the circle of Willis may also be present. Female coarctation is uncommon but occurs in Turner's syndrome (XO).

In infancy

Severe obstruction is an important cause of heart failure presenting in the first 2 weeks of life. The diagnostic finding is absent or very much reduced femoral pulses. (There is no time for collateral vessels to develop so there is no radial–femoral delay.) Occasionally the coarctation involves the origin of the left subclavian artery and the left brachial artery pulse is also reduced. Murmurs are due to associated conditions and are not produced by the coarctation itself. Surgical treatment is recommended.

In adults

The presentation after infancy is less dramatic. The majority of patients are asymptomatic and are found to have hypertension or a murmur at a routine examination. The most important clue is diminished or delayed femoral pulses. The delay occurs as a result of the development of a collateral circulation which supplies the femoral arteries. There are two murmurs; a midsystolic murmur over the anterior chest due to flow through the narrowed segment; and systolic or continuous murmurs over the scapulae due to flow in collateral vessels (Table 12.12).

The mechanism of hypertension is uncertain but is most likely

Table 12.12

FEATURES OF ADULT COARCTATION OF THE AORTA

Symptoms	Usually none Legs ache on exertion Backache due to intercostal aneurysms
Physical signs	Increased development of the upper body Hypertension in upper limbs Reduced blood pressure in lower limbs Diminished or delayed femoral pulses Bounding carotid pulses Collateral vessels over the scapula Left ventricular hypertrophy Apical click from dilated ascending aorta Systolic murmur maximal over the back Associated signs of bicuspid aortic valve and aortic stenosis
Electrocardiogram	Left anterior hemiblock Right or left bundle brach block Left ventricular hypertrophy
Chest X-ray	The common appearances of the aorta include Double aortic knuckle (Figure 12.3 appearance) The bulge is formed by the left subclavian artery and aortic arch. The lower bulge is due to poststenotic dilatation of the descending aorta Flat aortic knuckle due to inconspicuous left subclavian artery, a small aortic arch, narrow isthmus and absent poststenotic dilatation The heart is usually enlarged Notching of the inferior border of the ribs (4–8 posteriorly). If the coarctation involves the left subclavian the rib notching will occur only on the right

to be mechanical due to increased resistance in the aorta and collateral vessels. There are inconsistent changes in renal blood flow and plasma renin activity.

Surgical correction should be done before the age of 15 and will improve long-term prognosis. Hypertension is usually reduced but if surgery is delayed until later life secondary structural changes tend to maintain the high pressure. In uncorrected coarctation, there is a high mortality in middle age from left ventricular failure, aortic rupture, cerebral haemorrhage from rupture of a berry aneurysm and infective endocarditis (most common on an associated defect).

Drugs

Oral contraceptive pill

A small increase in blood pressure occurs in most women taking oestrogen containing oral contraceptive pills. In some there is a very marked rise and the accelerated phase of hypertension has been reported. Oestrogens increase the synthesis of renin substrate in the liver and this may be the underlying mechanism. Progesterone-only pills have also been associated with hypertension but this appears to be more unusual.

Blood pressure usually falls to normal when the oral contraceptive is stopped but if the high level of pressure is left unchecked for months or years it may cause structural changes which maintain hypertension even after stopping treatment.

The practical implications are:

(i) Hypertensive women should use alternative methods of contraception.
(ii) Blood pressure should be checked before initiating treatment.
(iii) Blood pressure should be checked after 6 months and a rising pressure requires careful observation or cessation of treatment.

Pregnancy

Hypertension may pre-date pregnancy and be either essential or secondary, or it may be induced by pregnancy.

Pre-existing hypertension

Intensive antenatal care and drug treatment will usually ensure a successful outcome for both mother and baby (Table 12.13).

Table 12.13

THE MATERNAL AND FETAL RISKS WITH PRE-EXISTING HYPERTENSION

Increase in maternal blood pressure with advancing gestation
Increase in the incidence of superimposed pre-eclampsia
Acute and/or chronic fetal compromise
Increase in maternal and perinatal mortality

Methyldopa is still the most extensively used drug in pregnancy and has been shown to be safe and free from serious side-effects in both short-term and long-term followup studies of infants born to mothers taking treatment. More recently beta-adrenoceptor blocking agents have been used, but in high doses these may result in infants being born with signs of beta-adrenoceptor blockade.

Secondary hypertension may be caused by pre-existing renal disease. Phaeochromocytoma is occasionally first diagnosed when the gravid uterus presses on the tumour and causes a catecholamine crisis. Surgical removal is recommended. Coarctation of the aorta is occasionally first recognised in pregnancy. Fetal growth is normal because the collateral supply to the uterus is under normal pressure. Resection can be undertaken but is usually deferred until after delivery.

Pregnancy-induced hypertension (PIH)

Definition

Pregnancy-induced hypertension is a blood pressure of greater than 140/90 mmHg after the 20th week of gestation in a previously normotensive woman.

Measurements should be made on two occasions in standard conditions because of the lability of blood pressure. Korotkoff phase IV sounds are used, as definition of phase V is often imprecise in pregnant women.

Incidence

Pregnancy-induced hypertension is commonest in the first pregnancy when 10% of women are affected. Patients at increased risk are those with pre-existing hypertension, diabetes, twin pregnancies, rhesus immunisation and hydatidiform mole.

Aetiology

The cause is unknown but appears to be associated with increased production of thromboxane A_2, a potent vasoconstrictor, by the placenta and platelets. This possibility is the rationale for trials of low dose aspirin to restore the prostacyclin/thromboxane imbalance.

Complications

The risk of developing hypertension in later life is not increased if the blood pressure rise is only with the first pregnancy.

Pre-eclampsia

This is hypertension with proteinuria greater than 0.3 g/litre protein. Fluid retention is frequently manifest by oedema and may become very severe in pre-eclampsia.

Eclampsia

A rapid rise in blood pressure associated with headaches, visual disturbance, oliguria and striking periorbital oedema with generalised convulsions and occasionally coma. It is usually but not always preceded by pre-eclampsia.

The management of pregnancy-induced hypertension is summarised in Table 12.14 (*see* p 366).

Pathology of hypertension

The consequences of hypertension are a combination of adaptive changes as a result of high pressure and damage due to increased mechanical stress.

Adaptive changes

Medial hypertrophy and duplication of the internal elastic lamina of the smaller arteries and arterioles develop in response to the increased load. These changes increase resistance to flow even when the vessels are fully dilated.

There is left ventricular hypertrophy with increase in wall thickness and mass. Eventually the left ventricle cannot sustain

Table 12.14

MANAGEMENT OF PREGNANCY-INDUCED HYPERTENSION

Mild to moderate pregnancy-induced hypertension, blood pressure 140/90–140/100 mmHg.

Admit to hospital; 4 h blood pressure measurement; 24 h urine protein estimations. Fetoplacental assessment. Aim for conservative management unless there is evidence of worsening hypertension and/or fetal compromise.

Severe pre-eclampsia/eclampsia, blood pressure 140/110 mmHg with proteinuria and symptoms.

Admit patient to intensive nursing care area (via the obstetric flying squad)

Prevent convulsions with intravenous diazepam

Prevent complications of the illness such as disseminated intravascular coagulation (DIC), renal failure, cardiac failure, adult respiratory distress syndrome, cerebral haemorrhage, hepatic failure and intrauterine fetal death.

When the mother is 'stable' deliver as expeditiously as possible either by the vaginal route or by caesarean section

the cardiac output against the increased afterload and left ventricular failure occurs.

Damage

The arteries Hypertension accelerates the development of atheroma particularly at the sites in the arterial tree where there is turbulence or distorted blood flow. The mechanical stresses caused by high blood pressure produce focal endothelial damage in the large and medium-sized arteries.

This allows platelet aggregation and lipid accumulation which are the foundation of an atheromatous plaque. Atheroma is an important cause of cerebrovascular, coronary and peripheral vascular disease and is complicated by thrombosis and embolism (Table 12.15).

When the blood pressure is very high or rises rapidly there is focal damage to the small arteries, fibrinoid necrosis. The wall structure is destroyed and replaced by fibrin material. The vessel becomes narrowed and may occlude. Lesions are found in the kidney, brain, retina and the heart and are the hallmark of malignant hypertension.

Table 12.15

COMPLICATIONS OF HYPERTENSION

Target organ	*Pathology*	*Clinical complication*
The heart	Coronary atheroma	Angina pectoris Acute myocardial infarction Sudden death
	Increased vascular resistance ± ischaemic heart disease	Left ventricular hypertrophy Left ventricular failure Congestive heart failure Atrial fibrillation
The aorta	Aortic atheroma	Dissecting aneurysm
The peripheral blood vessels	Peripheral atheroma	Intermittent claudication Ischaemia of the feet
The brain	Atheroma of cerebral vessels—cerebral infarction	Transient ischaemic attacks Major stroke
	Charcot–Bouchard aneurysms cerebral haemorrhage	Major stroke
	lacunae	Minor stroke Multi-infarct dementia Pseudobulbar palsy
	Berry aneurysms on the circle of Willis	Subarachnoid haemorrhage
	Fibrinoid necrosis of arterioles	Hypertensive encephalopathy
The eye	Retinal artery and vein thrombosis due to atheroma	Blindness or partial field defect
	Papilloedema	Blurring of vision
	Fibrinoid necrosis	Haemorrhages and exudates
The kidney	Atheroma—renal artery stenosis	Worsening of hypertension
	Nephrosclerosis	Rise in blood urea
	Fibrinoid necrosis	Renal failure Microangiopathic haemolytic anaemia

Fibrinoid necrosis is associated with microangiopathic haemolytic anaemia. The red cells are damaged or destroyed as they pass through the fibrin deposits in the small arteries. These deformed or fragmented red cells (burr cells) are seen in the peripheral blood film and increased fibrin degradation products are present in the plasma and urine.

The heart In hypertension 65% of deaths are due to heart disease. Ischaemic heart disease due to coronary atheroma increases with the level of the blood pressure. Hypertrophy of the left ventricle due to the increased afterload eventually leads to left ventricular failure.

The brain Hypertension is the most important risk factor for cerebrovascular disease. The commonest pathology in major stroke is cerebral infarction (60–80% of cases). The causes are either thrombosis of an atheromatous cerebral artery or embolism from atherosclerotic carotid, vertebral or innominate arteries. The aorta is a less common source.

Transient ischaemic attacks are four times more common in hypertensives and result from dislodgement of platelet emboli from atherosclerotic plaques in the extracranial arteries to the brain.

Cerebral haemorrhage is responsible for about 25% of strokes and is caused by rupture of a Charcot–Bouchard aneurysm. These focal aneurysms develop on the small intracerebral vessels in the basal ganglia and subcortical regions of the brain and are only associated with increasing age and high blood pressure. There is a loss of the arterial media at the small 1–2 mm aneurysm.

Thrombotic occlusion of the small arteries at the sites of Charcot–Bouchard aneurysms gives rise to lacunar infarcts of the brain. Lacunae, small cavities in the basal ganglia, internal capsule and pons, are associated with minor strokes. These are distinguished from transient ischaemic attacks because they take days or weeks to recover. Multiple lacunar infarcts result in progressive dementia or pseudobulbar palsy.

Berry aneurysms occur on the larger vessels of the circle of Willis and are due to a congenital weakness of the vessel wall. High blood pressure increases the chance of rupture and subarachnoid haemorrhage.

When the arterial pressure is very high or rises rapidly there is a breakdown in the intrinsic autoregulation of the cerebral vessels. The physiological response is for the vessel to constrict to protect the brain from high perfusion pressure. In hypertensive encephalopathy there are areas of abnormal arterial dilatation where autoregulation is no longer apparent. These sections are abnormally permeable and cerebral oedema results.

The kidney There is hyperplastic thickening, nephrosclerosis, of the small arteries and particularly the afferent arterioles. Conventional renal function tests are normal in mild or moderate essential hypertension but as the arterial changes worsen there is a reduction in renal blood flow and the glomerular filtration rate.

Extensive atheroma may develop in the large renal arteries. It occasionally causes renal artery stenosis rendering the kidney sufficiently ischaemic to stimulate the renin–angiotensin system.

Of patients with the accelerated phase of hypertension 75% have fibrinoid necrosis affecting the renal arterioles. Obliteration of the afferent glomerular arterioles leads to the loss of the glomeruli and renal failure. Ischaemia of the juxtaglomerular apparatus stimulates renin release which accentuates the high pressure. Blood urea rises and urinalysis shows proteinuria, red cells and casts.

Clinical consequences of hypertension

Symptoms

Mild or moderate hypertension is an asymptomatic condition until it causes complications (Table 12.14). Headaches, nosebleeds and episodes of dizziness are usually unrelated to the height of the blood pressure. However, these symptoms make patients consult doctors and lead to the measurement of the blood pressure. The implications of this are:

(i) Screening of healthy people is necessary to identify hypertension before it causes a serious complication.
(ii) People who feel well should only be given treatment when there is sufficient evidence that this is going to do more good than harm.
(iii) Treatment should be tailored for each patient so that symptomatic side-effects are avoided.

Table 12.16

HIGHER BLOOD PRESSURE SHORTENS LIFE EXPECTANCY

Age	*Blood pressure*		*Projected life span (years)*	
	Systolic	*Diastolic*	*Men*	*Women*
45	120	80	77	82
	130	90	74	80·5
	140	95	71	77
	150	100	65	73·5
55	120	80	78·5	82·5
	130	90	77·5	82
	140	95	74·5	79·5
	150	100	72·5	78·5

The accelerated phase of hypertension is associated with symptoms. Visual disturbance occurs and a morning occipital headache is clearly related to the high level of blood pressure. Hypertensive encephalopathy is a rare complication of severe hypertension, usually with papilloedema. Headache, clouding of consciousness and vomiting are early symptoms which may lead to generalised convulsions.

Reduction in life expectancy

Insurance statistics show that life span decreases with increasing blood pressure. Casual blood pressure measurements appear to predict prognosis in population studies (not necessarily for an individual). Examples from these statistics are shown in Table 12.16.

Assessment of the hypertensive patient

Once sustained high levels of blood pressure are confirmed it is necessary to assess the patient both for a cause of hypertension and for evidence of end organ damage. Intensive investigation to find a cause should be reserved for young patients, patients who fail to respond adequately to medical treatment or when there are strong clinical indications of secondary hypertension.

Urinalysis, blood urea and electrolytes, electrocardiogram and chest X-ray are the routine baseline investigations.

Table 12.17

CLINICAL ASSESSMENT OF THE HYPERTENSIVE PATIENT

	Assessment	*Implication*
History	Family history	Essential hypertension
For the cause	Recurrent urinary infections, nocturia, loin pain	Renal hypertension
	Muscle weakness, paraesthesiae, tetany	Primary aldosteronism
	Paroxysmal headache, sweating, palpitations and tremor	Phaeochromocytoma
	Oral contraceptive pill, liquorice, carbenoxalone, MAOI, sodium-retaining drugs	Drug-induced
For complications	Angina, claudication, transient ischaemic attacks (TIA)	Atheroma
	Shortness of breath	Heart failure
	Visual change	Retinal disease
For cardiovascular risk profile	Smoking habit	
	Early cardiovascular events in first-degree relatives	
Examination		
For a cause	Abdominal examination	
	for renal mass	Polycystic kidneys
	renal bruit	Renal artery stenosis
	Truncal obesity, bruising	Cushing's syndrome
	Infantilism	Adrenocortical enzyme deficiency
	Palpation of femoral pulses	Coarctation of aorta
For end organ damage	Fundi	Grade of retinopathy
	Heart	Left ventricular hypertrophy
		Heart failure
	Peripheral arteries	Carotid or peripheral atheroma
		Aortic aneurysm
	Central nervous system	Stroke
		Dementia

Retinal appearances

The prognostic importance of the retinal appearances was recognised by Keith *et al.* in 1939. It is now clear that not only papilloedema but retinal haemorrhage and exudates are an immediate indication that the patient's life is at serious risk from hypertension. The World Health Organisation has recommended a new definition of malignant hypertension to include patients with haemorrhages and exudates as well as those with papilloedema.

(i) *Grade I retinopathy:* increased light reflex due to thickening of the arterial wall (silver or copper wiring), increased tortuosity.
(ii) *Grade II retinopathy:* arteriovenous nipping (distortion of the retinal veins at the points where they are crossed by arterioles). These changes may be associated with ageing as well as with a significant rise in blood pressure.
(iii) *Grade III retinopathy:* haemorrhages and exudates.
(iv) *Grade IV retinopathy:* papilloedema.

Treatment of hypertension

Guidelines

Patients with the accelerated phase of hypertension, hypertensive heart failure and hypertensive crises must be treated as medical emergencies.

Patients under the age of 70 with a sustained blood pressure of greater than 175/110 mmHg should be offered treatment. The benefits of treatment in such patients is undisputed. The incidence of strokes, the risk of a further stroke and the incidence of cardiac failure are reduced. The development of the accelerated phase of hypertension is prevented.

Mild hypertension has been defined by the Medical Research Council (MRC) working party as a phase V diastolic pressure of between 90 and 109 mmHg. Similar figures have been used for other large studies. The evidence suggests that the incidence of stroke particularly in men is reduced by treatment. There is no clear effect on the incidence of coronary events. The overall conclusions of the MRC study are that if 850 mildly hypertensive patients are given active antihypertensive drugs for 1 year about one stroke will be prevented. Treatment did not appear to save lives. To achieve this benefit a substantial proportion of patients suffered side-effects as a result of treatment. At present there is no overwhelming evidence that all mildly hypertensive patients should be treated with drugs. Other risk factors like cigarette smoking should be tackled vigorously, weight reduction encouraged and perhaps dietary salt restriction applied. Heavy alcohol consumption should be discouraged.

Treatment of the elderly

The European Working Party on High Blood Pressure in the Elderly has reported benefits of treating patients aged 72 ± 8 years (SBP 183 ± 17 and DBP 101 ± 7). It is sensible to judge physiological as well as chronological age and initiate treatment if there are no contraindications. With care old people will tolerate treatment well and the approach is similar to younger patients.

Hypertensive crises

There are very few indications for rapid reduction of blood pressure with intravenous therapy. Special circumstances are:

(i) Hypertensive encephalopathy.
(ii) Dissection of the aorta.
(iii) Acute hypertension with a phaeochromocytoma.
(iv) Monoamine oxidase inhibitor—tyramine interaction.
(v) Clonidine withdrawal rebound hypertension.

Rapid reduction of blood pressure to a 'normal' value can be dangerous. Autoregulation of the cerebral circulation in sustained severe hypertension is reset to an increased pressure range. It is no longer effective at normal levels and cerebral ischaemia with neurological damage or death can result.

Nifedipine is the agent of first choice in most crises because it increases cerebral blood flow. It can be given orally, by buccal absorption or intravenously. Other drugs used included intravenous sodium nitroprusside, hydralazine and labetalol.

Treatment of chronic essential hypertension

The aims are:

(i) To lower the blood pressure to the normal range.
(ii) To use as few tablets as possible.
(iii) To tailor treatment to avoid side-effects.

Non-pharmacological management

It may be helpful to lose weight and to reduce salt intake. Some patients can learn relaxation techniques which have a beneficial effect on their blood pressure. However, it has been shown that in studies of patients with moderate to severe hypertension drug treatment is considerably more effective than any of the above measures. Cigarette smoking has a major adverse influence on the prognosis of untreated and treated hypertension.

Drug treatment

A stepped approach to treatment is recommended (Table 12.18). Each treatment should be assessed, in non-emergency treatment, after 2 weeks on the drug. The decisions at each assessment are:

(i) Adequate fall in pressure (no side effects): continue with long term followup.
(ii) Useful but insufficient fall in pressure: add a second agent.
(iii) Little or no fall in pressure: withdraw and substitute a second agent.
(iv) Side effects: withdraw.

There are two recent advances in medical treatment.

Table 12.18

SUGGESTED THERAPEUTIC APPROACH ASSUMING NO SPECIFIC CONTRAINDICATIONS

Step (1)	Beta-blocker or thiazide diuretic (low dose)
Step (2)	Combination tablet of above
Step (3)	Add vasodilator, such as nifedipine, enalapril
Step (4)	Add centrally acting agent, such as methyldopa
Step (5)	Consider non-compliance ? Admit for observation, further investigation

(i) The calcium antagonists: nifedipine and verapamil.
(ii) The angiotensin-converting enzyme (ACE) inhibitors: captopril and enalapril.

The exact place in the treatment regime for these drugs is not yet fully established. However, both types of agent have proved to be very effective and will undoubtedly become increasingly important in the management of hypertension.

Withdrawal of treatment

The majority of patients with proven sustained hypertension need long-term or lifelong treatment. If a decision is made to try without treatment then observation must be continued for some months because the rise in pressure does not always happen at once. Myocardial infarction may be a complication of hypertension which reduces blood pressure and allows withdrawal of treatment.

Failure to control blood pressure

The commonest cause is non-compliance. Even 'sensible' patients sometimes do not take the prescribed treatment.

FURTHER READING

Davies R., Kapila, H. (1983). Investigation of hypertension. *British Journal of Hospital Medicine*, **29,** 5, 428–439.

Keith N. M., Wagener H. P. and Barker N. W. (1939). Some different types of essential hypertension: their course and prognosis. *American Journal of Medical Sciences*, **197,** 332–343.

Lever A. F. (1986). Slow pressor mechanisms in hypertension: a role for hypertrophy of resistance vessels? Editorial review. *Journal of Hypertension*, **4,** 515–524.

McInnes G. T. (1986). Antihypertensive drugs: new developments and new agents. *Current Opinion in Cardiology*; **1,** 594–602.

Medical Research Council Working Party (1985). Medical Research Council trial of treatment of mild hypertension: principal results. *British Medical Journal*, **291,** 97–104.

Vann Jones J., Graham, D.I. (1983). The cerebral circulation and high blood pressure. In *Scientific Foundations of Cardiology*, Chapter 24 (Vann Jones J., Sleight, P., eds). London: Heinemann.

Zanchetti A., Ledingham J. G. G. (eds) (1985) Symposium on decision-making in the management of hypertension. *Journal of Hypertension*, **3,** Suppl. 2.

Chapter Thirteen

Infective Endocarditis

Definition

Infective endocarditis is the disease caused by infection of the heart valves or endocardium. It is usually bacterial but the infecting organism may be a rickettsia or a fungus. The bacteria are often of low virulence and the illness is typically subacute.

Background

Each year 21 cases per million population are diagnosed and the numbers are increasing (Table 13.1). Infective endocarditis was fatal until penicillin was discovered in 1943. The mortality rate is still greater than 20%. Three reasons account for the persisting high mortality.

(i) Antibiotic prophylaxis is not given to all patients at risk.
(ii) The illness is difficult to recognise and treatment may not be started until complications have occurred. Diagnosis is delayed because infective endocarditis presents with only vague symptoms and signs. It may mimic

Table 13.1

REASONS FOR THE INCREASED INCIDENCE OF INFECTIVE ENDOCARDITIS

Life expectancy has increased and there is more degenerative valvular disease
Children with congenital heart disease now survive into adult life
There are more patients with prosthetic heart valves
There is an increased number of surgical and therapeutic procedures

other diseases, in particular renal or cerebrovascular disease.

(iii) The haemodynamic deterioration due to valve destruction is not always fully appreciated. Patients can die because valve replacement is not undertaken in time.

Pathogenesis

Vegetations are thought to develop in three stages.

(i) *There is damage to the endothelium:* this can be initiated by abnormalities in blood flow. Infective endocarditis is most common when there is a regurgitant stream of blood from a high pressure source into a low pressure sink, especially when this is through a narrow orifice. Vegetations develop on the low pressure side of the orifice where the mechanical stresses are greatest. These haemodynamic conditions are most commonly found in aortic regurgitation, a ventricular septal defect, a patent ductus arteriosus and coarctation of the aorta.

(ii) *Platelets adhere to the damaged surface* because of the loss of endothelial prostacyclin which normally prevents adhesion and aggregation of platelets. Fibrin is deposited and a platelet-fibrin thrombus is formed.

(iii) *Circulating organisms enter the thrombus*, colonise it, and multiply to produce an infective vegetation. These are often bacteria of low virulence which normally reside on mucosal surfaces. They appear in the circulation after minor trauma to the gums, gastrointestinal or genito-urinary tracts. It is likely that the causative organisms have specific properties which make them more liable to adhere to the thrombus. For instance streptococci, the most common infective organism, produce the polysaccharide dextran which encourages adhesion. In contrast this is not produced by Gram-negative bacteria which quite often cause a transient bacteraemia but rarely produce infective endocarditis.

Although the classic development of subacute infective endocarditis involves abnormal endocardium it is clear that in many cases infection develops on apparently normal valves. The mechanisms involved are not understood.

When antibiotic treatment is effective the vegetations shrink and endothelium gradually covers the surface. However, the valve may be scarred and damaged. Haemodynamic deterioration can continue after the infection is cured.

Autoimmune changes

Specific agglutinating antibodies to the bacteria are produced and may enhance adherence. Depending on the duration of the illness, the bacteria in the vegetation stimulate the body's immune system to produce a generalised increase in gamma-globulins. These explain the false-positive serological tests for syphilis and positive rheumatoid factor found in some patients. The excess antigen, antibodies and serum complement join together to make immune complexes. These pass through capillary walls into the subendothelial tissues and induce damage. The focal nephritis and diffuse glomerulonephritis complicating infective endocarditis are the result of immune complex deposition. Serum complement is often increased in subacute infective endocarditis but the C3 component falls when nephritis develops. The other manifestations of infective endocarditis which may be related to immune complex deposition are the vasculitic skin lesions, splinter haemorrhages, Roth spots, Osler's nodes and arthralgia. Autoimmune changes are not seen in acute infective endocarditis.

Microbiology

Table 13.2 shows the causative organisms. The teeth and gums are the commonest source. The risks are increased if there is poor oral hygiene; this is as important as dental manipulation. Other foci of infection are:

(i) Pharynx and tonsils.
(ii) Gastrointestinal tract.
(iii) Genitourinary tract.
(iv) Respiratory tract.
(v) Skin.
(vi) Intravenous injections.

Often a source cannot be identified.

Some 5–10% of cases are culture-negative. The possible reasons are listed in Table 13.3. The commonest is the recent use

Table 13.2

ORGANISMS WHICH CAUSE INFECTIVE ENDOCARDITIS

Organism	*Percentage of cases*
Oral streptococci	60
Strep. sanguis	
Strep. mitior	
Strep. mutans	
Strep. salivanius	
Lancefield group D streptococci	10
Strep. bovis	
Strep. faecalis	
Staphylococci	25
Staph. aureus	
Staph. epidermidis	
Haemophilus	5
Coliforms	
Chlamydia psittaci	
Coxiella burneti	
Fungi	
candida (commonest)	
aspergillus	
histoplasms	

Table 13.3

REASONS FOR NEGATIVE BLOOD CULTURES

Recent antibiotic treatment
Long illness and renal failure—antibodies develop and lead to negative cultures
Technical problems such as inadequate number of cultures or quantity of blood, failure to culture in anaerobic conditions
Wrong diagnosis
Unusual organisms
- *Coxiella*
- *Chlamydia*
- Fungi

of antibiotic treatment. Sometimes this effect can be neutralised in the laboratory by adding penicillinase to the blood cultures.

Pathology

The heart

Vegetations are always present. There may be evidence of underlying acquired or congenital heart disease. Vegetations develop along the line of closure of the valve leaflet on the low pressure side of the defect and vary in size from small nodules to large friable masses. The infection causes progressive damage and there may be perforation of the valve leaflets or rupture of a chordae tendineae producing rapid haemodynamic deterioration. Abscesses can develop in the fibrous valve ring and spread into the myocardium. Pericarditis is a serious complication and is caused by direct spread. Myocarditis with areas of monocytic infiltration (Bracht–Wachter bodies) is sometimes found. Myocardial infarction may result from embolism into a coronary artery.

The kidney

About 15% of cases have evidence of important renal involvement. Focal segmental nephritis or a diffuse glomerulonephritis with renal failure is caused by immune complex deposition. Renal infarction and abscess formation are rarer.

Emboli

Systemic emboli are a major threat in infective endocarditis. They may cause infarction of the brain, spleen, kidney or bowel. Embolisation of the vasa vasorum of a major artery leads to the formation of a mycotic aneurysm.

Pulmonary emboli occur with right-sided endocarditis and left-to-right shunts.

Causes of death

These are listed in Table 13.4. Acute infective endocarditis is a much more aggressive illness than the subacute form and valve destruction is an early complication.

Table 13.4

CAUSES OF DEATH IN INFECTIVE ENDOCARDITIS

Cause	*Mechanism*
Heart failure	Destruction of the aortic valve
	Destruction of the mitral valve
	Myocarditis
	Coronary artery embolism
Renal failure	Nephritis due to immune complex deposition
Stroke	Cerebral artery embolism
Haemorrhage	Ruptured mycotic aneurysm

Patients

There is a male:female ratio of 2:1. This is because of a higher incidence of bicuspid aortic valves and calcific aortic stenosis in males. Rheumatic fever, which was commoner in females, has diminished in importance.

The age of infected patients has altered; 35 years ago, when rheumatic fever was still common, the mean age of presentation was 32 years. In a recent survey the mean age was 52 years.

The patients who are most at risk from subacute infective endocarditis are those with a known cardiac defect (Table 13.5). However, it is now realised that about 30% of patients are unaware of a pre-existing heart lesion and in most cases the heart was probably normal.

Drug addicts

Drug addicts are at high risk because they inject pathogenic bacteria directly into their veins. The tricuspid and pulmonary valves become infected. *Staphylococcus aureus* accounts for about two-thirds of infections while the remainder are caused by other Gram-positive cocci (20%), *Pseudomonas* (5%), other Gram-negative organisms and candida. The patient is often very ill at presentation and has evidence of tricuspid or pulmonary regurgitation. Pneumonia or septic pulmonary emboli occur in 95% of cases.

Table 13.5

PATIENTS AT RISK OF INFECTIVE ENDOCARDITIS

High risk	Prosthetic heart valves (mechanical and heterografts) Surgical arteriovenous shunts Patients with a past history of infective endocarditis
Moderate risk	Aortic stenosis and regurgitation Mitral regurgitation (including mitral valve prolapse with mitral regurgitation) Most congenital heart defects, especially ventricular septal defect patent ductus arteriosus (PDA) bicuspid aortic valve coarctation of the aorta Surgically corrected congenital heart disease (except atrial septal defect (ASD) and PDA) Hypertrophic obstructive cardiomyopathy
Negligible risk	Atrial septal defect (ASD) Pure mitral stenosis Mitral valve prolapse without regurgitation (systolic click or echocardiographic evidence only) Postcoronary artery vein grafts

Table 13.6

CLINICAL FEATURES OF INFECTIVE ENDOCARDITIS

Clinical feature	*Mechanism*
Features of heart disease	
Heart murmur	Pre-existing heart disease
Changing murmurs (less than 10% of cases)	Vegetations and destruction of the valve Dehiscence of prosthetic heart valve
Heart failure	Haemodynamic consequences of valve destruction Myocarditis Myocardial infarction

Table 13.6

CLINICAL FEATURES OF INFECTIVE ENDOCARDITIS

Clinical feature	*Mechanism*
General features of infection	Response to infection—'flu-like' symptoms
Fever—usually low grade and may be absent in elderly patients	
Malaise	
Night sweats	
Loss of weight	
Myalgia	
Low back pain	
Headache	
Confusion	
Anaemia	
Splenomegaly	
Complications of emboli	
Stroke	Cerebral infarction
Loin pain	Renal or splenic infarction
Frank haematuria	Renal infarction
Abdominal pain	Bowel infarction
Peripheral gangrene	Major limb vessel embolism
Mycotic aneurysm	Embolism of vaso vasorum of major arteries
Immunological phenomena	Immune complex deposition
Nephritis—microscopic haematuria renal failure	
Skin petechiae	
Splinter haemorrhages in nail beds	
Osler's nodes (small red, raised and painful lesion in the pulp of the terminal phalanges)	
Janeway lesions (flat, red but painless lesions on the palms or soles)	
Roth spots (canoe-shaped fundal haemorrhages)	
Arthralgia	

Clinical features

Subacute infective endocarditis develops insidiously and there should be a low threshold of suspicion in any unwell patient with a heart murmur. Unexplained heart failure is always a reason to take blood cultures. The clinical features fall into four groups (Table 13.6). Symptoms and signs may be vague and can lead to referral to other than a cardiologist i.e. cerebral symptoms to either a neurologist or psychiatrist and renal failure to a renal unit. Absence of a raised temperature should not rule our the diagnosis and if in doubt, blood cultures should be taken.

Investigations

Most culture-positive cases of infective endocarditis can be diagnosed by the first three blood cultures taken over a period of 12 h. The bacteraemia is usually continuous and there is no need to wait for a spike of fever. Other useful investigations are listed in Table 13.7.

Table 13.7

INVESTIGATION OF INFECTIVE ENDOCARDITIS

Investigation	*Comment*
Blood cultures	90% are positive
Special cultures for fungi	Candida
Serological tests	For coxiella and chlamydia
Immunological tests	
Serum complement	Low C3 with glomerulonephritis
Circulating immune complexes	Present in 75% of cases
C-reactive protein	Usually elevated
Rheumatoid factor	Positive in 50% of cases
Haematological indices	
Anaemia	Normochromic, normocytic
Raised plasma viscosity	Usual
Raised white cell count	In 25–50% of cases
Urine	
Microscopic haematuria	Glomerulonephritis
Proteinuria	
Echocardiography	

Echocardiography

This is an important investigation for both the diagnosis and monitoring of the disease. Two-dimensional echocardiography will detect vegetations in 80% of cases of infective endocarditis. Vegetations of only 2 mm in size can be visualised but failure to image them does not exclude the diagnosis. The diagnostic accuracy is least when there is calcific aortic stenosis. Echocardiography will also show perivalvular abscesses. It provides information about the pre-existing cardiac defect and serial examinations will demonstrate any increase in size of the cardiac chambers. Doppler echocardiography is particularly useful in the diagnosis of a perivalvular leak in a patient with dehiscence of a prosthetic heart valve.

Prophylaxis

All patients with susceptible heart disease should be told about the risk of infective endocarditis. They should be aware of the

Table 13.8

PROCEDURES WHICH REQUIRE ANTIBIOTIC PROPHYLAXIS

All patients	*Dental procedures* Extractions Scaling Operations involving the gums
	Tonsillectomy and adenoidectomy
	All genitourinary surgery Urethral catheterisation Instrumental childbirth
	Other major surgery
High risk patients Prosthetic heart valves Surgical arteriovenous shunts Previous infective endocarditis	As above and the following: Endoscopy Colonoscopy Sigmoidoscopy Barium enema Normal vaginal delivery Inserting intrauterine contraceptive device (IUCD) Bronchoscopy

need for prophylactic antibiotics and carry a card which give information about their heart condition and recommended antibiotic treatment. This advice must be reinforced regularly. They should maintain good dental hygiene and should be encouraged to report any unexplained fever or illness to their doctor. Table 13.8 lists the procedures which require antibiotic prophylaxis and Table 13.9 the recommended prophylactic antibiotics.

Table 13.9

ANTIBIOTIC PROPHYLAXIS FOR DENTAL PROCEDURES

Under local anaesthesia		*Under general anaesthesia*		
Not allergic to penicillin	*Allergic or recently treated with penicillin*	*No special risk*	*Special risk*	
Amoxycillin 3 g orally	Erythromycin 1.5 g orally		Refer to hospital	
			Not allergic to penicillin	Allergic to penicillin
	Orally 0.5 g after 6 h	Amoxycillin 1 g intramuscularly	Amoxycillin 1 g intramuscularly	Vancomycin 1 g slow intravenous injection
		Orally 0.5 g after 6 h	Gentamicin 120 mg	Gentamicin 120 mg intravenously
			Amoxycillin 0.5 g orally after 6 h	

For genitourinary procedures, tonsillectomy, obstetric and gastrointestinal manipulation	
At induction of anaesthesia	Amoxycillin 1 g intramuscularly + gentamicin 120 mg intramuscularly
6 h later	Amoxycillin 0.5 g orally or intramuscularly

These are the recommendations of a working party of the British Society for Antimicrobial Chemotherapy (1982)

Timing of antibiotics

Oral amoxycillin should be given under supervision 1 h before dental procedures undertaken with a local anaesthetic. Patients who are allergic to penicillin should be given oral erythromycin 1–2 h before the procedure and again 6 h later. When a general anaesthetic is necessary intramuscular antibiotics should be given before induction of anaesthesia.

Referral to hospital

Special risk patients should be referred to hospital for dental treatment. These are patients:

(i) Who need a general anaesthetic.
(ii) With a prosthetic heart valve.
(iii) Who have had infective endocarditis in the past.
(iv) Who are allergic to penicillin and need a general anaesthetic.

Pregnancy and infective endocarditis

The risk of infective endocarditis after a normal vaginal delivery is very small. Routine antibiotic prophylaxis for women with heart murmurs is not recommended. Antibiotics should be given to high risk patients (with prosthetic heart valves or previous infective endocarditis) in the second stage of labour.

Instrumental delivery, caesarean section and manual removal of the placenta should be covered with antibiotics in all patients at risk.

Management of infective endocarditis

Three sets of blood cultures should be taken over 12 h. If possible treatment should be delayed until the results of the cultures are available. In ill patients, with complications or with acute infective endocarditis, treatment should be started after the first blood culture is taken. Intravenous antibiotic treatment is essential and it is best given through a central intravenous subclavian line inserted under aseptic conditions.

Length of treatment

Intravenous antibiotic treatment should be given for a minimum of 4 weeks in uncomplicated cases. In patients with prosthetic heart valves or complicated cases the treatment should be maintained for at least 6 weeks. (Selection of patients for referral for surgery must always be considered.)

Initial treatment

Strep. viridans is the most likely organism in subacute infective endocarditis. Until culture results are available treatment can be started with benzyl penicillin 2 megaunits (MU) (1.2 g) by intravenous bolus injected every 4 h, *plus* gentamycin 80 mg by intravenous bolus injected every 8 h. In elderly patients or where renal function is impaired netilmicin should be used.

If staphylococcal infection is suspected the initial treatment should be flucloxacillin and gentamicin or fusidic acid.

Further treatment

There must be a close liaison between clinician and bacteriologist. Suggested regimes are outlined in Table 13.10.

The laboratory control of treatment is essential and should include:

(i) Determination of the minimum bactericidal concentration (MBC) of penicillin for the streptococcus:
MBC $<$ 1 mg/l = sensitive streptococcus
MBC $>$ 1 mg/l = moderately resistant streptococcus.

(ii) Measurement of the effectiveness of antibacterial activity. Serum collected 20 min after administration should kill the bacteria at a dilution of one in eight or more.

(iii) Blood levels of gentamicin twice weekly should be measured in blood taken 20 min after a dose and 20 min before the next dose (peak and trough). A trough level of $>$2 mg/l may lead to toxicity so reduce or stop gentamicin.

Table 13.10

ANTIBIOTIC TREATMENT

Organism	*Treatment*
Penicillin-sensitive Streptococci	Benzylpenicillin and gentamicin together for 2 weeks for the maximum bactericidal effect. Then penicillin alone for at least 2 more weeks
Less sensitive Streptococci	Benzylpenicillin for 4–6 weeks
Staphylococci	Flucloxacillin 2 g intravenous bolus injection every 4 h *plus* fusidic acid 500 mg every 8 h by mouth or gentamicin 80 mg by intravenous injection according to blood levels Treat for 6 weeks
Candida	Intravenous amphotericin *plus* oral flucytosine

Dental treatment in infected patients

The teeth and gums should be X-rayed in all patients with infective endocarditis. Even an edentulous patient may have a hidden infected root. An oral surgeon should be asked to undertake necessary dentistry immediately after admission or at the end of treatment under different antibiotic cover (for example, vancomycin 1 mg intravenously over 60 min).

Followup

The fall in temperature to normal will reflect effective antibiotic control of the infection. Occasionally a secondary fever develops which is due to penicillin allergy.

Despite antibiotics the haemodynamic consequences of the valvular damage may progress and patients must be carefully observed throughout the course of treatment. Chest X-ray and echocardiography are essential investigations. X-ray screening of a prosthetic heart valve can be used to detect an abnormal rocking movement when dehiscence is occurring.

INDICATIONS FOR VALVE REPLACEMENT

Valve replacement should never be delayed if valvular regurgitation is causing haemodynamic deterioration. Most patients die as a result of heart failure due to valvular destruction and the onset of heart failure is an indication for urgent surgery. This is more likely to occur in acute staphylococcal endocarditis but can complicate any type of infection. The other indications are listed in Table 13.11.

Table 13.11

INDICATIONS FOR SURGERY IN INFECTIVE ENDOCARDITIS

Refractory congestive cardiac failure usually due to valve cusp perforation or destruction
Systemic embolism
Failure of the infection to respond to antibiotics
Prosthetic valve endocarditis
Relapse of endocarditis (3 months or less after antibiotic 'cure')
Recurrence of endocarditis (6 months or more after antibiotic 'cure')
Intracardiac spread of infection with abscess formation
Tricuspid valve replacement in some drug addicts with pulmonary emboli

ACUTE INFECTIVE ENDOCARDITIS

Acute infective endocarditis attacks previously normal hearts as a complication of septicaemia. Immunologically compromised patients are particularly susceptible. The infective organism is a pathogen, often a *Staphylococcus*.

At an early stage there may be no cardiac signs but rapidly advancing destruction of the valve leads to gross regurgitation. Severe heart failure can develop within a week, particularly if the aortic valve is involved. Emboli from the large vegetations are common.

Early recognition with urgent valve replacement under appropriate antibiotic cover is essential for survival.

COXIELLA (Q FEVER) ENDOCARDITIS

About 1–2% of patients infected with *Coxiella burneti* develop chronic illness with endocarditis. There may be a delay of months or years between the acute infection, which is often undiagnosed, and the presentation with endocarditis. Patients with an underlying heart lesion or prosthetic heart valve are most at risk.

Primary or acute Q fever is an influenza-like illness which is often accompanied by pneumonia and normally follows a benign course. The reservoir of infection resides in sheep and cattle which are symptomless but excrete the organisms at parturition. Airborne spread accounts for most cases. One large outbreak in the United Kingdom was due to contamination of urban roads by farm vehicles.

Clinical features

Clinically Q fever endocarditis presents as culture negative endocarditis with patients showing signs of fever, tachycardia, heart murmurs and splenomegaly. The vegetations are often small and may not be detected with echocardiography. The diagnosis must be made serologically. There will be seroconversion or a significant rise in phase II antibody titres and a phase I antibody titre of greater than 1 in 200 is consistent with Q fever endocarditis.

Treatment

Tetracycline or doxycycline should be given for at least 12 months but valve replacement is often necessary.

CHLAMYDIA ENDOCARDITIS

Diseased birds are the source of infection with *Chlamydia psittaci*. Endocarditis is rare and the diagnosis is confirmed by a positive complement fixation test. Long-term doxycycline may be effective but valve replacement is usually necessary.

FUNGI

Endocarditis may be caused by candida, histoplasma and aspergillus. The infection gains access during surgery or by direct injection (drug addicts). The vegetations are very large and friable and are easily detected by echocardiography. Repeated blood cultures and special culture will confirm the diagnosis. Treatment is intravenous amphotericin and surgical excision of the infected valve.

PROSTHETIC VALVE ENDOCARDITIS

Both tissue valves and mechanical valves may become infected. The increased risk is due to the endothelial damage and exposure to bacteraemia during surgery. Valve replacement for native valve endocarditis carries an increased risk of further infection which is probably due to patient susceptibility to endocarditis rather than persisting infection.

Infective endocarditis can occur early after surgery (within 2 months) or later. The incidence of infection has been found to be 2.7% for early endocarditis and the cumulative risk is about 5% at 10 years.

Early Onset Cases

These patients have a mortality rate of between 30 and 90%. *Staphylococcus epidermidis* accounts for 30% of cases and other important organisms are Gram-negative bacilli, *Staph. aureus* and fungi. Sources of infection include carrier members of staff, contamination of the blood by the oxygenator or instruments at operation, infected sternal wounds and postoperative drains and catheters.

The patients are seriously ill and often have rigors. Prompt surgical replacement is indicated in most cases.

Late Onset Cases

The microbiological pattern is similar to that found in native valve endocarditis. Most may be initially treated with antibiotics but valve replacement is often necessary.

FURTHER READING

Bayliss R., Clarke C., Oakley C., Somerville W., Whitfield A. G. W. (1983). The teeth and infective endocarditis. *British Heart Journal*, **50,** 506–512.

Bayliss R., Clarke C., Oakley C., Somerville W., Whitfield A. G. W., Young S. E. J. (1983). The microbiology and pathogenesis of infective endocarditis. *British Heart Journal*, **50,** 513–519.

British Society for Antimicrobial Chemotherapy (1985). Antibiotic treatment of streptococcal and staphylococcal endocarditis. Report of a working party of the BSAC. *Lancet*, **2,** 815–817.

Gray I. R. (1981). Management of infective endocarditis. *Journal of the Royal College of Physicians of London*, **15,** 173–178.

Palmer S. R., Young S. E. J (1982). Q-fever endocarditis in England and Wales, 1975–81. *Lancet*, **2,** 1448–1449.

Robbins M. J., Soeiro R., Frishman W. H., Stom J. A. (1986). Right-sided valvular endocarditis: Etiology, diagnosis and an approach to therapy. *American Heart Journal*, **111,** 128–135.

Varma M. P. S., McCluskey D. R., Khan M. M., Cleland J., O'Kane H. O., Adgey A. A. J. (1986). Heart failure associated with infective endocarditis. A review of 40 cases. *British Heart Journal*, **55,** 191–197.

Westaby S., Oakley C., Sapsford R. N., Bentall H. H. (1983). Surgical treatment of infective endocarditis with special reference to prosthetic valve endocarditis. *British Medical Journal*, **3,** 320–323.

Chapter Fourteen

Prevention of Heart Disease

CORONARY HEART DISEASE

Background

Coronary heart disease is the commonest cause of death in the United Kingdom. It accounts for 31% of male and 23% of female deaths, a total of 160 000 deaths per year.

The British Heart Study shows that by the age of 40–44 one in six men has clinical evidence of coronary heart disease and by the

Table 14.1

DEATHS FROM CORONARY HEART DISEASE
WORLD HEALTH ORGANISATION STATISTICS FOR 1986

Country		*Deaths per 100 000 population*
	Scotland, Northern Ireland	298
	Czechoslovakia	290
	Irish Republic	282
Highest	Finland	264
	England and Wales	243
	Hungary	238
	United States	230
	Greece, Yugoslavia	85
	Portugal	82
Lowest	Spain	79
	France	74
	Japan	45

age of 55–59 one in three is affected; 20 million working days are lost due to this cause.

In world ranking Scotland and Northern Ireland have the highest incidence (Table 14.1).

The United Kingdom has not experienced the same decline in mortality which has been seen in a number of countries (1972–82, United States of America: 35%; Australia: 32%; Belgium: 27%). There is clearly the potential for a reduction in coronary disease but all the reasons are yet to be understood. In the United States the greatest fall has occurred in non-white women which suggests that reduction in risk factors and improvement in health care are not the only factors.

The majority of deaths occur outside hospital and within 2 h of the onset of symptoms. Advances in cardiopulmonary resuscitation and early coronary care will have an impact and it has been calculated that 9000 lives a year could be saved if prehospital defibrillation were readily available. Only primary prevention will have a greater impact.

Risk factors

These are shown in Table 14.2.

Table 14.2

RISK FACTORS FOR HEART DISEASE

Major factors
Cigarette smoking
High serum cholesterol
Hypertension
Family history of premature coronary heart disease
Increasing age
Male sex
Others
Obesity, ? development of a paunch in men
Lack of exercise
Stress and type A behaviour
Oral contraceptives
Diabetes
Softness of drinking water

Cigarette smoking

The association between smoking and coronary heart disease is established. Current smokers have a three-fold risk compared to those who have never smoked. There is no definite dose response—light smokers carry a considerable excess risk.

Smoking cigarettes causes atherosclerosis, induces spasm in the coronary arteries, alters platelet function and liability to thrombosis and may produce arrhythmias. Increased levels of carboxyhaemoglobin, associated with cigarette smoking, aggravate exercise-induced angina.

People who stop smoking have a lower risk of developing coronary heart disease than those who persist; 10 years after the cessation of smoking their risk is similar to that of people who have never smoked. Most evidence supports benefit from stopping smoking even after myocardial infarction and a mortality ratio of about 2:0 in favour of survivors who stop is consistently reported in secondary prevention studies.

General practitioners have so far obtained success rates of 5–10% in persuading patients to stop smoking.

Objective tests of smoking are required to be absolutely certain of smoking status. Detection of the nicotine metabolite, cotinine, in a random sample of urine is a simple and inexpensive test for smoking.

Serum cholesterol

This is the best biochemical indicator for increased risk. There is a continuous and marked trend of increased risk with increased serum cholesterol. A treatment trial of symptomatic men aged 35–59 years in the top 5% of frequency distribution of serum cholesterol showed benefit from reduction in cholesterol (Lipid Research Clinics Coronary Primary Prevention Trial, 1984). Treatment with diet and cholestyramine 24 g/day reduced the incidence of death and heart attacks by 19%, the incidence of angina by 20% and of a positive exercise test by 24%.

HDL-cholesterol

Low levels are associated with increased risk.

Serum triglyceride

The importance of hypertriglyceridaemia is less well established. Some studies suggest it is a risk factor while others have not shown it to be independent of levels of total cholesterol.

Hypertension

Hypertension is an independent risk factor. A systolic pressure of greater than 160 mmHg and a diastolic pressure of greater than 100 mmHg carries a considerable risk (the Framingham, USA study found a 24 year incidence of coronary disease in men aged 30–39 years of 157 per 1000 with systolic pressure 120–139 mmHg and 444 per 1000 with systolic pressure greater than 180 mmHg). There is no definite evidence that antihypertensive treatment will prevent coronary events.

Family history

Coronary heart disease clusters in families. This results in part from the association of other accepted risk factors. The Denver Risk Index suggests that there is increased risk if a first-degree relative suffers myocardial infarction before the age of 55.

Obesity

This is a relatively unimportant risk factor. Fears of weight gain should not deter smokers from ceasing to smoke. A body mass index of over 30 (acceptable range 20–25) only equates to the risk of smoking 20 cigarettes a day (body mass index is the relationship of weight, kg/height, metres). The distribution of fat may be important. A middle-aged man's paunch size has been suggested as a better prediction of coronary heart disease than other measures of obesity.

Exercise

Physical fitness increases the sense of wellbeing. Whether it reduces the incidence of coronary heart disease is controversial. Regular exercise helps prevent weight gain. Vigorous dynamic exercise may have a protective effect by increasing HDL cholesterol and fibrinolytic activity as well as improving cardiopulmonary function.

Stress

There is some evidence that coronary heart disease occurs more frequently in people who have an excessive sense of time-urgency, preoccupation with deadlines, aggressiveness and competitive drive (type A behaviour). A recent study has suggested that social isolation and life stress, in particular the lack of a job and financial difficulties, were of prognostic importance of survivors of acute infarction.

It has not been established that reducing stress lowers the risk of coronary heart disease. People who are undertaking hard and responsible work with care and effort should not be discouraged.

Acute stress such as extreme fright may be the setting of acute myocardial infarction.

Oral contraceptives

The greatest risks are in women who are also cigarette smokers and in those older than 40 years. The use of oral contraceptives in these groups should be discouraged. Oral contraceptives may elevate the blood pressure and should not be prescribed in patients with hypertension. The blood pressure should be checked prior to prescription and during the first 12 months of treatment. If a significant rise occurs then the oral contraceptive should be discontinued. In most patients blood pressure will then fall back to normal.

Diabetes

Diabetes confers a two-fold increase in the risk of coronary heart disease independently of other risk factors. There are often associated risk factors which influence the development of atherosclerosis, such as hyperlipidaemia, hypertension and obesity.

Softness of drinking water

Evidence from the British Regional Heart Study suggests that drinking very soft water increases the risk of a cardiovascular event by 10%. The risk is small but deliberate softening of drinking water should be discouraged.

Strategies for Primary Prevention

There are two approaches which should be complementary to each other.

Population strategy

This recognises that many people in western countries have moderately elevated risk factors. This strategy aims to improve health-oriented behaviour in the whole population.

Smoking should be discouraged. Dietary recommendations have been made by the Committee on Medical Aspects of Food Policy (COMA report) and the National Advisory Committee on Nutrition Education (NACNE report). Total fat intake should be reduced to provide less than 35% of total energy (currently more than 40%) and saturated fatty acids should provide less than 15% (currently 20%).

Health education, antismoking campaigns and screening for hypertension can have an impact. The World Health Organisation European Collaborative Group Study found that if risk factors are reduced then the incidence of coronary heart disease will also fall. In Belgium there was an overall reduction of 24%. A community programme in North Karelia, the most easterly county of Finland which had the highest death rate in the world, reduced mortality by 24% in men and 51% in women. These changes were significantly greater than those which occurred at the same time in the rest of Finland.

Individual or high risk strategy

The minority of people within the population who are at particular risk of coronary heart disease should be identified. The burden of 'case finding' will fall largely on general practitioners and the greatest efforts should be directed at younger people. Virtually all the population, in the United Kingdom, consults a doctor once in 5 years. This should provide an opportunity for measurement of each person's blood pressure. If it is not elevated the measurement

Table 14.3

SELECTION CRITERIA FOR SCREENING BLOOD CHOLESTEROL

A positive family history of cardiovascular disease occurring under the age of 50 years
Presence of xanthomas
Presence of xanthelasmas or corneal arcus under the age of 40 years
Diabetes
Hypertension

Table 14.4

CHOLESTEROL LEVELS FOR SELECTING ADULTS AT MODERATE AND HIGH RISK (NIH CONSENSUS CONFERENCE USA, 1985)

Age	*Moderate risk blood cholesterol*		*High risk blood cholesterol*	
	mm/l	mg/dl	mm/l	mg/dl
30–39 years	>5·69	(220)	>6·21	(240)
40 years	>6·21	(240)	>6·72	(260)

Conversion: plasma cholesterol into SI units: 1 mmol/l = 39 mg/dl

need not be repeated for a further 5 years. Screening for hypercholesterolaemia should be mainly restricted to people under 55 years. Particular attention must be paid to patients with criteria listed in Table 14.3.

The levels of cholesterol considered to be of moderate and high risk are given in Table 14.4. Details of some large trials of high risk intervention are given in Table 14.5.

Treatment of hypercholesterolaemia

Patients should be screened for a possible *secondary cause* such as diabetes, hypothyroidism, nephrotic syndrome and primary biliary cirrhosis—measurement of blood sugar, serum thyroxine, blood urea and liver function tests.

Diet

Diet is the initial treatment. Obese patients should have restricted

Table 14.5

TRIALS OF PRIMARY PREVENTION IN HIGH RISK MEN

Oslo heart study (1981): 16 202 well men aged 40–49 years were screened; 1232 high risk men were randomised.
Mean cholesterol 7·5–9·8 mmol/l, 80% smoked.
Result: Intervention group 5 year coronary events 3·2%; placebo group 5·7%; significant reduction in coronary events ($P=0{\cdot}03$)

Lipid Research Clinic's coronary primary prevention trial (1984): 480 000 men aged 35–59 years were screened; 18 000 had a serum cholesterol 6·85 mmol/l. If the cholesterol fell with diet alone the man was excluded; 3806 men were randomised into two groups: one received 24 g cholestyramine/day. The trial was double-blind
Result: Intervention over 7 years showed coronary events were reduced by 20%.

Multirisk factor intervention trial (1982) USA (MR FIT): 361 662 men were screened; 12 866 were randomised because they were the upper 15% of risk score (cholesterol, blood pressure, smoking).
Result: Intervention for 6 years was associated with a fall in coronary events but not significantly different from controls. However, the control group showed a reduction in smoking, blood pressure and cholesterol levels. Over the study period the mortality from coronary disease in the United States fell by 20% and both groups fared better than predicted

calories. All patients should have a reduced intake of total fat and saturated fatty acids. The proportion, but not the absolute quantity, of polysaturated fats should be increased. An increase in fibre-rich carbohydrates can be recommended. The effects should be assessed after 3–6 months and then drug treatment should be considered.

Lipid-lowering drugs

The aim in patients younger than 55 years should be to lower the blood cholesterol to below 5.2 mmol/l (200 mg/dl). If the initial level is greater than 7.8 mmol/l (300 mg/dl) it is unlikely that diet alone will suffice. It is often necessary to combine drugs acting in different ways to achieve a satisfactory fall in cholesterol (Table 14.6). Cholestyramine is the most widely used agent but its use is

Table 14.6

DRUGS USED IN THE TREATMENT OF HYPERCHOLESTEROLAEMIA

Drug	*Mode of action*	*Side-effects*
Bile acid-binding agents Cholestyramine Colestipol	Binds to bile acids in the gut and prevents their reabsorption. To compensate cholesterol, their major precursor is oxidised at an increased rate in the liver. Plasma cholesterol falls	Constipation Abdominal discomfort Nausea Binds to warfarin and digitoxin
Fibrates Clofibrate Bezafibrate Gemfibrozil	Probably increase activity of lipoprotein lipase which increases catabolism. Gemfibrozil elevates HDL	Clofibrate causes an increased incidence of gallbladder disease and large bowel malignant neoplasms The other agents are under scrutiny

Probucol	Unclear	Gastrointestinal disturbance
Nicotinic acid	? Inhibits lipolysis in adipose tissue ? Increases activity of lipoprotein lipase Elevates HDL	Severe skin flushing and pruritus. (This is prostaglandin-mediated and reduced by aspirin or by using low initial doses) Gastrointestinal disturbance.
HMGCoA *reductase inhibitors* Simvastatin	Specific competitive inhibitor of 3 hydroxy-3 methyl glutaryl (HMG) (coenzyme A reductase) rate-controlling enzyme in cholesterol synthesis	Not fully established ? Cataracts ? Reduced testosterone

HDL = high density lipoprotein
HMGCoA = 3 hydroxy-3-methyl glutaryl (HMG) coenzyme A reductase inhibitor

limited by troublesome side-effects. Clofibrate is no longer generally prescribed because of adverse effects with long-term use.

A new group of drugs which are specific competitive inhibitors of 3 hydroxy-3 methyl glutaryl (HMG) coenzyme A reductase are under trial. Simvastatin is one of these drugs. HMG-COA reductase is the enzyme which catalyses the conversion of HMG-COA to mevalonate. This is an early step in the biosynthetic pathway of cholesterol. Simvastatin therefore lowers cholesterol. They are highly effective and can lower plasma cholesterol levels by 40%.

Drugs and Prevention of Coronary Heart Disease

This is shown in Table 14.7. Reduction in the level of cholesterol with cholestyramine and diet, in high-risk patients, has been shown to reduce the risk of a heart attack.

Table 14.7

DRUGS AND PREVENTION OF CORONARY HEART DISEASE

Drug	Trial	Result
Primary prevention		
Clofibrate	WHO Primary Prevention Trial using clofibrate (1980)	Adverse effects increased overall mortality
Cholestyramine	Lipid Research Clinic's Coronary Primary Prevention Trial (CPPT) (1984)	Positive benefits in high risk men (top 5% of frequency distribution of cholesterol)
Propranolol/bendrofluazide	Medical Research Council Trial of Mild Hypertension (1985)	No overall effect on coronary events
Oxprenolol	International Prospective Primary Prevention Study in Hypertension (1985)	Inclusion of a beta-blocker had no influence on the incidence of heart attacks

Table 14.7

DRUGS AND PREVENTION OF CORONARY HEART DISEASE

Drug	Trial	Result
Secondary prevention		
Antiplatelet agents		
Sulphinpyrazone	Anturane Reinfarction Trial (ART) (1978)	Positive result but much criticised for flaws in trial design
Dipyridamole	Persantin Aspirin Reinfarction Study (PARIS) (1980)	Favourable trend but not statistically significant
Aspirin	Many trials including Aspirin Myocardial Infarction Study (AMIS) (1980)	No benefit
	Overall assessment	Favourable trend but not statistically significant.
Anticoagulants	Sixty Plus Reinfarction Group (1980)	Stopping anticoagulants may increase risk
Beta-blockers	Many trials including Beta-blocker Heart Attack Trial (1981) (propranolol) Norwegian Multicentre Trial (1982) (timolol)	
	Overall assessment	Positive benefit in first year after infarction in selected patients

Secondary prevention trials are easier to do because there will be more endpoints—deaths or heart attacks. At present there is a trend in favour of aspirin after infarction but there is no hard proof of benefit either in secondary or primary prevention. There is some evidence that anticoagulation is useful or at least that withdrawal may be harmful after a heart attack. However, there are strong disadvantages to long-term anticoagulation which must be considered. Beta-blockers give undoubted benefit in the first year after infarction in selected patients.

Proposals for Preventing Coronary Disease

These can be summarised as follows.

General advice

(i) Stop smoking.
(ii) Sensible eating:
  (a) reduce fat intake;
  (b) avoid obesity.
(iii) Treat sustained hypertension.

Additional advice to patients under 55 at high risk

(i) As above.
(ii) Screen serum cholesterol—intervene if high:
  (a) with diet
  (b) with cholestyramine and diet.
  The ideal to aim for is 5·0–5·5 mmol/l as this is associated with a minimum incidence of coronary heart disease.

HYPERTENSIVE HEART DISEASE

Mild hypertension is common. One-fifth of the adult population have a diastolic pressure (phase V) between 90 and 110 mmHg. Treatment is discussed in Chapter 10. It is established that the higher the blood pressure, the worse is the cardiovascular prognosis.

Primary prevention

Salt

The physiological requirement for sodium is no more than 20 mmol sodium/day (1 g of NaCl). The average consumption in the West is 170–250 mmol/day (8–12 g NaCl). There is some evidence that a high salt intake increases the likelihood of hypertension:

(i) Epidemiological: the blood pressure of populations can

be correlated with the mean salt intake. Pacific islanders ingest about 2 g of salt a day and do not have hypertension. In north Japan the salt intake is high, 25 g daily and there is a high incidence of hypertension and stroke.

(ii) The Kempner rice and fruit diet (10 mmol Na/day) was an early (1948) effective but unpleasant treatment of hypertension.

(iii) Animal experiments show that high levels of sodium intake increase blood pressure.

However, blood pressure and salt intake have not been correlated in individuals. People may vary in susceptibility. A generally recommended dietary goal for most adults is 6 g salt/day (100 mmol Na); 70% of salt intake is in the food and only 30% is added at the table. 'Fast foods' contain large quantities of salt and food labelling will help individual choice.

Obesity

Blood pressure is correlated to obesity—3 mmHg elevation for 10 kg overweight. Weight reduction is associated with a statistically significant fall in blood pressure.

Excess alcohol

Consistent heavy drinking (780 g/day) increases blood pressure. Abstention results in a fall. Moderate alcohol intake has no adverse cardiovascular effects.

Secondary prevention

Hypertension is usually asymptomatic so screening programmes are required to detect patients at risk before they develop cardiovascular complications.

It is now established that effective drug treatment of moderate or severe hypertension will reduce the risk of stroke and hypertensive heart failure.

CONGENITAL HEART DISEASE

About eight in every 1000 babies born alive have a congenital heart defect. The incidence in stillborn or spontaneously aborted fetuses is very much higher.

Prevention

Methods of prevention are:

(i) Genetic counselling in any family with a parent or one child with a congenital heart defect.
(ii) Identification and elimination of environmental teratogens.
(iii) Antenatal diagnosis with the possibility of termination of pregnancy.

The aetiology and incidence of congenital heart disease are discussed in Chapter 5.

Investigations

(i) *Fetal echocardiography* at 18 weeks will detect hypoplastic left hearts and termination may be considered. Other lesions will be revealed at 22 weeks. If pregnancy is allowed to continue the baby should be delivered in a paediatric surgical centre.
(ii) *Amniocentesis* to identify Down's syndrome and Ehlers–Danlos syndrome.

FURTHER READING

The British Cardiac Society Working Group (1987). Coronary prevention: conclusions and recommendations. *British Heart Journal*, **57,** 188–189.

Committee on Medical Aspects of Food Policy (COMA) (1984). *Diet and Cardiovascular Disease.* London: HMSO.

Consensus Conference National Institutes of Health (1985). Lowering blood cholesterol to prevent heart disease. *Journal of the American Medical Association*, **253,** 2080–2086.

Lipid Research Clinics Programme (1984). The Lipid Research Clinic's coronary prevention that results. 1 Reduction in incidence of coronary heart disease. *Journal of the American Medical Association*, **251,** 351–64.

Mulcahy, R. (1983). Review: Influence of cigarette smoking on morbidity and mortality after myocardial infarction. *British Heart Journal*, **49,** 410–415.

National Advisory Committee on Nutritional Education (NACNE) (1983). A discussion paper on proposals for nutritional guidelines for health education in Britain. London: The Health Education Council.

Nemura K., Pisa Z. (1985). Recent trends in cardiovascular disease mortality in 27 industrialised countries. *World Health Statistics Quarterly*, **38,** 142–162.

Shaper A. G., Pocock S. J., Walker M., Phillips A. M., Whitehead T. P., Macfarlane P. W. (1985). Risk factors for ischaemic heart disease: the prospective phase of the British Regional Heart Study. *Journal of Epidemiology and Community Health*, **39,** 197–209.

Study Group, European Atherosclerosis Society (1987). Strategies for the prevention of coronary heart disease: a policy statement of the European Atherosclerosis Society. *European Heart Journal*, **8,** 77–88.

Chapter Fifteen

Diseases of the Pericardium

Background

The pericardium surrounds the heart and the roots of the great vessels. The outer layer is strong fibrous tissue. Inside this is a single layer of mesothelial cells which form the sac. One surface of this sac covers the fibrous pericardium and together they are called the parietal pericardium. It is continuous with an inner layer attached to the epicardial surface of the heart, the visceral pericardium. The two serosal layers are separated by a small volume of serous fluid (about 50 ml).

The pericardium is not essential to life. It can be congenitally absent or surgically removed. The most common defect is a partial absence of the left-sided pericardium and this is detected as a bulge of the left heart border on a chest X-ray. Pericardial cysts occur in one in every 100 000 people (spring water cysts). Their only importance is that they mimic mediastinal tumours on X-ray.

Four important clinical syndromes are recognised:

(i) Acute pericarditis.
(ii) Pericardial effusion.
(iii) Cardiac tamponade.
(iv) Pericardial constriction.

ACUTE PERICARDITIS

Pericarditis is most frequently secondary to acute myocardial infarction. Most cases of transmural infarction are associated with localised pericarditis and in about 10% of patients it

Table 15.1

CAUSES OF ACUTE PERICARDITIS

- liopathic
- nfection
  - Viral
  - Bacterial
  - Mycoplasma
  - Legionella
  - Fungi
  - Parasitic
- Malignant
- rradiation of mediastinum
- Acute myocardial infarction
- Postmyocardial and postpericardial injury
- Pleural disease, extension from pulmonary embolism, pneumonia
- Uraemia
- Myxoedema
- Connective tissue disease
  - Rheumatic fever
  - Rheumatoid arthritis
  - Systemic lupus erythematosus
  - Scleroderma
- Drugs
  - Hydralazine
  - Procainamide
  - Isoniazid
  - Penicillin

produces symptoms and signs. The next commonest variety is idiopathic or viral pericarditis. Other causes are listed in Table 15.1.

Idiopathic Pericarditis

The diagnosis is made when no infective agent can be isolated or underlying cause identified. Some 40% of patients are young men aged between 11 and 30 years. The clinical presentation and course are similar to viral pericarditis and it is likely that many cases are viral in aetiology. A seasonal incidence in spring and autumn, when there is an increase in viral epidemics, supports this.

Viral Pericarditis

Viruses which cause acute pericarditis include coxsackie A and B ECHO virus, influenza, adenovirus, mumps, varicella and Epstein–Barr.

There is often a history of malaise, upper respiratory infection, diarrhoea or skin rash in the preceding 3 weeks. The clinical course is usually benign with complete resolution in 1–2 weeks. A pericardial effusion is not uncommon but tamponade and constriction are rare. One recurrence during the next 3 months occurs in about a quarter of patients, and multiple repeated attacks are seen in a few patients.

Bacterial Pericarditis

Common organisms include *Staphylococcus aureus*, *Pneumococcus*, *Streptococcus and Haemophilus influenzae*. Infection of the pericardium occurs by direct extension from intrathoracic infection or is blood-borne from suppurative foci like osteomyelitis.

Bacterial pericarditis presents as an acute illness with rigors and a high spiking fever. Pericardial effusion and tamponade are frequent complications.

Tuberculous Pericarditis

This may result from early dissemination following the primary infection or from direct involvement from peritracheal and mediastinal lymph nodes. The illness is insidious with vague initial symptoms. Pericardial effusion develops in the majority of cases and progresses to constriction over a period of months in two-thirds of cases.

Fungal Pericarditis

Immunosuppressed patients and drug addicts are particularly susceptible. Histoplasmosis can cause a massive effusion. Other fungal infections are blastomycosis, coccidiomycosis, aspergillosis and candidiasis. Tamponade and constriction are frequent complications.

Malignant Pericarditis

The most common neoplasms to metastasise to the heart and pericardium are carcinomas of the lung in men and of the breast in women. Pericardial involvement also occurs in lymphoma and leukaemia. The effusion is usually bloodstained.

Irradiation Pericarditis

Transient pericarditis is an occasional complication of chest irradiation and can occur during the course of radiotherapy or within a few months of treatment.

Pericarditis with Acute Myocardial Infarction

Pericarditis with a friction rub is common in the first 4 days after acute transmural infarction. It clinically resolves within 48 h and complications are rare.

Postmyocardial Infarction and Pericardiotomy Syndrome

A syndrome of pericarditis, fever and often pleural effusion and pulmonary infiltration following myocardial infarction was described by Dressler in 1959. Symptoms usually start 10 days to 6 weeks after acute infarction. The cause is unknown but hypersensitivity to antibodies developed in necrotic heart muscle has been suggested. Pericardial effusion and tamponade may be complications. The ESR is nearly always raised and there may be a moderate elevation in the white cell count.

About 5% of patients who have undergone cardiac surgery develop a similar illness. Haemopericardium is a common complication due to the concurrent use of anticoagulants following surgery.

Uraemic Pericarditis

This continues to cause significant morbidity and mortality

among patients undergoing renal dialysis. Pericarditis with ef fusion often develops after adequate dialysis and the level o blood urea and creatinine do not predict the patients who wil develop this complication.

Connective Tissue Disease

Pericarditis is the most common cardiac manifestation of systemic lupus erythematosus, and occurs in about a quarter of patients at some time during the course of the disease. Effusion is uncommon and pericarditis usually goes as the disease activity remits.

Pericardial effusions have been found in one-third of patients with rheumatoid arthritis. Secondary infection, tamponade and constriction are rare complications.

In acute rheumatic fever, pericarditis accompanies myocarditis and endocarditis.

Clinical presentation of acute pericarditis

Most patients complain of chest pain. There is a pericardial friction rub and the electrocardiogram shows typical changes.

Pericardial pain

This is retrosternal, usually sharp and stabbing and worsened by inspiration, movement or lying flat. It is often relieved by sitting upright and leaning forward. The pain can radiate widely. Occasionally it is a more oppressive pain which is difficult to distinguish from myocardial infarction (Table 15.2). The patient takes shallow breaths to minimise pain and sometimes perceives this as shortness of breath.

Pericardial friction rub

This is caused by the grating of the visceral and parietal pericardial surfaces but may be heard even if there is a pericardial effusion. It is usually loudest at the left sternal edge, when the patient leans forward and breathes in. The noise is superficial and sounds nearer to the stethoscope than the heart sounds. It may have two or three components. In sinus rhythm there is a rub in

Table 15.2

DIFFERENCES BETWEEN PERICARDIAL AND ISCHAEMIC HEART PAIN

	Pericarditis	*Myocardial infarction*
Typical pain	Sharp	Crushing or constricting
	Worse on breathing, swallowing	No effect
	Relieved by sitting forward	No effect
ECG	S-T segment elevation concave upwards	Convex upwards
	Diffuse distribution of S-T segment changes	Confined to one area of myocardium
	No Q waves	Q waves

atrial systole and a rub in ventricular systole. There may also be a diastolic component due to rapid ventricular filling. Rubs frequently come and go.

Investigations

Electrocardiogram

Electrocardiographic changes usually occur within a few hours of the onset of chest pain. The changes are transient and are due to involvement of the subepicardial myocardium adjacent to the involved pericardium. The sequence of changes are listed in Table 15.3.

It is important to recognise that several millimetres of ST segment elevation (particularly in chest leads V_2–V_4) can be a

Table 15.3

SEQUENCE OF ELECTROCARDIOGRAPHIC CHANGES IN ACUTE PERICARDITIS

Elevated S-T segments involving the limb and chest leads, usually concave upwards and lasting hours to days
Depression of S-T segments and flattening of T waves
T wave inversion lasting days or weeks
Return of the electrocardiogram to normal

normal variant in 2% of healthy adults. This is commonest in young and particularly black patients. The elevated ST segments are similar to changes of pericarditis and serial electrocardiograms may be required to differentiate.

Other investigations

Echocardiography is often unhelpful in acute pericarditis but is invaluable in detecting pericardial effusion and tamponade. Investigations to establish the aetiology of pericarditis are listed in Table 15.4.

Table 15.4

INVESTIGATIONS IN ACUTE PERICARDITIS

Investigation	*Aetiology*
Blood tests	Coxsackie, ECHO virus, influenza
Viral titres: acute and after 2 weeks	
Cold agglutinins	Mycoplasma
Paul Bunnell	Infectious mononucleosis
Blood culture	Bacterial
White blood cell count	Elevated in bacterial pericarditis Leukaemia
Blood urea	Uraemia
Thyroid function	Myxoedema
Rheumatoid factor	Rheumatoid
Antinuclear factor	Systemic lupus erythematosus (SLE)
Antistreptolysin O titre	Rheumatic fever
Throat swab and stool culture	Viral
Chest X-ray	Tuberculosis, neoplasm, lymphoma
Pericardiocentesis	Bacterial
Examination and culture of fluid	Tuberculosis Malignant

Differential diagnosis

The main features which distinguish acute pericarditis from myocardial infarction are listed in Table 15.2. The symptoms of epidemic pleurodynia (Bornholm disease) resemble pericarditis but there is no pericardial friction rub or electrocardiographic change. Pulmonary infarction and spontaneous pneumothorax can also present with similar symptoms.

Management

Acute idiopathic or viral pericarditis

(i) *Pain relief:* aspirin or a non-steroidal anti-inflammatory agent (NSAID) is usually effective. Corticosteroids relieve pain but do not alter the course of the disease and should only be given in exceptional cases when pain has proved refractory.

(ii) *Bed rest:* patients should be rested in bed until the pain and fever have resolved.

(iii) *Treat complications:* a careful watch for the development of a large effusion and tamponade is essential.

Other causes

Specific antibiotics should be given to patients with other infective causes. Antibiotics attain high levels in pericardial fluid. Patients with malignant disease may respond to systemic cytotoxic chemotherapy after pericardiocentesis. Corticosteroids are useful in the postmyocardial infarction and pericardiotomy syndromes and in patients with systemic lupus erythematosus. Uraemic pericarditis is treated by continued dialysis after relief of tamponade.

Pericardial effusions, tamponade, reaccumulation of the effusion and constriction are frequent complications in patients with pericarditis of non-viral (or idiopathic) origin. Many will require pericardectomy.

PERICARDIAL EFFUSION

Causes

(i) *Small effusions:* these are frequently present in any case of acute pericarditis. They also occur in patients with heart failure and hypoalbuminaemia.

(ii) *Large effusions:* the most common causes are tuberculosis, malignancy, cardiac trauma, uraemia and myxoedema.

Clinical signs

A small pericardial effusion produces no clinical signs if intrapericardial pressure is normal. The signs of a large pericardial effusion are listed in Table 15.5 and the signs of cardiac tamponade are described on page 420.

Investigations

(i) *Chest X-ray:* this will show globular enlargement of the cardiac silhouette but no evidence of pulmonary vascular congestion. Table 15.6 lists the differential diagnosis.

(ii) *Electrocardiogram:* QRS voltage is reduced and there may be electrical alternans (due to the swinging motion of the heart within the effusion).

(iii) *Echocardiogram:* this is very helpful in diagnosis, quantifying volume and in serial assessment. An echo-free

Table 15.5

CLINICAL SIGNS OF A LARGE PERICARDIAL EFFUSION

Sign	*Explanation of sign*
Faint heart sounds	Large amount of fluid surrounding the heart
Pericardial friction rub	May still be audible despite effusion
Dullness to percussion beneath left scapula (Ewart's sign) Bronchial breathing in same area	Backward displacement of the heart by a large effusion compresses the left lung base
Râles over the lung fields	Compression of lung parenchyma

Table 15.6

CAUSES OF A HUGE HEART ON CHEST X-RAY

Pericardial effusion
Cardiomyopathy
Chronic rheumatic mitral and aortic disease
Atrial septal defect
Ebstein's anomaly

space appears behind the posterior left ventricular wall but disappears behind the left atrium. Small to moderate-sized effusions are imaged only posteriorly. Volumes greater than approximately 300 ml are imaged both anteriorly and posteriorly.

(iv) *Pericardiocentesis:* the fluid is either an exudate or transudate.
- (a) exudates (protein $>3{\cdot}0$ g/100 ml) occur with infection, uraemia, neoplasia and connective tissue disorders;
- (b) transudates (protein $<2{\cdot}0$ g/100 ml) are due to heart failure, hypoalbuminaemia or myxoedema.

Culture of the pericardial fluid will reveal bacterial or tuberculous infection and cytological examination malignant disease.

Haemorrhagic effusions are caused by malignancy and trauma and are also found in postpericardiotomy and renal dialysis patients being treated with anticoagulants. Rarely the effusion may be chylous due to trauma to the thoracic duct or neoplastic lymph obstruction.

CARDIAC TAMPONADE

Definition

Cardiac compression here is due to increased intrapericardial pressure secondary to pericardial effusion, resulting in raised intracardiac pressures, restriction of ventricular diastolic filling and a reduction of stroke volume.

Pathogenesis

The speed of development of a pericardial effusion is importan[t] A slow accumulation of fluid gradually stretches the fibrou[s] pericardium and up to 3 litres may be present without causin[g] tamponade. If the effusion is acute, as little as 300 ml may stretc[h] the pericardium to its limit and the intrapericardial pressure wil[l] rise. When this happens diastolic ventricular filling is reduced Compensatory measures, to maintain cardiac output and systemic blood pressure, are a rise in right and left atrial pressures, a reflex tachycardia and vasoconstriction. Eventually these become inadequate, cardiac output falls and there is circulatory collapse.

Clinical features

Patients present with evidence of a low cardiac output. They are usually distressed, have a tachycardia, a small pulse volume and cold sweating skin. The effusion makes the heart sounds soft and the apex beat impalpable. Stretching of the pericardium causes chest discomfort and the patient may prefer to sit upright or adopt a knee–chest position.

Pulsus paradoxus

Pulsus paradoxus is an important physical sign. It is the abrupt reduction in pulse volume or even disappearance of the pulse during inspiration. It is an exaggeration of the normal variation in pulse volume during respiration. The 'paradox' described by Kussmaul is the finding of a constant heart beat at the apex associated with disappearance or reduction in the arterial pulse volume during inspiration.

The explanation for pulsus paradoxus in cardiac tamponade is the restriction of the heart in a finite space. Right ventricular filling is maintained at the expense of left ventricular volume. In inspiration venous return to the right heart increases due to negative intrathoracic pressure. The interventricular septum is shifted from right to left. The diaphragm moves downwards in inspiration, pulls on the tense parietal pericardium and further increases pressure. These effects reduce left ventricular filling causing stroke volume and pulse pressure fall. It can be appreciated why removal of as little as 100 ml of fluid (one stroke olume) may produce a dramatic improvement in haemodynamics.

Pulsus paradoxus (usually a fall in blood pressure of not more han 30 mmHg during inspiration) is also found in conditions where there is a marked alteration in intrathoracic pressure, such s severe asthma and laryngeal stridor.

Jugular venous pulse (JVP)

The jugular venous pulse is always elevated due to restriction of ight atrial filling. There may be a further rise during inspiration when intrapericardial pressure is further raised (Kussmaul's ign). There is a rapid X (systolic) descent. This is due to systolic ejection of blood and reduction of the volume of the heart with tamponade. This allows blood to flow into the right atrium with a fall in venous pressure.

Treatment

Cardiac tamponade is a medical emergency and should be treated by pericardiocentesis.

The safest approach is from the angle between the xiphoid process and the left costal margin. The patient should be sat up in bed at a 45° angle. After skin preparation and injection of local anaesthetic an aspiration needle is advanced in the direction of the left shoulder and at an angle of 45° to the abdominal wall. The needle is attached to a large syringe by a three-way tap and gentle suction should be maintained, while the needle is advanced, until freeflowing fluid is obtained. The needle should be also attached to the V-lead of an ECG machine. This lead is monitored throughout and if the needle touches the myocardium sudden S-T segment elevation and ventricular ectopic beats will occur. If this happens the needle should be withdrawn until the electrocardiographic changes disappear. An alternative is to monitor the procedure with two-dimensional echocardiography.

If the pericardial aspirate is bloody it is essential that it is immediately differentiated from blood withdrawn from the right ventricular cavity. Venous blood and aspirate should both be sent for urgent haemoglobin estimation. Pericardial fluid may also be distinguished by its failure to clot because it is defibrinated.

When the effusion is large it is often useful to advance a

catheter over the needle into the pericardium. This can remain *i*
situ for longer periods of pericardial drainage.

PERICARDIAL CONSTRICTION (PICK'S DISEASE)

Definition

This is gross fibrosis (and calcification) of the pericardium causing restriction of ventricular filling and interference with ventricular systole. This results in a major haemodynamic disturbance.

Causes

In the majority of cases the cause is unknown although many are assumed to be due to tuberculosis. (Until the development of antituberculous chemotherapy, tuberculosis was the commonest cause.)

Constriction can complicate pericarditis of other aetiology, most likely bacterial or fungal infection, haemopericardium, malignant and rheumatoid pericarditis.

Pathophysiology

The thickened and fibrotic pericardium holds the ventricles in a rigid shell. Both ventricles are usually restricted and the reduced output from the right ventricle helps to prevent a great rise in left atrial pressure. Dyspnoea at rest is therefore not a prominent symptom. The considerable increase in mean venous pressure due to obstruction of right ventricular filling results in hepatic enlargement, ascites and peripheral oedema. The abnormal haemodynamics are reflected in the venous pulse. Stroke volume is reduced because of the restriction to diastolic filling and the inability of the heart to shorten its long axis in systole. The cardiac output can only be increased by a rise in heart rate. This is inadequate during exercise and only slight exertion may cause considerable shortness of breath. The pulse volume and systolic blood pressure are usually reduced.

In addition to restriction there is often a myocardial abnormality. The muscle becomes involved in the disease process and atrophies.

Clinical features

Constriction develops insidiously. The early symptoms are shortness of breath on exertion and fatigue due to a low cardiac output. At the time of presentation the clinical picture is dominated by the obstruction of right ventricular filling (Tables 15.7 and 15.8). The patient will complain of abdominal swelling and discomfort and gross peripheral oedema.

Investigations

The underlying cause should be considered and similar investigation as outlined in acute pericarditis may be appropriate. The investigations confirming pericardial constriction are listed in Table 15.9.

Table 15.7

JUGULAR VENOUS PULSE IN PERICARDIAL CONSTRICTION

Abnormality	*Explanation of abnormality*
Very raised (often to 20 cm) so the patient may have to stand upright to appreciate the waveform)	High right atrial pressure due to restriction of filling
A further rise with inspiration (Kussmaul's sign)	The right heart is unable to accommodate the increased flow during reduced intrathoracic pressure
Rapid Y (diastolic) descent and trough (Friedreich's sign)	Abrupt filling of the right ventricle when the tricuspid valve opens. Pressure rises again when filling is stopped by the rigid pericardium
Rapid X (systolic) descent. This is less common. It is not seen if the ventricle is atrophic or if constriction is severe and atria cannot accommodate increased volume	Quick ejection of stroke volume which reduces volume of blood within rigid pericardium and allows flow into the heart

Table 15.8

OTHER PHYSICAL SIGNS IN PERICARDIAL CONSTRICTION

Sign	*Explanation of sign*
Gross peripheral oedema Ascites Hepatomegaly	Increased venous pressure due to restriction of right heart filling
Small volume pulse Tachycardia	Low cardiac output
Atrial fibrillation (30% of cases)	High atrial pressure
Pulsus paradoxus (in less than 50% of cases and less prominent than in tamponade)	See cardiac tamponade
Impalpable cardiac impulse but diastolic shock at same time as Y descent	Constriction of ventricles and rapid filling of non-distensible ventricle
Pericardial 'knock'; a very loud third sound 0·1 s after aortic valve closure	Expansion of ventricles is terminated by constricted pericardium

Differential diagnosis

The diagnosis of pericardial constriction is clear if the classical signs of an elevated jugular venous pulse with rapid Y descent, gross ascites and oedema and a calcified pericardium on chest X-ray are present.

In other patients it has to be distinguished from congestive heart failure and restrictive cardiomyopathy. Features of congestive heart failure are a history of orthopnoea, a dilated heart on X-ray and echocardiogram, reduced ventricular function with functional tricuspid and mitral regurgitation and a response to diuretic treatment which lowers the jugular venous pulse. Restrictive cardiomyopathy (see Chapter 4) is more difficult and sometimes not possible to differentiate without either an endomyocardial biopsy or thoracotomy. This is because the haemodynamic changes in both conditions may be identical. Some contrasting features are listed in Table 15.10.

Table 15.9

INVESTIGATIONS FOR PERICARDIAL CONSTRICTION

Investigation	*Abnormality*
Electrocardiogram	Decreased QRS voltage with non-specific T wave changes. Atrial fibrillation (30%)
Chest X-ray (posteroanterior, posteroanterior penetrated and left lateral films)	Normal or enlarged cardiac silhouette. Calcification of the pericardium is the most important finding and is present in 50% of cases. Widened superior vena cava and azygos vein. Pleural effusion
Chest screening	Reduced cardiac pulsation
Echocardiogram	Pericardial thickening. Diastolic flattening of left ventricular posterior wall. Abnormal septal motion. Premature pulmonary valve opening
Computerised axial tomography (CAT)	High density fibrous pericardium
Cardiac catheterisation pressures	Elevation and identity of diastolic pressures in all chambers
	Rapid early diastolic dip followed by a high diastolic plateau (square root sign) in right ventricular and left ventricular pressure tracings
Angiography	Right atrial cineangiography shows pericardial thickening. Left anterior descending coronary artery is within the cardiac silhouette and not on the surface

Table 15.10

FEATURES DIFFERENTIATING PERICARDIAL CONSTRICTION AND RESTRICTIVE CARDIOMYOPATHY

	Pericardial constriction	*Restrictive cardiomyopathy*
Signs		
Pulse	Pulsus paradoxus	Narrow pulse pressure, no paradox
Apex beat	Impalpable	Usually palpable
Heart sounds	Early pericardial knock	Third or fourth sound; often a gallop rhythm
Murmurs	None	Sometimes mitral and tricuspid regurgitation due to distortion of valves
Investigations		
Chest X-ray	Normal size heart Pericardial calcification	Mild cardiac enlargement Occasionally endocardial calcification in endomyocardial fibrosis
Electrocardiogram	No conduction defect	Right bundle branch block or left bundle branch block are common
Echocardiogram	Previous pericardial effusion Thickened pericardium	Increased ventricular wall thickness Bright myocardial echoes in amyloid disease
Cardiac catheter	High and equal right and left ventricular end diastolic pressures	Left ventricular end diastolic pressure raised more than right
Angiography	No valvular regurgitation	Mitral and tricuspid regurgitation

Treatment

Once pericardial constriction is established the prognosis without surgery is poor. The pericardium must be removed to release the heart. Operative mortality is related to the degree of constriction and the sooner diagnosis is made and pericardiectomy performed the better the outlook. Surgery should not be delayed in tuberculous pericardial constriction but antituberculous drugs should also be given.

The surgeon normally removes the parietal pericardium from the anterolateral and inferior right ventricle and from the anterolateral and diaphragmatic surface of the left ventricle extending across the atrioventricular groove. The visceral pericardium is also stripped if cardiac constriction does not improve satisfactorily after removal of the parietal layer. This is necessary in the majority of cases.

Postoperative recovery is not always complete because of the myocardial atrophy due to immobilisation and involvement of the ventricles in the disease process. Continued treatment with digoxin and diuretics is often required.

FURTHER READING

Dressler W. (1959). The post-myocardial infarction syndrome: a report of forty-four cases. *Archives of Internal Medicine*, **103,** 28.

Haskell R. J., French W. J. (1985). Cardiac tamponade as the initial presentation of malignancy. *Chest*, **88,** 70–73.

Kirk J., Cosh J. (1969). The pericarditis of rheumatoid arthritis. *Quarterly Journal of Medicine*, **38,** 397–423.

Permanyer-Miralda G., Sagrista-Sauleda J., Soler-Soler J. (1985). Primary acute pericardial disease: a prospective series of 231 consecutive patients. *American Journal of Cardiology*, **56,** 623–630.

Seifert F. C., Miller D. C., Oesterle S. N., Oyer P. E., Stimson E. B., Shumway N. E. (1985). Surgical treatment of constrictive pericarditis: analysis of outcome and diagnostic error. *Circulation*, **72** (Suppl. 2), 264–273.

Spodick D. H. (1983). The normal and diseased pericardium: current concepts of the pericardial physiology, diagnosis and treatment. *Journal of American College of Cardiology*, **1,** 240–251.

Woodruff J. F. (1980). Viral myocarditis: a review . *American Journal of Pathology*, **101,** 428–478.

Chapter Sixteen

Miscellaneous Heart Conditions

AORTIC DISSECTION

Background

Aortic dissection occurs when a tear in the aortic intima allows a column of blood at systemic pressure to separate the intima from the adventitia, destroying the media. The dissection may tear the intima distally thus re-entering the true aortic lumen.

Dissection occurs twice as often in men as in women and is commonest between 50 and 70 years of age.

Pathology

The pathological substrate of aortic dissection is cystic medial necrosis, a degenerative condition of medial muscle, collagen and elastic tissue with prominent cystic change. Additional factors predisposing to dissection are shown in Table 16.1. Dissections are classified by their site of origin, a factor which also determines the definitive management of choice (Table 16.2).

Table 16.1

AORTIC DISSECTION: PREDISPOSING FACTORS

Systemic hypertension
Marfan's syndrome
Pregnancy
Aortic stenosis
Aortic coarctation

Table 16.2

CLASSIFICATION AND MANAGEMENT OF AORTIC DISSECTION BY SITE OF ORIGIN

Classification	*Site of origin*	*Management*
Type A (proximal)	Ascending aorta, just above the aortic valve	Surgical
Type B (distal)	Descending aorta, distal to origin of left subclavian artery	Medical

Symptoms

(i) *Pain* is almost invariable. Abrupt onset, extreme severity and a 'tearing' quality are typical. The pain migrates as the dissection extends. Anterior chest pain favours a type A dissection while posterior interscapular pain is commonest in type B dissection.

(ii) *General symptoms* include nausea, vomiting, profuse sweating, fear, faintness and syncope.

(iii) *Physical signs* depend on the path and extent of the dissection:

- (a) *absent or diminished peripheral pulses* result from direct compression or occlusion of the arterial orifice by a flap of intima;
- (b) *aortic valvular regurgitation* occurs in one half of type A dissections due to dilatation, distortion or dissection of the aortic valve ring;
- (c) *neurological deficits* include syncope, stroke and paraplegia;
- (d) signs of *pericardial tamponade* or *left haemothorax* result from rupture of the dissection through the adventitia into the pericardial or left pleural cavities respectively, the commonest sites of rupture.

Investigations

(i) *The chest X-ray* shows a widened mediastinum. The

'calcium sign', if present, is almost diagnostic—if the aortic knuckle is calcified a gap of more than 1 cm between the calcified intima and the outer aortic border is seen.

(ii) *Two-dimensional echocardiography/CT scan* both offer sensitive, non-invasive methods of diagnosis and followup where available.

(iii) *Aortic angiography* is the single most useful investigation. It is performed by retrograde catheterisation from the femoral artery and confirms the diagnosis, the site of origin and the extent of the dissection.

Treatment

A management plan is shown in Table 16.3. Haemodynamic factors influencing the initiation and propagation of aortic dissection are the systolic blood pressure and the force and velocity of left ventricular contraction. The aims of initial management are therefore pain relief, urgent reduction of systolic blood pressure and beta-adrenergic blockade for its negative inotropic effect. When the patient is stable aortic angiography is performed.

Surgical management includes transection of the aorta to excise the intimal tear, oversewing the aortic circumference to obliterate the false lumen and reconnection of the two ends by direct suture or insertion of a prosthetic graft. Aortic valve replacement is indicated for aortic valvular regurgitation.

Definitive *medical* management continues the initial aims of maintaining the lowest tolerated systolic blood pressure including the use of negatively inotropic drugs, usually propranolol. The same long-term medical management is indicated for patients successfully treated by surgery.

Prognosis

Without treatment aortic dissection is generally fatal—one-quarter of patients die within 24 h, one-half by 1 week and almost all by 1 year from the onset of dissection.

For proximal dissection surgical treatment results in clearly superior hospital survival. Patients discharged from hospital following successful surgical or medical management have a good long-term prognosis.

Table 16.3

MANAGEMENT PLAN FOR ACUTE AORTIC DISSECTION

Initial	
All cases	Admit to intensive care unit Reduce systolic blood pressure to 100–120 mmHg (for example, nitroprusside infusion, 25–50 μg/min) Reduce force and velocity of cardiac contraction (propranolol 1 mg intravenously every 5 min until heart rate is 60–70 beats/min) Aortic angiography
Definitive	
Indications	
Surgical	Proximal (type A dissection) Aortic regurgitation Progressive dissection Aortic rupture Failed medical management
Medical	Distal (type B) dissection Chronic dissection (> 2 weeks from onset)
Long-term	
All cases	Systolic blood pressure control < 140 mmHg Beta-adrenergic blockade Regular non-invasive assessment by chest X-ray, two-dimensional echocardiogram and/or CT scan

NEOPLASTIC DISEASE OF THE HEART

Background

Primary tumours of the heart are rare, being found in about 0·1% of autopsies. Three-quarters of primary cardiac tumours are benign of which the majority are myxomas. Metastatic tumours are much more common and are found in 6% of autopsies on patients with malignant disease. The histological types of cardiac tumour in approximate order of frequency are shown in Table 16.4.

Table 16.4

CARDIAC TUMOURS: RELATIVE INCIDENCE

Metastatic
Bronchogenic carcinoma
Breast
Malignant melanoma
Lymphomas
Leukaemia

Primary
Benign
- Myxoma
- Lipoma
- Papillary fibroelastoma
- Rhabdomyoma

Malignant
- Angiosarcoma
- Rhabdomyosarcoma
- Fibrosarcoma

Clinical features

Metastatic tumours are often silent but may cause pericardial effusion, a variety of cardiac arrhythmias, heart block and congestive cardiac failure.

Primary tumours produce a variety of systemic, embolic and cardiac features. Systemic abnormalities include malaise, fever, weight loss, joint pains, Raynaud's phenomenon, clubbing, raised erythrocyte sedimentation rate (ESR), anaemia, increased red, white or platelet cell counts and hypergammaglobulinaemia. Systemic or pulmonary tumour emboli may occur. Cardiac manifestations depend mainly on the mechanical effects caused by the anatomical location of the tumour, for example, obstruction of valves, and conduction disturbances.

MYXOMAS

Background

Myxomas are benign tumours of the heart. They account for up o half of all primary cardiac tumours and occur at all ages, although the majority are reported in the fourth to sixth decades. Some 90% are found in the atria, favouring the left atrium in a ratio of 4:1. Multiple atrial and ventricular myxomas occur especially if there is a family history of myxoma.

Pathology

The left atrial myxoma is usually a mobile, lobulated, pedunculated mass attached by a fibrovascular stalk to the interatrial septum. The stalk is often long enough to allow the myxoma mass to prolapse through the mitral valve into the left ventricle during diastole. They average 4–8 cm in diameter. Light microscopy reveals uniform polygonal cells in a myxomatous matrix containing a high proportion of glycosaminoglycan. Other constituents include elastic and smooth muscle cells, collagen, calcium, lymphocytes, plasma cells, mast cells and bone. Haemorrhagic areas within the tumour and surface thrombus are common.

Clinical presentation

The diagnosis of left atrial myxoma is often missed because it is rare and often simulates more common conditions, especially mitral valve disease. The clinical features are those common to other primary cardiac tumours (page 432) while the mechanical effects of mitral valve obstruction result in effort breathlessness, orthopnoea, paroxysmal nocturnal dyspnoea and pulmonary oedema. Syncope, especially related to certain body positions, is characteristic of left atrial myxoma but rare in mitral valve disease. Presenting features of left atrial myxoma in approximate order of frequency are shown in Table 16.5.

Table 16.5

PRESENTING FEATURES OF LEFT ATRIAL MYXOMA

Presenting features
Symptoms and signs of mitral valve disease
Systemic embolism
Asymptomatic: incidental finding, especially on echocardiography
Syncope, sudden death
Pericarditis
Malaise, night sweats, pyrexia (mimics infective endocarditis)
Myocardial infarction

Cardiac physical signs

These commonly mimic mitral stenosis (Table 16.6). Postura variation is a characteristic distinguishing feature of left atria myxoma.

Investigations

(i) *Two-dimensional echocardiography* is the pre-eminent diagnostic test. It is highly sensitive and provides accurate information regarding the size of the tumour, its motion pattern and site of attachment. A technically satisfactory two-dimensional echocardiogram which has imaged all four cardiac chambers provides sufficient information to undertake surgery without cardiac catheterisation.

(ii) *M-mode echocardiography* is an adequate though slightly less sensitive screening test but does not provide information on the size or site of attachment of the tumour. Dense tumour echoes are seen behind the mitral valve leaflets and in the left atrial cavity during diastole.

(iii) *Cardiac catheterisation* usually reveals elevated pulmonary capillary wedge and pulmonary artery pressures due to

Table 16.6

CARDIAC PHYSICAL SIGNS ASSOCIATED WITH LEFT ATRIAL MYXOMA

Physical sign	*Explanation of sign*
Loud, widely split first heart sound	Delayed mitral valve closure
Tumour 'plop'	Tumour motion abruptly halted by stalk, or impact against heart wall. Simulates opening snap
Fourth heart sound (in sinus rhythm)	Atrial contraction against mitral valve obstruction
Mid-diastolic murmur	Mitral valve obstruction
Systolic murmur	Mitral regurgitation; tumour interferes with mitral closure
Postural variation in signs	Tumour position shifts with posture

Table 16.7

ECG, CHEST X-RAY AND LABORATORY FINDINGS IN LEFT ATRIAL MYXOMA

ECG	Usually sinus rhythm, left atrial abnormality. Atrial arrhythmias
Chest x-ray	Can mimic mitral stenosis: left atrial enlargement, pulmonary venous congestion, tumour calcification, pulmonary arterial hypertension
Laboratory findings	
Haematology	Raised ESR Anaemia Polycythaemia Leucocytosis Thrombocytopenia Thrombocytosis
Biochemistry	Hypergammaglobulinaemia
Immunology	High titre of antimyocardial antibodies

mitral valve obstruction. Left heart catheterisation is unnecessary and, especially in the case of transseptal catheterisation, positively hazardous since tumour emboli may result from catheter damage to the friable tumour mass. The myxoma is visualised by injecting contrast medium into the pulmonary artery and following it through to the left atrium where a mobile filling defect is demonstrated.

(iv) *ECG, chest X-ray and laboratory findings* are never diagnostic for left atrial myxoma but provide confirmatory evidence. More importantly, an unexpected abnormality in these investigations may provide the first clue to the diagnosis. Common findings are summarised in Table 16.7.

Differential diagnosis

An atrial ball-valve thrombus or a different histological type of intracardiac tumour may give similar investigational findings. More important are those commoner conditions which may be simulated by left atrial myxoma or its embolic complications and which therefore cause the diagnosis to be missed, a sometimes fatal error (Table 16.8).

Table 16.8

MISTAKEN DIAGNOSES IN PATIENTS WITH LEFT ATRIAL MYXOMA

Mitral valve disease
Infective endocarditis
Collagen diseases
Tricuspid valve disease
Ischaemic heart disease
Cerebrovascular disease
Pulmonary hypertension
Peripheral vascular disease
Malignant neoplastic disease

Treatment

Surgical removal using direct vision under cardiopulmonary bypass is imperative. Additional tumours are finally excluded during the procedure.

Prognosis

Surgery is curative. Recurrence of the tumour has been reported in up to 5% of cases following apparently successful removal of the initial myxoma.

FURTHER READING

Braunwald E. (1984). *A Textbook of Cardiovascular Medicine*, p. 1457. Philadelphia: Saunders.

Fabian J. T., Rose A. G. (1982). Tumours of the heart. *South African Medical Journal*, **61,** 71.

Heath D. (1968). Pathology of cardiac tumours. *American Journal of Cardiology*, **21,** 315.

Roberts W. C. (1981). Aortic dissection: anatomy, consequences and causes. *American Heart Journal*, **101,** 195.

Rowlands D. J. (1983). Left atrial myxoma. *British Journal of Hospital Medicine*, **30,** 415.

Vecht R. J., Bestermann E. M. M., Bromley L. L., Eastcott H. H. G., Kenyon J. R. (1980). Acute dissection of the aorta: long-term review and management. *Lancet*, **1,** 110.

Wolfe W. G., Moran J. F. (1977). Editorial: The evolution of medical and surgical management of acute aortic dissection. *Circulation*, **56,** 503.

Index